ANCIENT EGYPTIAN
MEDICINE

'A splendid book. Here we have an author who is not only a clinical consultant but also an authority on the texts themselves ... Unique in our generation ... it will surely be the definitive work on the subject.'   *Antiquity*

'Comprehensive in scope, well researched, thoroughly documented ... this work reflects the careful scholarship of England's recently retired premier anaesthesiologist ... Well illustrated throughout.'
Journal of the American Research Center in Egypt

'It is rare for a book on Egyptian medicine to be written by someone whose knowledge of medicine is matched by expertise in Egyptology ... Dr Nunn more than fulfils the claim that this book is the most comprehensive and authoritative of general books on the subject for many years.'
Journal of the Royal Society of Medicine

'Well researched and very well written ... User friendly ... Highly recommended.'   *Palaeopathology Newsletter*

'A beautiful book ... The illustrations are stunning ... John Nunn is one of the great scholar-scientists.'   *Anaesthesia*

ANCIENT EGYPTIAN
MEDICINE

JOHN F. NUNN

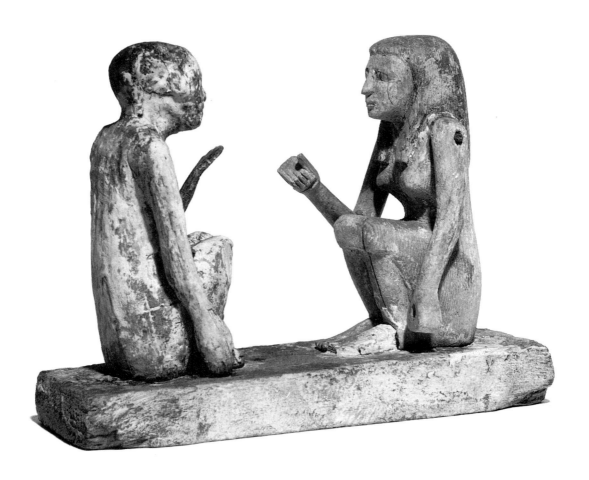

BRITISH MUSEUM PRESS

Figure acknowledgements

The following museums have kindly provided photographs of objects in their collections: The Trustees of the British Museum (cover, 1.5, 2.3, 4.1, 4.10, 5.1, 5.3, 5.4, 5.5, 5.6, 5.7, 6.2, 6.9, 7.1, 7.5); British Museum (Natural History), London (4.9); Petrie Museum, University College London (7.2, 8.5); Hunterian Museum of the Royal College of Surgeons of England (8.10); Ashmolean Museum, Oxford (6.12); Manchester Museum, University of Manchester (frontispiece); Metropolitan Museum of Art, New York (5.8); Musée du Louvre, Paris (6.13); Carlsberg Glyptotek, Copenhagen (4.5); State Museum of Berlin (4.12); Vatican Museum (6.11); Egyptian Museum of Turin (1.2, 1.3, 1.4, 1.7, 8.1).

The Griffith Institute of the Ashmolean Museum provided 5.2, and the Werner Forman Archive 4.6 and 9.1b from the Egyptian Museum, Cairo. I am grateful for computed tomography scans by Dr Clive Baldock (4.2), and for photographs taken by Miss Carol Andrews (5.10, 6.4, 6.6), Mrs Frances Welsh (6.3 and 8.2), Mrs Rosalind Park (4.14), and the photographic departments of the Institute of Archaeology, University of London (7.4) and Northwick Park Hospital (8.9).

I am especially indebted to Richard Parkinson for drawing 1.6, 3.6, 4.11, 4.13, 4.15, 6.14, 8.3, 8.4 and 9.3, and to Louise Perks for 2.2, 3.3 and 3.4. Other drawings are by the author.

First published in 1996 by British Museum Press
A division of The British Museum Company Ltd
46 Bloomsbury Street, London WC1B 3QQ

First published in paperback 1997

A catalogue record for this book
is available from the British Library

ISBN 0-7141-0981-9 (cased edition)
ISBN 0-7141-1906-7 (paperback edition)

Designed by Harry Green

Phototypeset in Times and Gill by Southern Positives
and Negatives (SPAN), Lingfield, Surrey
Printed in Great Britain by The Bath Press

Frontispiece: 'The consultation', Middle Kingdom, provenance unknown. (Manchester Museum)
Cover: Vignette from the *Book of the Dead* papyrus of Ani. 19th Dynasty, *c.* 1250 BC. Ht 8 cm. (EA 10470/5)

Contents

Preface

Graeco-Roman medicine is widely accepted as the origin of clinical practice as we know it today. However, the works of the Hippocratic School, Galen and others have been favoured by many factors which ensured that they were not lost to the medical historian. Copious writings have survived intact, written in languages which were never lost to scholars; many items of surgical equipment from the Roman Empire have survived in excellent condition, and there are clear representations of medical treatment. We can thus form a very good picture of medical practice in the early Roman Empire (Jackson, 1988).

In contrast, our understanding of ancient Egyptian medicine is hampered by many factors which do not apply to the Graeco-Roman period. Knowledge of the Egyptian scripts was totally lost from the early Christian period until the decipherment of the hieroglyphs began with Champollion in 1822, after preliminary contributions by Åkerblad (1802) and Thomas Young (1819). To this day there is uncertainty as to how the language was spoken, and the meaning of many words remains unresolved. The second problem is that the medical writings which have survived from pharaonic times are sparse in comparison with those from Greece and Rome, and there are very few accounts of medical treatment from the point of view of the lay person or patient, and certainly nothing to compare with the writings of Celsus, Pliny, the account of the extirpation of Marius' varicose veins (Plutarch) or the diaries of Aelius Aristides. No Egyptian medical equipment has survived from earlier than the Roman period, and there are very few representations of medical treatment. Whilst Jackson has stressed the difficulty of selection from the vast amount of medical material available from the Roman Empire, the problem with Egyptian medicine is one of interpretation of very limited material. The main bonus for study of pharaonic medicine is the excellent preservation of human material.

Additional difficulties arise from the immense time span of Egyptian civilisation, the Old Kingdom being as many centuries before Hippocrates as we are after him. Medical practice is now changing very rapidly, and the rate of change is itself increasing. Indeed, the medical advances of the last century have been far greater than the changes between pharaonic times and the beginning of the Victorian era. Thus it is becoming progressively more difficult to comprehend the medicine of ancient times.

The geographical and historical isolation of the ancient Egyptians, the loss of their language and the magnificence of their monuments have all encouraged the belief that Egypt must have been the repository of arcane knowledge, particularly in the field of the occult. Attempts to unravel these secrets have been pursued with immense enthusiasm, alongside the strict academic discipline of Egyptology. In the field of medicine, improbable claims have been made, whether on the basis of surmise or over-imaginative interpretation of the medical papyri. Such speculations tend to receive the wider publicity and have greatly confused the picture. In truth, there is no need to exaggerate the medical skills of the ancient Egyptians. What they accomplished in the three millennia before the Christian era is outstanding, and a match for their achievements in so many other fields of endeavour.

A major difficulty in writing this book has been the range of specialised knowledge of those who might be tempted to read it. They could include doctors, biologists, medical historians and Egyptologists. Some other readers may be unfamiliar with any of these subjects and I have, therefore, tried to make the text intelligible to all.

The meaning of Egyptian words lies at the very heart of attempting to understand their medicine. So many words cannot be translated with confidence that it seemed impossible to avoid the use of some Egyptian terms. To minimise disruption of the text, I have used the anglicised version of their supposed vocalisation, realising that consistency is impossible and we do not know how most Egyptian words were pronounced. Such words, other than proper names, appear in italics and, for the benefit of the serious student, the more important are listed with their hieroglyphs and transliterations in Appendix D. All citations are attributed and it should be possible to pursue any subject I have mentioned through the *Grundriss*. I have hyphenated some proper names to make them easier to pronounce and to read.

Any writer on Egyptian medicine must be in awe of the scholarship of his or her predecessors, and the range of disciplines they encompass. This work would have been quite impossible without the help so freely given from many quarters. First and foremost I am indebted to the late Mr Cyril Spaull and then to Miss Carol Andrews, who have laboured for almost a quarter of a century teaching a medical scientist the elements of the Egyptian language, and directing him towards a study of the medical papyri. No one could have better teachers. The staff of the British Museum, particularly Miss Carol Andrews, Dr Stephen Quirke, Dr Ralph Jackson, Dr Richard Parkinson and Dr John Taylor, have been unstinting in the help they have given me by supplying new information which I would otherwise have missed.

Members of other institutions have also given most generous help, in particular, Dr Theya Molleson, Dr David Rollinson and Dr Colin McCarthy of the Natural History Museum, London, Dr Elizabeth Allen of the Royal College of Surgeons of England, Mrs Rosalind Janssen of the Petrie Museum, University of London, Dr Vivian Nutton of the Wellcome Institute for the History of Medicine, Professor K A Kitchen of the University of Liverpool, Dr Rosalie David of the University of Manchester, Dr Jaromir Malek of the Griffith Institute, Oxford, Madama Donadoni and Dr Elizabeth Valtz of the Museo Egizio, Turin, the late Professor Ghaliounghui of Cairo University, Dr James Allen of the Metropolitan Museum of Art, New York, Dr de Meulenaere of the Fondation Egyptologique Reine Elizabeth, Brussels, Professor Jan Quaegebeur of the Catholic University, Leuven, and Dr Robert Miller of the Bioanthropology Foundation, Northport, New York.

My friend Dr Benson Harer has provided much information and valued criticism in his capacity as both a doctor and an Egyptologist. I could not have attempted an interpretation of the Brooklyn Papyrus on snake bite without the guidance of Professor David Warrell of the University of Oxford. Mrs Jeanette McKenna gave much help in translations from German texts. I have had valuable correspondence with Dr John Stevens, Mr J Thompson Rowling FRCS, Dr Guido Majno, Dr Ian Conacher, Dr Lise Manniche and Dr Renate Germer. Many more friends have also made very helpful contributions, including Dr Richard Loveday, Mr Theo Welsh FRCS, Mrs Frances Welsh, Mr Michael Muller, Dr Walter Loebl, Dr Malcolm Thomas, Dr Judith Maconochie, Mr John Evans, Mr Pierre Querinci, Mr George King, Mrs Rosalind Park and my son Dr Geoffrey Nunn. I would particularly like to express my gratitude to Professor Wolfhart Westendorf, who kindly criticised an earlier manuscript on a related topic, and my indebtedness to the authors of the *Grundriss der Medizin der alten Ägypter*. Without their work, the task would have been impossible.

I am especially grateful for the support of the British Museum Press and of Gillian Clarke, who has been correcting my English grammar for over thirty years. Finally, my dear wife has yet again borne, without complaint, the burden of a preoccupied husband immersed in the trials of writing a book.

CHAPTER ONE

The land of the Nile

Egyptian medicine evolved in a unique environment. The geography of Egypt is like that of no other country in the world, and it underlay the historical and cultural events which allowed a sophisticated system of medicine to develop and be recorded from the third millennium BC.

Geography

Throughout much of its recorded history the heartland of Egypt, from the first cataract to the Mediterranean, was similar to that contained within its present political boundaries (fig. 1.1). To the east and west the Nile Valley was enclosed by deserts which were very difficult for an army to cross in the second and third millennia BC. This enabled the Egyptians to concentrate their defences on the southern frontier and the land bridge into Asia; to a lesser extent they had to guard against intrusions from Libya. Nevertheless, their geography favoured defence to an extent which was exceptional for a continental country. This resulted in long-term stability and engendered a powerful sense of national identity, mingled with considerable xenophobia. Foreigners were often represented in the official record as corpses, prisoners or tribute bearers.

The Nile was the second decisive geographical factor which shaped the destiny of the Egyptians. The desert savanna of the Neolithic Period, with its flora and fauna, gave way to increasingly arid conditions, and rainfall alone was never adequate for agriculture. However, the river brought unlimited supplies of water, and the silt built up as a fertile valley along the river banks. Nevertheless, it would have been difficult to transport large quantities of water from the river banks uphill and across the valley floor. Were it not for the annual inundation, this limitation would have restricted cultivation to narrow strips on either side of the river.

The inundation resulted from summer rains in Ethiopia which still cause the Blue Nile and the Atbara to rise during May, June and July. The Nile in Egypt formerly rose during July, August and September by an average of about nine metres at Aswan, and seven metres at Cairo, some 650 km to the north. The inundation had two major effects on agriculture. First, it carried the water across the cultivated lands to the edge of the desert. This saved an enormous labour in the transportation of water, although much work was still needed to retain it. Secondly, it deposited vast quantities of silt, which renewed the fertility of the land. When the waters had subsided, it was necessary to resurvey the fields, and this played a part in the stimulation of mathematical expertise. The height of the inundation was crucially important. Too high a water level might flood the villages, which could result in loss of life, animals and buildings. Too low a level would result in poorer crops, if not actual failure. The height of the inundation was so critical that it was measured in the Late Period by stone-built nilometers, some of which have survived. The whole process has, of course, now been arrested by the construction of the Aswan dams and a series of barrages, the length of the valley down to north of Cairo.

These factors resulted in a sharp differentiation of Egypt into two zones, still sharply divided into the Black Land (*Kemet*) and the Red Land (*Deshret*). The former was the land previously covered by the inundation, and comprised strips along the two banks of the Nile with a width varying from almost nothing where the river passes

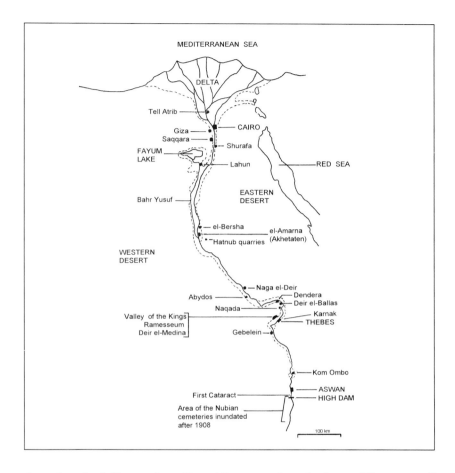

1.1 Map of Egypt showing locations mentioned in the text.

through rocky defiles, to about fifteen kilometres where the desert cliffs are set well back from the river. Two areas depart from this generalisation. An effluent branch of the Nile, the Bahr Yusuf, leaves the mainstream just south of Hermopolis and runs parallel to the west bank for some 170 km as far as Heracleopolis where it turns to the west to drain into the lake of Fayum, an important area of settlement in Pre-dynastic times (fig. 1.1). The second special area is the delta which is the alluvial out-wash fan of the Nile. This is an area some 250 km east to west and 150 km north to south, which is interlaced with the outflow channels of the Nile and is virtually all arable. The total cultivated area at the end of the Predynastic Period has been esti-mated at about 16,000 sq. km, which would support 100,000–200,000 inhabitants with the prevailing intensity of agriculture (Butzer, 1976). Before the high dam was built at Aswan, the cultivated area had increased to only 23,000 sq. km but was supporting a population in excess of 36,000,000 (Darby, Ghaliounghui and Grivetti, 1977).

The Nile was also extremely important for transportation. The prevailing wind blows from the north and ships could therefore travel upstream under sail, and drift downstream with sails lowered. The determinative hieroglyphs for faring upstream and downstream are boats with sails hoisted or lowered, respectively. Progress may have been slow but it required minimal human work and made possible the trans-portation of enormous loads such as monolithic granite obelisks from the quarries of

Aswan to temples far to the north. During the inundation, the breadth of the Nile increased greatly in certain areas and this enabled Tura limestone to be easily shipped from quarries on the east bank to the pyramids of Giza on the west bank. This would have been possible when the farmers were unable to work on their fields and so became available for building and transportation.

The ease and reliability of water transport inhibited the development of land transport. Horses were not imported into Egypt until the Fifteenth (Hyksos) Dynasty (*c.* 1650–1550 BC). There was minimal development of roads, and no major highway linked the two ends of the country, partly because of the obstacles caused by irrigation dykes and canals.

Egyptian history in relation to food and medicine

Stone artefacts indicate that parts of Egypt were inhabited by man in the Palaeolithic Period, at least as early as 200,000 years ago, and it may be presumed that they were hunters, fishers and gatherers (Saffirio, 1972; Spencer, 1993). An Upper Palaeolithic/Mesolithic site (*c.* 10,000 years ago) near Kom Ombo was described by Vignard (1923). This site showed early signs of settlement, including middens with food residues, and stone implements for grinding wild cereals. These finds indicated a diet including molluscs, fish and a variety of herbivores in addition to cereals.

From the late sixth millennium BC, Neolithic cultures appeared in various parts of Egypt, particularly in the Fayum (fig. 1.1). These people, in settled communities, engaged in agriculture and stock raising, though continuing with hunting, fishing and gathering. They grew barley (*Hordeum* species) and emmer (*Triticum dicoccum*) which remained the staple cereals of Egypt until the Late Period when wheat was introduced. They made bread, and the discovery of spoons and ladles suggests that they had developed a type of porridge. Beer was brewed and it seems likely that they would have enjoyed a good balanced diet. Pottery made its appearance, and sheep, goats, pigs and perhaps dogs were domesticated. Copper first appeared among Predynastic Badarian grave-goods in the fifth millennium BC, and the technology of its use developed steadily thereafter. Flint working reached its highest development in the fourth millennium BC. Little is known of the medicine during this time, apart from what we can learn from skeletons and naturally desiccated bodies. Of the various Neolithic cultures, the Predynastic Badarian and Naqada I and II people may be considered the predecessors of the Pharaonic civilisation, and the Neolithic comprises the Predynastic Period of Egyptian history (Appendix A).

The beginning of recorded history is marked by the unification of Upper and Lower Egypt under the first king of the First Dynasty (*c.* 3100 BC), Narmer being the earliest king depicted wearing the crowns of both parts of the country. The Early Dynastic Period (*c.* 3100–2686) comprised the first three dynasties and, for most of this time, the country remained under centralised control from the Delta to Aswan. Writing, an important marker of the Dynastic Period, appeared at the same time, and most of the pre-Ptolemaic hieroglyphs were already used in the First Dynasty. Bronze goods first appeared at the end of the Second Dynasty, with two bronze vessels found in the tomb of King Khasekhem (*c.* 2700 BC). The reign of Netjerkhet (Djoser) in the Third Dynasty saw the first major stone building in the world, the step pyramid of Saqqara, and the first recorded doctor, Hesy-ra (see Chapter 6). Imhotep was the royal chamberlain to Netjerkhet and was subsequently revered as a god of healing (p. 122). As early as the Second Dynasty trade was established with Lebanon, and sea-going vessels were employed at least by the early Fourth Dynasty. This trade was important for the supply of wood and certain drugs.

The Old Kingdom comprised the Third to Sixth Dynasties (c. 2686–2181 BC) and was a period of spectacular achievement. The building of the great pyramids at Giza provides irrefutable evidence of an astonishing level of competence in mathematics, astronomy, stonework, transport and organisation. The hieroglyphs assumed their canonical form early in the Old Kingdom, and a wealth of texts in this script, mostly funerary and religious, have survived. Most of the methods of food production described in the following section were already developed and recorded in the Old Kingdom, and the population was estimated to have increased to between one and one and a half million (Butzer, 1976).

Almost half of all known pharaonic doctors practised during the Old Kingdom, and specialisation was already well advanced. It is thought by many that parts of some of the medical papyri, the Edwin Smith in particular, were first written during this time (Breasted, 1930; Westendorf, 1992; see Chapter 2). However, only copies from later periods have survived. The earliest medical writings seem to contain less magic than in later periods, and Westendorf (1992) has suggested that the spectacular achievements of the early Old Kingdom must have engendered a feeling of immense confidence in the powers of mankind, and particularly the king. A people who could raise the pyramids must have felt that everything was within their power. Turning at a later date towards magic for the cure of disease may have reflected a loss of confidence in mankind and the ability of the king to control their destiny. It may not be coincidental that, in the Fifth Dynasty, all kings acknowledged in the cartouche of their nomen that they were the sons of Ra, and their pyramids were much smaller. At the end of the Dynasty, the pyramid texts featured in the pyramid of Unas and the role of magic became dominant.

During the Old Kingdom, many large tombs of high officials were constructed at Giza and Saqqara, usually surrounding the pyramid of the king they had served. It was believed that anything portrayed on the walls would, by magic, be available to the deceased in the hereafter, and this has provided great insight into the management of estates, hunting, food production and certain aspects of medicine, including the only complete representation of a circumcision (Chapter 8).

The brilliance of the Old Kingdom ultimately faded, and the country lapsed into instability during the First Intermediate Period (c. 2181–2040 BC). This was followed by reassertion of central authority and another period of great splendour known as the Middle Kingdom (c. 2040–1795 BC). This was the classical period of the Egyptian language, and many of the important medical papyri are written in middle Egyptian. Extant copies of two medical papyri, the Kahun and Ramesseum, date from this period or shortly afterwards.

The Second Intermediate Period was again a time of loss of central control and, this time, foreign domination by the Hyksos from Palestine, who ruled parts of Egypt for about a hundred years. Towards the end of this period, the death and embalmment of the pharaoh Seqenenra provided a unique record of injuries from weaponry of the period (see fig. 8.6). Central authority was restored in the New Kingdom which lasted from c. 1550 to 1069 BC, and comprised the Eighteenth to Twentieth Dynasties. This was also a period of great brilliance when Egypt became an international power, fighting major overseas battles at Megiddo under Thutmose III and at Qadesh under Ramses II. Trigger et al. (1983) argued that the population might have been three million rising to perhaps four million by the end of the New Kingdom.

The New Kingdom pharaohs abandoned pyramid building and their tombs were constructed in the Valley of the Kings at Thebes. Excavation of the necropolis workmen's village and their tombs at Deir el-Medina has provided valuable information about food and way of life (Janssen, 1975; Bierbrier, 1982; Kitchen, 1982). In particular, the undisturbed tomb of Kha, the supervisor of works, excavated and described by Schiaparelli (1927), has given unique insight into the possessions of a privileged and highly placed royal artisan. The extant copies of the most important medical papyri date from the New Kingdom.

The heretical pharaoh Akhenaten (Amenhotep IV, c. 1352–1336 BC) interrupted the New Kingdom, creating the Amarna Period, so called after the modern name of his new capital city. Its unorthodox and naturalistic styles of art have provided insight into certain aspects of royal domestic life which are otherwise lost in the strict canon of conventional ancient Egyptian art. It has also raised very difficult questions about the pathology of Akhenaten himself (p. 83). The reign of Tutankhamun saw the return to orthodoxy and his tomb remained intact until modern times after early resealings following robberies soon after interment. The tomb contained many items of medical interest, particularly the botanical specimens. It is widely believed that the New Kingdom covered the period of the Hebrews in Egypt, and Merenptah (c. 1213–1203 BC) may have been the pharaoh of the biblical oppression.

The New Kingdom was followed by yet another period of loss of central control, eventually leading to foreign intrusions. The Third Intermediate Period (Twenty-first to Twenty-fifth Dynasties) lasted from c. 1069 to 656 BC and included both Libyan and Nubian dynasties. In 671 and 667 BC, the Assyrians invaded Egypt and sacked Thebes but allowed Psamtek to govern Lower Egypt on their behalf. In due course, as Psamtek I, he became ruler of all Egypt and the first king of the Twenty-sixth (Saite) Dynasty (664–525 BC), which featured a revival of aspects of the ancient Egyptian civilisation, looking backwards to emulate many of the glories of the past. However, Egypt of the Late Period was perforce more outward looking and maintained close relations with Greek mercenaries and traders, who were permitted to establish their own city at Naucratis in the Delta.

Assyria fell to the Babylonians at the end of the reign of Psamtek I, but independence lasted only until 525 BC when Psamtek III was defeated by Cambyses (Cambyses II of Persia), who established the Twenty-seventh (Persian) Dynasty. The Egyptian chief physician Wedja-hor-resnet held high office under both Cambyses and his successor Darius I (p. 129). Greek medicine was already challenging Egyptian medicine and there were strong Greek schools at Croton, Cyrene and Cnidus: the great Hippocratic medical school flourished in Cos from c. 430 to 330 BC. Herodotus made his celebrated visit to Egypt in about 450 BC and so was well placed to comment on the complex interaction of Egyptians, Persians and Greeks. He also wrote about Egyptian medicine of the Twenty-seventh Dynasty and referred to the challenge of Greek medicine (p. 206). Meteoric and probably some imported iron were known and worked in the New Kingdom (Lucas and Harris, 1989), but the use of iron did not become widespread until the Twenty-seventh Dynasty.

A second brief period of Persian rule was terminated abruptly in 332 BC by the Macedonian invasion under Alexander the Great. Chapter 10 describes how this led to the establishment of the great Alexandrian medical school and its profound influence on Egyptian medicine during the Ptolemaic, Roman and Coptic periods. Diodorus Siculus wrote about Egypt on the basis of a visit in the middle of the first century BC, when he estimated the population to have been 'seven million in antiquity and remained no less down to our day'.

The production of food

As a result of the favourable climate and geography, food production was never a major problem in Egypt provided that the inundation of the Nile occurred each year

1.2 Loaves from the undisturbed tomb of Kha, Deir el-Medina, 18th Dynasty. (Egyptian Museum, Turin)

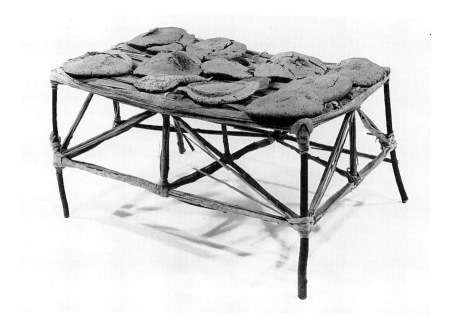

and the population did not exceed the capacity of the available land. The Egyptian year comprised twelve months divided into three seasons each of four months. The year commenced with the rising of Sirius before sunrise, an event which heralded the inundation, occurring during the season of *akhet* corresponding to July to October. As soon as the flood had receded, usually in September or October, the fields were remeasured and assessed for their likely productivity. Ploughing and sowing then took place during the four-month season November to February, known as *peret* (time of emergence). The four-month period March to June was known as *shemu* (harvest).

The main cereal crops were barley (*it*) and emmer (*bedet*), wheat being introduced only in the Late Period. Loaves (*te*) were the staple form of carbohydrate intake, and there were many different types and flavours (Samuel, 1993). Figure 1.2 shows loaves from the undisturbed tomb of Kha (Eighteenth Dynasty). Barley was also used to make beer (*henqet*). Loaves were baked, soaked in water, fermented and strained (Samuel, 1993), the yeast converting the cereal grains into many valuable nutritional components (Katz and Voigt, 1986) and might have been a source of dietary tetra-cyline (see Chapter 7). Beer was much valued and the offering formulae in countless tombs commence with a request for 'thousands of bread and beer'. This typical example is from the stela of Tjetji (BM 614):

An offering which the king gives and Osiris, lord of Busiris, foremost of the westerners (i.e. those in the necropolis), lord of Abydos in all his shrines. Invocation offering of one thousand loaves and beer, one thousand flesh of cattle, one thousand of fowl, one thousand of alabaster vessels and linen garments, one thousand of all things beautiful and pure.

Vegetables were grown on a large scale, including many familiar varieties (Table 1.1). There was a profusion of fruit available (Table 1.2): pomegranates are shown in fig. 1.3 from the tomb of Kha. Grapes were fermented to produce wine (*irep*): many

13

Table 1.1 Vegetables and marsh plants in use in pharaonic Egypt

COMMON NAME	LINNEAN NAME	EGYPTIAN NAME	FIRST RECORDED USE AS FOOD	MEDICAL USE
Vegetables				
bean	*Vicia faba*	*iuryt*	Fifth Dynasty	extensive
cabbage	*Brassica oleracea*	uncertain	Nineteenth Dynasty[1]	–
celery	*Apium graveolens*	*matet*	Roman	extensive
chickpea	*Cicer arietinum*	*heru bik*	Twentieth Dynasty	none
cos lettuce	*Lactuca sativa*	*abu*	Old Kingdom	not for *abu*[2]
cucumber	*Cucumis sativus*	*bendet*	New Kingdom at least	none
		shespet		occasional
garlic	*Allium sativum*	*kheten*?	New Kingdom	not for *kheten*
leek	*Allium kurrat / porrum*	*iaqet*	Twentieth Dynasty ?	occasional
lentil	*Ervum lens*	*aarshan*	Predynastic	unlikely
melon	*Cucumis melo*	*shespet*	unclear	occasional
onion	*Allium cepa*	*hedju*	Fifth Dynasty	extensive
pea	*Pisum cepa*	*tehua*	Twelfth Dynasty	extensive
radish	*Raphanus sativus*	uncertain	Twelfth Dynasty	–
Marsh plants				
Eg. bean	*Kyamon aegytion*	*neheb*	Herodotus II, 92	none
papyrus	*Cyperus papyrus*	*mehyt*	Herodotus II, 92	occasional
sedge	*Cyperus esculentus*	*gyu*	Predynastic[3]	extensive
white lotus	*Nymphaea lotus*	*seshen*	Old Kingdom	occasional

First recorded use as food depends both on texts and on archaeological findings (Darby, Ghaliounghui and Grivetti, 1977). Accounts of medical use are based on the appearance of the Egyptian word in the medical texts (*Grundriss* VI, 1959). Egyptian names are usually very difficult to relate to Linnean names, and many of the identifications in these and the following tables must be accepted with caution.

1 According to Breasted, if *shawt* is the correct Egyptian word for cabbage.

2 *Afet / afay* is now believed to be the wild lettuce (*Lactuca virosa*) which had considerable medical use; *afet* was alternatively thought to mean clover (*Melilotus officinalis*). See Table 7.5.

3 The roots of *Cyperus esculentus* bear edible and nutritious 'earth almonds' or 'tiger nuts' (*wah*), which also had extensive medical use.

tomb reliefs show the cultivation of vineyards, gathering the grapes and expressing the juice. Alcoholic intoxication (*tekh*) was well described and illustrated. Vegetable oils were obtained from the linseed plant and nuts of the moringa tree, *Moringa pterygosperma* (*baq*). This oil (*ben* oil) was used not only for cooking but also in medical remedies. Sweetening was with dates or honey. Although beekeeping was actively developed, honey remained a relatively precious commodity and this tended to protect the ancient Egyptians from dental caries (Chapter 9). There was a modest range of herbs and spices, many of which were used in medicine (Table 1.3).

The consumption of a very wide variety of animal products was enjoyed by at least the wealthier Egyptians (Darby, Ghaliounghui and Grivetti, 1977). Cattle (*menmenet*) were raised on a large scale. Tomb paintings, reliefs and models show the counting of large herds, and the *Tale of Two Brothers* commences with intimate scenes of animal husbandry. There was also portrayal of delivery of calves and butchery: the epithet 'one who knows the bulls' (*rekh kaw*) seems to describe those with veterinary skills. Cattle were included in the usual offering formula for the dead and there can be no doubt that joints of beef were a much prized item of diet. Milk was highly valued

Table 1.2 Fruit in use in pharaonic Egypt

COMMON NAME	LINNEAN NAME	EGYPTIAN NAME	FIRST RECORDED USE AS FOOD	MEDICAL USE
apple	*Malus sylvestris*	*depeh(t)*	Nineteenth Dynasty	not known
carob	*Ceratonia siliqua*	*djaret*	Twelfth Dynasty	extensive
date	*Phoenix dactylifera*	*bener*	Predynastic	extensive
doum palm	*Hyphaene thebaica*	*mama / ququ*	Predynastic	not known
fig	*Ficus carica*	*dab*	Second Dynasty	frequent
grape	*Vitis vinifera*	*iarret*	Third Dynasty	extensive[1]
jujube	*Zizyphus spina-Christi*	*nebes*	Third Dynasty	frequent
olive	*Olea europaea*	*djedet?*	Eighteenth Dynasty[2]	not known
persea	*Mimusops schimperi*	*shawabu*	Third Dynasty	?
plum	*Cordia myxa*	uncertain	Eighteenth Dynasty	not known
pomegranate	*Punica granatum*	*inhemen*	Twelfth Dynasty	occasional
sycomore fig	*Ficus sycomorus*	*nehet*	Predynastic	extensive
watermelon	*Citrullus vulgaris*	*beddu-ka*	New Kingdom	frequent

First recorded use as food depends both on texts and on archaeological findings (Darby, Ghaliounghui and Grivetti, 1977). Accounts of medical use are based on the appearance of the Egyptian word in the medical texts (*Grundriss* VI, 1959).

1 Wine was used extensively as a vehicle for medicines.

2 Olive stones were reported by David Jeffreys from late Middle Kingdom levels, perhaps Thirteenth Dynasty, at Memphis (provisional identification by Maryanne Murray).

Table 1.3 Spices and herbs in use in pharaonic Egypt

COMMON NAME	LINNEAN NAME	EGYPTIAN NAME	FIRST RECORDED USE AS FOOD	MEDICAL USE
aniseed	*Pimpinella anisum*	*inset* ??	Pliny	considerable[1]
cinnamon	*Laurus cinnamonum* (*Cinnamonum zeylanicum*)	*ti-shepes*	Twentieth Dynasty[2]	considerable
conyza	*Erigeron aegypticus* (*Conyza aegypticus*)	*innek* ??	uncertain	considerable[3]
coriander	*Coriandrum sativum*	*shaw*	Eighteenth Dynasty[4]	considerable
cumin	*Cuminum cyminum*	*tepnen*	Eighteenth Dynasty[2,4]	considerable
dill	*Anethum graveolens*	*imset*	Eighteenth Dynasty[4]	occasional
fenugreek	*Trigonella foenum-graecum*	*hemayt*	unclear	extensive
safflower	*Carmathus tinctorius*	*kata* ??	unclear	none
thyme	*Thymus acinos*	*innek* ??	unclear	considerable[4]

First recorded use as food depends both on texts and on archaeological findings (Darby, Ghaliounghui and Grivetti, 1977). Accounts of medical use are based on the appearance of the Egyptian word in the medical texts (*Grundriss* VI, 1959).

1 This is based on the word *inset*, for which the meaning is still uncertain.

2 Presented by Ramses III to the gods on many occasions, but found earlier in non-specific contexts.

3 Medical use is based solely on the word *innek*, which cannot be translated with any certainty.

4 Found in tomb of Tutankhamun (Hepper, 1990).

both as a food and as an important component of medical remedies. There are representations of children and adult royalty feeding directly from the udders of cows.

'Small cattle' (*awet*) was a term describing sheep, goats and pigs (*sha*). Large flocks of sheep were kept, and some sheep were revered as manifestations of specific deities. However, there is no clear evidence that their meat was either a favoured item of diet or that it figured in offerings. Diodorus Siculus (I, 87), writing in the first century BC,

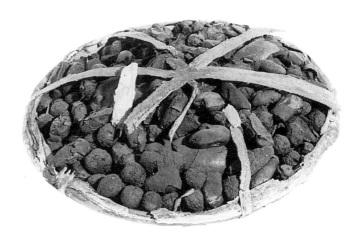

1.3 Pomegranates from the undisturbed tomb of Kha, Deir el-Medina, 18th Dynasty. (Egyptian Museum, Turin)

mentions the value of sheep in producing wool, milk and cheese but makes no mention of their meat. Herodotus (II, 47) reported in the fifth century BC that the pig was considered unclean, but Darby and his colleagues reviewed the evidence that pigs were eaten throughout the Dynastic Period. For example, pig bones, particularly skulls, were found in the waste deposits of Deir el-Medina. Pigs were included in the inventory of the possessions of Nemtynakht which were forfeit to the hero in the Middle Kingdom *Tale of the Eloquent Peasant*. Products of pigs were also included in some medical remedies. Many species of wild animals were hunted and some of these were presumably used for food.

Birds feature in the offering formula above, where they probably refer to ducks (*aped*). The ideogram for 'fear' (Gardiner sign-list F 54) is a trussed duck or goose ready for the oven. Dressed and cooked ducks were found within an amphora in the tomb of Kha (fig. 1.4). Every stage of the husbandry and preparation of fowl has been shown on tomb paintings. These include force feeding (cranes and geese), penning, plucking, dressing, cooking and eating (Darby, Ghaliounghui and Grivetti, 1977). Ducks can be seen carried by a doctor as a funerary offering in fig. 6.7. There are many representations of netting wildfowl or killing them with a throwstick. The eating of quail is known from the early Old Kingdom, and the quail chick is perpetuated in the phonetic hieroglyph representing '*w*'. The position of the domestic fowl (*Gallus domesticus*) is less well documented, although a single find of skeletal remains and eggs was dated to the Eighteenth Dynasty (Darby *et al.*, 1977). However, hens were probably not kept on a large scale until the Ptolemaic Period. Over all, there is ample evidence that fowl represented a very welcome component of the diet.

The Nile abounded in fish and there are many representations of fishing techniques with a wide range of hooked lines, harpoons, spears, nets and traps (Brewer and Friedman, 1989). There are also illustrations of the preparation of fish, clearly with

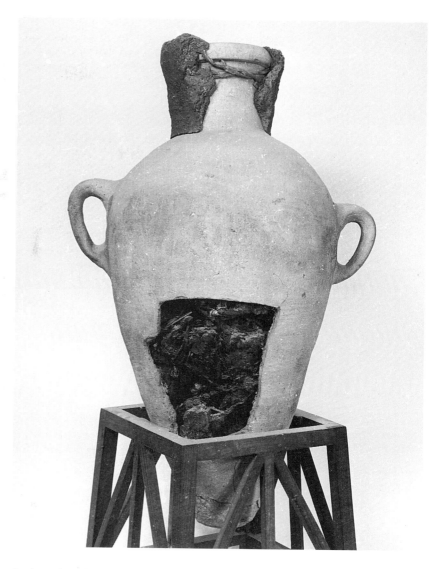

1.4 Cooked ducks in a jar from the undisturbed tomb of Kha, Deir el-Medina, 18th Dynasty. Preparation is shown in the Theban tomb of Rekhmire (Wilson, 1988). (Egyptian Museum, Turin)

the intention that they should be cooked and eaten. The acceptability of fish is, however, less clear. Again, Darby *et al.* (1977) amassed ample evidence to show that fish were consumed in quantity by large sections of the population. However, it seems likely that some priests were forbidden to eat certain fish, particularly the Oxyrhynchus, Lepidotus and Phagrus which fed on the phallus of Osiris after his murder and dismemberment by Seth, according to the late account of Plutarch (Isis and Osiris, 358, 18 B).

Relatively pure samples of salt (*hemat*) have been found from the Sixth Dynasty (Wilson, 1988), but the method of preparation is unknown. The absence of sulphates and carbonates in the samples makes it unlikely that salt was extracted from natron, and far more likely that it was obtained from the Mediterranean or Red Sea, either from natural salt deposits or by the use of salt pans. Pepper was unknown, but silicules of *Sinapis arvensis* (the mustard plant) are said to have been found in a Twelfth Dynasty tomb opened by Mariette (Aufrère, 1987). The likely Egyptian word is *senep*, which bears the same consonants as *Sinapi(s)*. It is improbable that the ancient Egyptians could have failed to discover vinegar, and Aufrère believes the word to be *ip-wer* or *pa-wer* (the great one).

Nutritional state

The preceding section indicates that there was a very large range of foodstuffs available to the ancient Egyptians. No doubt the privileged members of the community lacked for little, as shown by the funerary offerings for King Unas at the end of the Fifth Dynasty (*c*. 2494–2345 BC):

> … milk, three kinds of beer, five kinds of wine, ten loaves, four of bread, ten of cakes, fruit cakes, four meats, different cuts, joints, roast, spleen, limb, breast, tail, goose, pigeon, figs, ten other fruits, three kinds of corn, barley, spelt, five kinds of oil, and fresh plants …

Such a list accords with the foods which were shown heaped on offering tables in reliefs and paintings in innumerable tombs (fig. 1.5).

1.5 An offering table shown in a wall painting from the tomb of Nebamun, Thebes, 18th Dynasty. (British Museum, EA 37985)
1: Notched sycamore figs.
2: Lotus. 3: Loaves. 4: Heart.
5: Figs (*Ficus carica*).
6: Honeycombs.
7: Unidentified fruit. 8: Roast duck or goose. 9: Grapes.
10: Head of ox. 11: Leg of ox. 12: Gourd, ? cucumber. Wine jars are shown below.

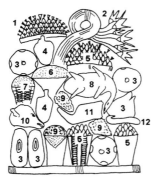

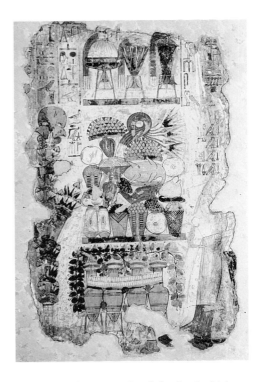

The undisturbed tomb of Kha provided a unique sample of the food which an important man in a supervisory capacity over the royal necropolis workers might have at his disposal in the reign of Amenhotep III (*c*. 1390–1352 BC). Examples listed above include loaves (fig. 1.2), pomegranates (fig. 1.3) and ducks (fig. 1.4). In addition there were oils, a wide variety of fruit and two large sacks of doum palm nuts.

Some idea of the variety of food available to 'Egyptians who live in the cultivated parts of the country' in the Late Period may be gained from Herodotus (II, 77) who said:

> They eat loaves . . . and drink wine made from barley . . . Some kinds of fish they eat raw, either dried in the sun or salted. Quails too they eat raw, and ducks and various small birds, after pickling them in brine; other sorts of birds and fish, apart from those which they considered sacred, they either roast or boil.

The basic source of calories was grain, and it is helpful to consider the energy balance of the population in these terms (Miller, 1991a). One *aroura* of land (2735 sq. m) yielded approximately 10 *khar* of grain (*c.* 765 litres) at each harvest. Assuming about 700 grams per litre of grain, and a calorific value of 3.6 kilocalories per gram, 1 *khar* would yield 192,780 kilocalories. Therefore one *aroura* of land would provide 5282 kilocalories for each day of the year, if all the produce was harvested, saved and eaten. If approximately half of this was lost to taxes and vermin, and saved for seed corn, the remaining value would be about 2641 kilocalories per day, sufficient to sustain one adult. In fact it was reckoned that one labourer could cultivate 20 *aroura*, which would provide the basic calorie requirement for twenty adults, and therein lay the essential basis for the economic strength of the country.

These calculations accord with estimates of arable land and population in pharaonic times (see above). If half of a cultivated area of (say) 20,000 sq. km was used for the production of grain, this could be expected to have supported a population up to about four million. This approximates to the estimated population in the New Kingdom (Trigger *et al.*, 1983).

It is not easy to determine the amount and variety of food available to different levels of society. Apart from the different esteem in which various trades and professions were held, their sustenance must also have depended on the quality of the harvest, the level of taxation and the relationship between the peasant and the

Table 1.4 Allocation of grain rations to various groups of necropolis workers (including their families) in Deir el-Medina, expressed in terms of the daily calorific value of the grain (from Cairo ostracon J 51518)

DESIGNATION	DAILY CALORIFIC VALUES (KILOCALORIES PER DAY)
chief of the workers	48,195
scribe	48,195
workman	35,343
guardian	28,917
female servant (*hemet*)	19,278
boy	12,852
porter	9,639
doctor (*swnw*)	8,033

3500 kilocalories/day is generally adequate for light manual labour.
2500 kilocalories/day is generally sufficient for sedentary work.

landowner. Such factors would inevitably change with time and also vary from one locality to another.

Some indication is given by the daily rations for working parties assigned to a specific task. Breasted (1906) calculated that a detachment of workers, sent by Seti I to the Silsileh quarries, received a daily allowance of 1.8 kilograms of bread, two bundles of vegetables and a roast of flesh. The bread alone would have yielded 6480 kilocalories, about double that required for light manual work. The 'Eloquent Peasant', during his enforced detention while making his repeated petitions, received a daily allowance of ten loaves and two jars of beer, the latter being perhaps generous to encourage his eloquence.

The Cairo ostracon J 51518 records rations for necropolis workers at Deir el-Medina (Cerny, 1927). These are an allocation of emmer and barley, part of which could no doubt be exchanged for vegetables, fruit, fish or meat. Money was not introduced until the Persian Period. Presumably the ration per man had to suffice for his wife and any children they might have had. Table 1.4 shows the rations calculated as total calories per day per family on the assumption that no exchanges were made. Light manual work would require about 3500 kilocalories per day, sedentary work 2500 kilocalories per day, and children would need less depending on their size. The very low rations for the doctor suggest that he also functioned as a workman, and received additional rations for his special duties, which could only have occupied a small fraction of his time (Janssen, 1975).

Physique

The ancient Egyptians were small by modern standards. Masali and Chiarelli (1972) found the mean skeletal length of Dynastic males to be 1.57 m (approx. 5 ft 2 in) and females 1.48 m (approx. 4 ft 10 in). Even the great Ramses II was only 1.73 m (approx. 5 ft 8 in) after mummification (Elliot Smith, 1912). The breadth of shoulders and pelvis of the men bore roughly the same proportion to height as that of modern Euro-

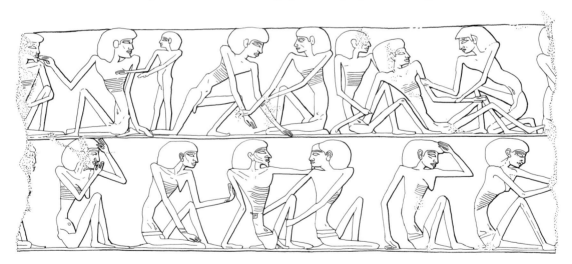

1.6 Scenes of famine shown on a stone block of the causeway leading to the pyramid of Unas at Saqqara, 5th Dynasty.

peans. However, the pelves of the women were considerably narrower in proportion to the shoulder girdle than is the case in modern women. In fact, their pelves bore the same proportion to height as those of their contemporary males. Therefore the graceful, slender proportions of so many Egyptian women in statues, reliefs and paintings were not merely idealising artistic license but based on sound anthropometric data.

There are many illustrations of obesity in stelae, reliefs and paintings (see fig. 4.11). However, it is often unclear whether they are factual representations or merely stylistic conventions to indicate affluence or high position. It was, furthermore, the custom to represent obesity as a normal characteristic of certain vocations such as male musicians. Wasting is less commonly shown but there are a few well known famine scenes (fig. 1.6). The Egyptian habit of squatting for various tasks, shown in many statuettes and reliefs, is confirmed by the 'squatting facets' on tibia and talus in over 90 per cent of 300 male and female skeletons studied by Satinoff (1972).

Clothing

The climate of Egypt required minimal clothing for most of the year. Workmen and peasants are commonly depicted wearing only a waistband or kilt. Well made clothing was available to the upper classes and Kha's tomb contains an elegant tunic with embroidered neck (fig. 1.7). The material was derived from flax (*Linum usitatissimum*), the stems producing flax or linen and the seeds producing linseed oil. Young plants produced a particularly fine linen which was made into the long and nearly transparent garments worn to such advantage by ladies of the court. There would have been little demand for woollen garments and there is almost no evidence for its use apart from the comment of Diodorus Siculus mentioned above. Cotton was unknown until the Coptic period (Stead, 1986). Children and female servants serving at banquets were almost always shown naked apart from girdles and jewellery, although it is unclear whether this represented their true state or was an artistic

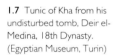

1.7 Tunic of Kha from his undisturbed tomb, Deir el-Medina, 18th Dynasty. (Egyptian Museum, Turin)

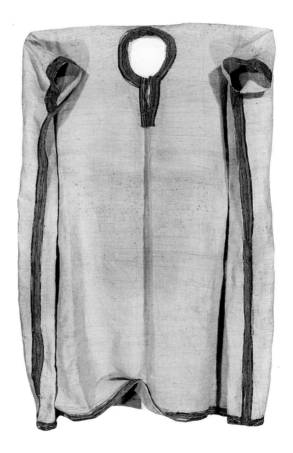

21

convention. Highly serviceable sandals were made of leather or papyrus, and are well represented in the tomb of Kha. Deficiencies of clothing are unlikely to have posed any threat to health.

Expectation of life

It is virtually impossible to determine the expectation of life in an ancient population. However, Masali and Chiarelli (1972) studied material from the Turin cemetery collections, comprising a Predynastic section from Gebelen and a Dynastic section from Gebelen and Asyut. The arithmetic mean age at death was thirty for the Predynastic Period, and thirty-six for the Dynastic Period. This accords well with the radiological age for royal burials (Seventeenth to Twentieth Dynasties) recorded by Krogman and Baer (1980) although royalty must have enjoyed a far more favourable life style (fig. 1.8). Masali and Chiarelli estimated that the population would be reduced to one-half at around twenty-five years for the Predynastics and at thirty

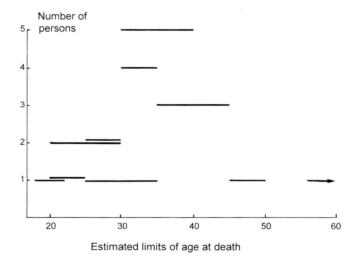

1.8 Estimated ages at death of royal personages from 17th to 20th Dynasties. (Data from Krogman and Baer, 1980)

years for the Dynastics. These values are not greatly different from other ancient populations, and some contemporary people without access to the benefits of modern medicine. There were very few burials of people over the age of sixty. Nevertheless, it should be noted that some commoners and at least two kings, Pepi ii and Ramses ii, survived well into their eighties according to the historical record.

Language and writing

The Egyptians were highly literate throughout the pharaonic period, and the preservation of texts on stone, wood, ostraca, sherds and papyrus is remarkably good whenever the material has remained dry. Black ink was carbon-based and red ink used ochre, both of which will last indefinitely. Some papyri have survived in mint condition. Although the language changed to a considerable extent during the three millennia of its existence, the degree of continuity was exceptional for such a long time span. Unfortunately, the script was lost about AD 450, although the spoken language survived in modified form in Coptic, which was written in Greek letters augmented by seven characters derived from demotic. Coptic was itself eventually replaced by Arabic but survived as the liturgical language of the Coptic church.

The language of ancient Egypt has been reconstructed laboriously from those texts which have survived, but the meaning of many words remains either unknown or uncertain. This is a particular problem with the medical texts which abound with words not found elsewhere. Furthermore, even when a word is familiar in non-medical contexts, there is always the possibility that it carried a special meaning when used in a medical sense. The full writing of most words contains phonetic signs, followed by a determinative which is a stereotyped representation of the word or group of words to which it belongs. Therefore, the determinative alone will usually give the general if not the specific meaning. Thus we can, for example, identify many drugs as plants, even though it may not be possible to identify the species.

The familiar hieroglyphs are cumbersome to write and their use was mainly confined to texts carved or painted on stone, plaster or wood. A simplified script, known as hieratic (literally: 'the writing of the priests'), came into use at least as early as the Old Kingdom, and was commonly used for writing on papyrus. However, certain religious texts, in particular the *Book of the Dead*, were written on papyrus in cursive or linear hieroglyphs. The Ramesseum v medical and the Kahun veterinary texts are unusual in being secular material written in cursive hieroglyphs (Chapter 2). Although hieratic was easier to write, it sometimes poses problems of legibility. The style of the hieratic characters evolved gradually and it is thus possible to date a text with considerable accuracy. This contrasts with the hieroglyphs which changed relatively little. Finally, during the Twenty-fifth and Twenty-sixth Dynasties there emerged a still more cursive script known as demotic ('the writing of the people') which was even faster to write. It evolved from hieratic and bore no obvious relation to the corresponding hieroglyphs. This replaced hieratic as the business and literary script on papyrus and was used in late medical papyri. Demotic was widely used in the Ptolemaic Period, when it was also a monumental script and appeared as one of the three texts on the Rosetta Stone.

An environment for development of a system of medical practice

The ancient Egyptians enjoyed a unique environment in which their medical practice could develop and be recorded. The Nile and its inundation ensured a supply of food which left ample time for activities unrelated to food production. The geography of Egypt ensured a relative freedom from foreign intrusions which was unusual for the time. Their conservatism ensured that favourable developments were retained, and used as a basis for further advances. Their early invention of writing and the durability of papyrus provided the means for codifying and propagating their medical practice. But perhaps the most important factor was the remarkable administrative, inventive and technical skills of the ancient Egyptians. It is not really surprising that a race which could build the pyramids in the third millennium BC should make major contributions to the early development of medicine.

CHAPTER **TWO**

The medical papyri

Some insight into the medical practice of ancient Egypt may be derived from human remains, from representations of bodies showing signs of disease and from occasional references to disease in the non-medical papyri and stelae. However, by far the most important sources of our knowledge are the medical papyri. According to Clement of Alexandria, writing in the second century AD, the forty-two books of human knowledge possessed by the ancient Egyptians included six of medical content:

37. The structure of the body	40. Remedies
38. Diseases	41. The eyes and their diseases
39. The instruments of doctors	42. Diseases of women

It is interesting to compare these six headings with the contents of the surviving pharaonic manuscripts, the first recalling sections of the Ebers papyrus (854 and 856 – see Chapter 3). For the second, there are extensive references to diseases in the Ebers, Hearst, Berlin and Chester Beatty papyri, but mainly in relation to remedies, and there are few specific accounts of the diseases themselves. Almost nothing has survived on the instruments of doctors and no unequivocally medical instruments can be identified from the pharaonic period. Remedies are listed in most of the medical papyri, but there is nothing corresponding to a pharmacopoeia except for a few passages such as Ebers 251 (see below and Chapter 7). Diseases of the eyes occupy a major part of the Ebers papyrus and this might perhaps relate to the fifth book to which Clement referred. Finally, one part of the Kahun papyrus is exclusively concerned with diseases of women and this might correspond with the material treated by the sixth book listed by Clement. The recto (front) of the Carlsberg papyrus concerns eye ailments, while the verso (back) covers gynaecological topics. Iversen (1939) noted the coincidence that these correspond to Clement's last two books.

The most important medical papyri were found during the last century or the early years of the present century and are listed in Table 2.1. In most cases they were offered for sale with little or no detail of their provenance. It seems plausible that some at least came from tombs of doctors, but in no case is it possible to link a medical papyrus with a known doctor. They are written on papyrus and, with the exception of Ramesseum V, in hieratic. The writing is horizontal from right to left, except for Ramesseum III, IV and V, which are written in vertical columns, a common practice in the Middle Kingdom. Although there is considerable repetition between some of the papyri, there is good reason to believe that we possess only a small fraction of the medical papyri, so many of which must have been lost by the ravages of time. Particularly serious losses were the disastrous fires in the library of Alexandria in 47 BC and AD 389, although there is no firm evidence that this essentially Greek institution would have held copies of Egyptian papyri. Many papyri would certainly have been destroyed during tomb robbing, some were used as fuel and a number were actually used to prepare magical remedies. Ebers 262 itself describes the use of 'an old book cooked in oil (or grease)' as a local application to be applied to the belly to help a child pass urine. A medical text might have been considered particularly effective.

The purpose of the present chapter is to give a general introduction to the medical papyri and provide an overall indication of their contents and their relationship to one another. Details of their contents are considered in the appropriate chapters.

Table 2.1 The most important medical papyri

TITLE	LOCATION	APPROXIMATE DATE OF COPY	CONTENTS
Edwin Smith	New York	1550 BC	surgical, mainly trauma
Ebers	Leipzig	1500 BC	general, mainly medical
Kahun (gynaecology)	University College, London	1820 BC	gynaecological
Hearst*	California	1450 BC	general medical
Chester Beatty VI*	BM 10686	1200 BC	rectal diseases
Berlin*	Berlin	1200 BC	general medical
London*	BM 10059	1300 BC	mainly magical
Carlsberg VIII	Copenhagen	1300 BC	gynaecological
Ramesseum III, IV, V*	Oxford	1700 BC	gynaecological, ophthalmic and paediatric
London and Leiden	BM 10072 and Leiden	AD 250	general medical and magical
Crocodilopolis	Vienna	AD 150	general
Brooklyn snake*	Brooklyn	300 BC	snake bite

*No English translation is available.
BM British Museum

The *Grundriss der Medizin der alten Ägypter*

The most comprehensive study of the medical papyri is enshrined in the *Grundriss der Medizin der alten Ägypter* (Outline of the medicine of the ancient Egyptians) produced from Berlin in the years 1954–73. No serious study is possible without consultation of these volumes. Table 2.2 (p. 31) lists the authors and titles.

A full hieroglyphic transcription of the most important medical papyri is to be found in volume v. Paragraphs are arranged according to the parts of the body in which disease occurs and not sequentially as the papyrus was written. Thus sections of different papyri appear together, particularly for parallel passages. Any section of a particular papyrus may be found by reference to the concordance at the back of volume v: this also indicates the page number of the corresponding German translation in volume IV 1. The commentary is in volume IV 2. Egyptian–German vocabulary for names of drugs is in volume VI, while all other Egyptian words are treated in volumes VII 1 and 2, which include citations for the more important appearances of the words in the various medical texts. The system is inevitably cumbersome to use, but the wealth of information is incomparable and unlikely to be surpassed in the foreseeable future. Both Gardiner's Egyptian grammar (1957) and Faulkner's Dictionary of Middle Egyptian (1962) make extensive reference to the medical papyri. Although the grammar is in most cases fairly standard, the vocabulary presents serious problems. Many words occur only in the medical papyri, and one suspects that others, with a well attested meaning elsewhere, may have a special interpretation in the medical context.

The Edwin Smith papyrus

This most important papyrus was offered for sale in 1862 by Mustafa Agha, the Egyptian merchant, dealer and Consular Agent in Luxor. It was purchased by Edwin

Smith, an American, who was resident in Luxor from 1858 until 1876, and on whom there are rather diverse views. Dawson and Uphill (1972) described him as an adventurer, money lender and antiquities dealer, and also noted that he was reputed to advise on, and even practise, the forgery of antiquities. However, Breasted (1930) took a far more charitable view of his countryman, and presented evidence of his extensive knowledge of hieratic, which was remarkable for the period and probably unique among Americans at that early date. It is greatly to his credit that he recognised the surgical nature of the papyrus when it was offered to him, and he later made a tentative translation. On his death in 1906, his daughter presented the papyrus to the New York Historical Society. It is now in the New York Academy of Medicine.

In 1930, Breasted, Director of the Oriental Institute in Chicago, published a facsimile reproduction, translation and extensive commentary, with medical advice from Dr Arno B. Luckhardt. This publication was a landmark, showing for the first time a medical text from ancient Egypt almost free from magic and following rational lines of diagnosis and treatment. The papyrus was subsequently translated into German by von Deines, Grapow and Westendorf (1958) in volume IV 1 of the *Grundriss* (Table 2.2), and again into German by Westendorf alone in 1966. Breasted's remains the only English translation of the whole papyrus.

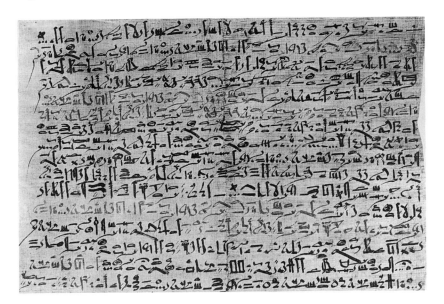

2.1 The start of column III of the Edwin Smith papyrus written in hieratic, from right to left as usual. Case 7 starts at the beginning of the second line. (From Breasted, 1930)

Nothing is known of the provenance of the Edwin Smith papyrus, but it is often assumed to have been taken from the tomb of a physician in the Theban necropolis on the west bank of the Nile opposite Luxor. It is possible that the Edwin Smith papyrus came from the same tomb as the Ebers papyrus which was also purchased by Edwin Smith in 1862 (see below). The dating of the scribes' hieratic script is similar for both papyri. The Rhind mathematical papyrus may have come from the same burial and it is entirely in keeping with the Egyptian view of the hereafter that a man should wish to have such texts with him in the netherworld.

The Edwin Smith papyrus is second only to the Ebers papyrus in length, comprising seventeen pages (377 lines) on the recto and five pages (92 lines) on the verso. The recto and most of the verso are in the same hand (fig. 2.1). It is well written in hieratic and the style of writing dates to approximately 1550 BC. There are several omissions, most of which have been corrected in the same hand. Both Breasted (1930) and Westendorf (1992) have expressed the view that the original must have been Old Kingdom on the grounds of some items of grammatical construction and vocabulary. This would be about 1000 years before the copy we possess. However, most of the text is written in classical Middle Egyptian and the early origin of the papyrus has recently been questioned by Collins, Parkinson and Quirke (personal communications, 1995). It would not be unusual if certain archaic features had been deliberately introduced into the text to give the appearance of antiquity, which was so revered by the ancient Egyptians. The original date is of great importance to our understanding of the time course of development of ancient Egyptian medicine.

The copy is unique, and almost none of the text is duplicated in any other medical papyrus. The suggested length of time between the original and the extant copy is not surprising because of the reverence in which the ancient Egyptians held old books. However, the New Kingdom physicians appeared to have had problems interpreting the meaning of many of the words and phrases used by the original author. Hence the papyrus is well provided with glosses, appended to most of the cases and following the general format: 'As for XXX, it means YYY'. These provide an invaluable medical dictionary for early surgical practice. Unlike the Ebers papyrus, most of the glosses are correctly located and there is no difficulty in relating the word or phrase which is explained to its original appearance in the text. Sometimes this has helped in the filling of a lacuna.

The contents

The recto, or 'front' side, of the roll comprises the surgical papyrus and is divided into seventeen pages describing forty-eight cases, nearly all the victims of trauma. It differs from most of the other medical papyri in its logical approach, being a *shesau* or 'instruction' book, rather than simply a compilation of remedies (a *pekhret* or remedy book). This enables us to visualise the ancient Egyptian doctor's examination of the patient, and we can gain considerable insight into the processes by which he arrived at a diagnosis. This contrasts with much of the Ebers papyrus, which usually assumes that the diagnosis has already been made and then follows with a remedy to eliminate the named disease. This is usually given without any indication of the symptoms of the disease and, in many instances, it is now impossible for us to know what was the disease.

The outside of a papyrus roll is more vulnerable to damage and it is therefore not surprising that the first page of the Edwin Smith is entirely missing and the second (numbered I) has many lacunae. The missing parts embraced the title, examination and part of the pronouncement for Case 1. These were largely reconstructed by Breasted and this was possible because of the highly structured format of the cases as described below. Fortunately Gloss A is preserved, which explains the phrase 'If you examine a man'. This gloss continues with the extremely important passage (quoted at the beginning of Chapter 6) as parallel to Ebers 854a. If the original of the Edwin Smith papyrus is Old Kingdom, this indicates the antiquity of this very important passage concerning examination of the pulse and the parallel roles of conventional doctors, priests of Sekhmet and magicians.

Each case is presented in four parts which are clearly differentiated.

The title is usually concise, a typical example being 'Instructions for a gaping wound in his head, penetrating to the bone and splitting his skull' (Case 4). The same words are usually repeated in the examination and the diagnosis.

The examination invariably starts 'If you examine a man having . . .' followed by the repetition of the title and then instructions for the examination of the patient as, for example, in Case 7, 'You should probe his wound [although] he fears it greatly. You should cause him to lift his face.' Then follow findings which were correctly recognised to be clinically important. Among the most striking of these are a cardinal sign of fractured base of skull – 'He discharges (literally 'gives') blood from his two nostrils and his two ears', and the most important sign of meningeal irritation – 'He does not find he can look at his two shoulders and his breast' (i.e. he cannot flex his neck). This section frequently includes the first stages of treatment even though the diagnosis has not been formally pronounced.

Diagnosis and prognosis. The next section invariably starts with the words 'You shall then say concerning him . . .'. This is normally followed by a repetition of the title and may be followed by a restatement of the more important clinical findings. Thus, for example, the two findings in the previous paragraph frequently reappear in the diagnosis. This is immediately followed by the prognosis, which was one of three stock phrases, quite close to the modern concept of triage for disaster victims:

An ailment which I will treat	(in 30 cases)
An ailment with which I will contend	(in 8 cases)
An ailment not to be treated	(in 14 cases)

In one case (number 9) there is no diagnosis or prognosis, but five other cases have two prognoses, based on two examinations. In general the prognoses seem very reasonable considering the therapeutic possibilities available at the time.

Treatment forms the final section and may be entirely omitted when the most unfavourable prognosis has been given as, for example, in Cases 24 (fractured mandible) and 44 (open fractured ribs). In other cases the unfavourable prognosis is followed by palliative treatment. Case 20 was an open fracture of the skull, perforating the temporal bone (see fig. 3.4) and with the patient unconscious. The patient was to be sat up, his head softened with grease and milk put into his ears. In most cases the physical treatment is quite logical by modern standards, such as stitching a flesh wound, setting a fracture, reduction of a dislocation or simply bandaging. Acute treatment is often followed by longer term therapy 'until he is well'.

Case 16 is cited in full as a brief, simple and very clear case to show the general format. The translation is literal but headings are for clarification and do not appear in the papyrus:

TITLE
Instructions for a split in his cheek.

EXAMINATION
If you examine a man having a split in his cheek and you find that there is a swelling, raised and red, on the outside of his split.

DIAGNOSIS AND PROGNOSIS
You shall say concerning him: One having a split in his cheek. An ailment which I will treat.

TREATMENT
You should bandage it with fresh meat [on] the first day. His treatment is sitting until his swelling is reduced. Afterwards you should treat it [with] grease, honey and a pad every day until he is well.

Several other examples of more involved cases are to be found in Chapter 8.

In certain more complicated cases there are repeated examinations which commence 'If you then find ...', followed by a declaration of the updated diagnosis and prognosis. It was not uncommon for treatment to be omitted after a less favourable prognosis was given following a second examination, for example Cases 7 (probably tetanus) and 37 (compound fracture of humerus, the bone of the upper arm).

Anatomical distribution of cases. The remarkably consistent structure of the individual case descriptions is matched by a highly systematic progression through different parts of the body. In general the papyrus starts with injuries to the top of the head and then works down through the face, jaw and neck to reach the upper part of the thorax, the spine and the arms (fig. 2.2). Working downwards from the top of the body to the feet follows the same pattern as for placing the different parts of the body under the protection of various gods in Spell 42 in the *Book of the Dead*, and also for the placing of parts of the body of a cat under divine protection after being stung by

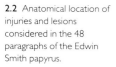

2.2 Anatomical location of injuries and lesions considered in the 48 paragraphs of the Edwin Smith papyrus.

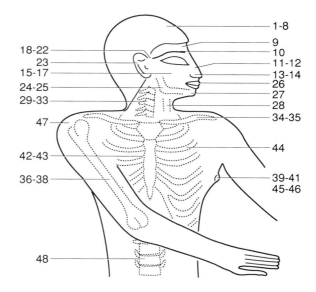

a scorpion (Metternich stela, Spell III). It is, furthermore, the order followed today in *Gray's Anatomy*. The extant copy of the Edwin Smith papyrus stops abruptly in the middle of Case 48, in the middle of a sentence and shortly after the scribe had dipped his pen in the ink and had retraced the last two signs he had written.

The Edwin Smith papyrus has an instant appeal to the doctor of today. It contains much that relates to current surgical practice and it is not difficult to see the workings of the pharaonic doctor. We can visualise him examining his patient, we can read his mind as he reaches a diagnosis and we can identify with him in his treatment of the patient. In keeping with the pragmatic approach, it is remarkably free of magic. There is only one spell, which occurs in Case 9 and will be considered in Chapter 5.

It is less clear what was the original purpose of the papyrus. Was it the personal record of patients treated by an earlier surgeon, whose work had become hallowed by tradition? Alternatively, were they idealised but typical accidents that might be encountered on the battlefield or in the work place, assembled to provide a manual of practice? Was it conceivably a surgical thesis? Whatever its original purpose, it seems clear that it had, over the time which had elapsed since it was written, become a standard reference work for the treatment of trauma, and the glosses testify to its practical use rather than as an object of historical curiosity.

The verso

Papyrus was an expensive commodity and it was common practice to write on the back. Although the first part of the verso appears to have been written by the same scribe who wrote the recto, no part of the surgical papyrus appears on the verso and the contents are totally different. First, there are eight incantations, some of which have relevance to the magical practice of medicine (see Chapter 5). Then follows a recipe for a woman with retained menstrual products (see Chapter 9) and two recipes to improve the complexion. There is then a recipe for transforming an old man into a youth, and the recto closes with a local application to relieve an obscure illness of the anus.

The Ebers papyrus

This papyrus was purchased in Luxor by Edwin Smith in 1862 at about the same time as the Edwin Smith papyrus. It is unclear from whom the purchase was made but the papyrus was said to have been found between the legs of a mummy in the Assassif area of the Theban necropolis on the west bank of the Nile opposite Luxor. However, when its importance was realised, the finders were dead and the tomb from which it was taken has never been identified. It can only be speculated that it came from the tomb of a doctor, and it is possible that it may have come from the same tomb as the Edwin Smith.

The papyrus remained in the possession of Edwin Smith until at least 1869 when there appeared, in a catalogue of antiquities, an advertisement for 'a large medical papyrus in the possession of Edwin Smith, an American farmer (sic) of Luxor' (Breasted, 1930). It was originally known as the Papyrus Smith and this appellation continued until at least 1873. The papyrus was purchased by Georg Ebers in 1872 and, in his publication of 1873, he referred to it for the first time as the Ebers papyrus. This served to distinguish it from what was to become known as the Edwin Smith papyrus (see above). The Ebers papyrus is now in the University Library of Leipzig.

In 1875, Ebers published a superb facsimile edition with Egyptian–Latin vocabulary and introduction. Joachim produced a German translation as early as 1890, a bold attempt in the state of linguistic knowledge of the time and well before Wreszinski published the hieroglyphic transcription in 1913. Bryan made an English translation in 1930, which was, in his own words 'a rendition into English of German and other translations of the Egyptian original'. Elliot Smith, in the introduction to Bryan's book, stated 'Dr Cyril Bryan is to be commended for giving us in English an interpretation based upon Dr Joachim's translation, though not slavishly following it'. The next major development was the translation into English by Dr Ebbell in 1937, and this remains at the time of writing the most easily available version of the Ebers papyrus to the English-speaking world. Unfortunately, Ebbell gave too free a rein to his imagination and medical insight, making many interpretations of obscure Egyptian words for which there is no firm linguistic basis. His book is often cited as giving evidence for the recognition by the ancient Egyptians of such conditions as angina, asthma, diabetes, hemiplegia, jaundice and a range of intestinal parasites which philological considerations cannot support. As an extreme example, Ebbell translated *shendet* (with a tree determinative!) as 'prepuce' instead of its well established meaning of 'acacia' (thorn in this case). Thus a passage dealing with injury from an acacia thorn was misrepresented as a complication of circumcision (Ebers 732).

The current definitive translation is by von Deines, Grapow and Westendorf (1958) in volume IV 1 of the *Grundriss* (Table 2.2). This is only available in German but Ghaliounghui (1987) made an English translation, based largely on the *Grundriss* translation, and with the support and encouragement of Wolfhart Westendorf, who wrote the foreword. Unfortunately, this book, although printed and bound, has not been placed on sale. I am indebted to Benson Harer for the sight of a copy given to him by the widow of Professor Ghaliounghui.

Table 2.2 Grundriss der Medizin der alten Ägypter

VOLUME	AUTHORS	YEAR	TITLE
I	Grapow, H.	1954	*Anatomie und Physiologie*
II	Grapow, H.	1955	*Von den medizinischen Texten*
III	Grapow, H.	1956	*Kranker, Krankheiten und Arzt*
IV 1	von Deines, H. Grapow, H. Westendorf, W.	1958	*Ubersetzung der medizinischen Texte*
IV 2	von Deines, H. Grapow, H. Westendorf, W.	1958	*Ubersetzung der medizinischen Texte Erläuterungen*
V	Grapow, H.	1958	*Die medizinischen Texte in Hieroglyphischer Umschreibung autographiert*
VI	von Deines, H. Grapow, H.	1959	*Wörterbuch der ägyptischen Drogennamen*
VII 1	von Deines, H. Westendorf, W.	1961	*Wörterbuch der medizinischen Texte, erste Hälfte (ȝ–r)*
VII 2	von Deines, H. Westendorf, W.	1962	*Wörterbuch der medizinischen Texte, zweite Hälfte (h–ḏ)*
VIII	Westendorf, W.	1962	*Grammatik der medizinischen Texte*
IX	von Deines, H. Grapow, H. Westendorf, W.	1973	*Ergänzungen (Drogenquanten, Sachgruppen, Nachträge, Bibliographie, Generalregister)*

All were published by Akademie-Verlag, Berlin.

The Ebers papyrus comprises 110 pages and is by far the longest of the medical papyri, in superb condition and written in a clear hand. It is dated by a passage on the verso to the ninth year of the reign of Amenhotep I, about 1534 BC, a date which is close to the copy of the Edwin Smith papyrus. One part of this papyrus shares with the Berlin the claim to ancient origin, in the typical format for such claims seen in many non-medical papyri. Paragraph 856a states that:

> The book of driving *wekhedu* from all the limbs of a man was found in writings under the two feet of Anubis in Letopolis and was brought to the majesty of the king of Upper and Lower Egypt Den (First Dynasty).

This reference, back to about 3000 BC, would have been intended to give the papyrus greatly added authority.

Contents

Unlike the Edwin Smith papyrus the Ebers is a collection of different medical texts which have been run together in a rather haphazard order. Two numbering systems are in general use. The basic method is by page and line, and this papyrus is unusual in being numbered on each page by the scribe, so that specific remedies could have been located in spite of the confused ordering. It is, however, generally more convenient to use the consecutive numbering of 'paragraphs' from 1 to 877. However, the lengthy and important paragraphs 854, 855 and 856 have been broken down to 854 a–o, 855 a–z and 856 a–h. The paragraph numbering system has been followed in this book. A full concordance is to be found in the *Grundriss*, volume v. Many paragraphs are out of order; seventeen are repeated and six pairs are almost identical. This suggests that more than one source had been copied onto the same roll.

Paragraphs 1–3 contain three spells considered in Chapter 5. They are followed by a section on diseases which mainly involve the belly (*khet*), with concentration on intestinal worms in paragraphs 50–85. Skin diseases feature in paragraphs 90–5 and 104–18, and diseases of the anus in paragraphs 132–64. Up to paragraph 187, the papyrus follows the general format of listing prescriptions which are to relieve a pathological condition of a part of the body. The latter can usually be translated with a high degree of certainty, and we recognise belly, stomach, anus, skin and so on. The diseases are often far more difficult to identify. Sometimes it takes the form of a recognisable symptom such as heat or obstruction, but may be a specific disease term, such as *wekhedu* of *aaa*, for which the meaning remains obscure (see Chapters 3 and 4). The names of the worms are a particular problem. The worm determinative at the end of the words is clear enough but identification of the species depends on inference from the symptoms, which are seldom defined. Thus, in general, this part of the Ebers papyrus assumes that the diagnosis has already been made and simply lists the recommended treatments. Many paragraphs are only headed 'another remedy' and one assumes that this relates to the last disease to be mentioned in the previous paragraphs. However, there is always the disturbing thought that the scribe may have confused the ordering of the paragraphs and the 'other' remedy may refer to a different disease. Some of the difficulties of these sections are illustrated in paragraphs 104–5:

> Beginning of ointments (*gesu*) to eliminate *wehau* skin rash: *iner-sepdu* mineral; milk; pure oil; smeared (*ges*) therewith for 4 days.

> Another ointment: acacia leaves; *sawer* resin, *iner-sepdu* mineral; *ta* liquid of laundryman; red natron; honey; oil/fat; smear therewith.

There is no clue which enables us to identify the *wehau* skin rash. The medicaments give no indication of the diagnosis and are probably intended to give only symptomatic relief. The *iner-sepdu* mineral appears in both paragraphs but we have no means of deducing its meaning, the only clue being the mineral determinative at the end of the word. Finally, there can be no certainty that the paragraphs have not become misplaced at one of the serial copyings of the original manuscript and therefore it is possible that the second paragraph does not relate to the *wehau* skin disease.

Paragraphs 188–207 comprise the 'book of the stomach' and show an abrupt change of style to something closer to that of the Edwin Smith papyrus (see above). Only 188 has a title, but all contain the phrase 'if you examine a man with a ...' or words to that effect, as in the examination section of the Edwin Smith papyrus. There follows a declaration of the diagnosis but usually in terms which are difficult to understand. There is, however, no declaration of the prognosis which was such a remarkable feature of the Edwin Smith papyrus. Treatment then follows the phrase 'You should then prepare for him ...'. Paragraphs 208–41 revert to the original style but include several paragraphs on conditions of the heart.

Paragraphs 242–7 contain remedies reputed to have been prepared by certain gods for their own use or sometimes prepared by one god for use by another. Only in paragraph 247 is the diagnosis mentioned:

A sixth remedy which Isis made for Ra himself to eliminate the disease that is in his head.

The following section continues with diseases of the head but without reference to use of the remedies by the gods. Paragraph 250 contains the celebrated reference to migraine (p. 93). This sequence is interrupted by paragraph 251 which is in a totally different format, with the emphasis on the drug rather than the disease. It seems to be an extract from something like a pharmacopoeia of which the rest is unfortunately lost. It commences as follows but is cited in full in Chapter 7:

Knowledge of what is made from *degem* (probably the ricinus plant yielding castor oil), as something found in ancient writings and as something useful to man.

Paragraphs 261–83 are concerned with the regulation of the flow of urine and are followed by remedies 'to cause the heart to receive bread' (284–93) and remedies for cough and the *gehew*-disease (305–35).

Diseases of the eyes comprise a large and compact section of the Ebers papyrus (336–431) and this may correspond to the book of the eyes and their diseases referred to by Clement. This section is our main source of information on treatment of eye disease in ancient Egypt and is considered in Chapter 9.

Treatment of bites, both by man and by crocodile, features in paragraphs 432–6 and the papyrus then returns to diseases of the head, but now with special attention to the hair. Paragraphs 477–81 relate to unspecified disease of the liver.

Paragraphs 482–529 are concerned with various injuries including burns, beating and flesh wounds. Paragraphs 530–42 comprise a mysterious section dealing with general suffering in relation to 'secretions' (*setja*). The following sections range widely in their scope to include a variety of conditions, some of which are uncertain (*akut*, *kakaut* and *benut* ulcers; see Appendix D) of teeth (553–4), legs (561–2 and 603–15), fingers and toes (616–26).

Paragraphs 627–96 are concerned with strengthening or relaxing the *metu*, a difficult word discussed at some length in Chapter 3. Whereas the *metu* can mean hollow vessels including blood vessels, they can also mean tendons and muscles which seem to be under consideration in this section.

Diseases of the tongue feature in paragraphs 697–704 and are followed by an important compact section on dermatology (708–21). There are other compact sections on teeth (739–50), diseases of the ear, nose and throat (761–81) and finally gynaecology (783–839). The content then changes abruptly to a section on household pests (840–53).

The next three paragraphs (854–6) are of great importance and provide the anatomical basis for consideration of the *metu* and what little is said about dysfunction of the cardiovascular system. These paragraphs are considered in detail in Chapter 3.

The final part of the Ebers papyrus is of a more surgical nature and is in the same style as paragraphs 188–207, rather like the Edwin Smith papyrus. Paragraphs 857–62 are concerned with ulcers and 863–75 with tumours and swellings. The 'knife treatment' is recommended in ten cases and this provides our main source of information on surgery other than trauma.

Most of the glosses cannot be related to their corresponding passages in the main text. Nevertheless, many of them provide important information. It will be clear that a simple classification of the Ebers papyrus is impossible. It is a compendium of many different original sources assembled in an order which often appears random. There are some eleven spells in addition to the three basic spells in the first three paragraphs. There are a very large number of parallels in other papyri, particularly the Hearst, Berlin and London, conveniently tabulated in volume IV 2 of the *Grundriss* (pages 241–8).

The verso has no medical content but provided the means of dating the whole papyrus to the reign of Amenhotep I.

The Kahun gynaecological papyrus

The so-called Kahun papyri were found in April and November 1889 by Flinders Petrie at the town-site near Lahun in the Fayum. Since then, they have been housed in University College London. The town flourished during the late Middle Kingdom, principally in the reigns of Amenemhat III and his successors. A note on the back of the gynaecological papyrus is dated year 29 of the reign of Amenemhat III (*c.* 1825 BC). Of the medical papyri, only the Ramesseum papyri (see below) are of similar age. The gynaecological treatise comprises three pages with respectively twenty-nine, thirty and twenty-eight lines. Unlike the Ebers papyrus, it was in a badly fragmented condition and, even after painstaking reassembly, there still remain many lacunae. Like all other medical papyri except Ramesseum V, it is written in hieratic but the accompanying veterinary text is written unusually in hieroglyphic script which, as a general rule, was used on papyrus only for religious texts such as the *Book of the Dead*.

The texts were published in facsimile, with hieroglyphic transcription and translation into English (certain indelicate passages being rendered into Latin) by Griffith in 1898. There was a further English translation by Stevens (1975). As for the other medical papyri, the definitive translation is (into German) in volume IV 1 of the *Grundriss* (Table 2.2).

Contents

The gynaecological text may be conveniently divided into thirty-four paragraphs, of which the first seventeen have a common format. They start rather like the Edwin Smith papyrus with the words 'Instructions for a woman suffering from ...' and are followed by a brief account of the symptoms, usually but not invariably relating to the reproductive organs. Unlike the Edwin Smith papyrus, there is no section suggesting how to examine the patient, although paragraph 2 suggests that certain questions should be asked. Undeterred by the lack of examination, there follows a formal declaration of the diagnosis, starting with the words 'You shall then say concerning her ...'. In some cases it is by no means easy to understand the logical progression from the instructions to the declaration. Paragraph 5 is an extreme example of the difficulties in understanding the logic of this section of the Kahun papyrus:

> Instructions for a woman suffering in her teeth and her gums who cannot open her mouth. You shall then say concerning her: This is acute pain of the womb ...

The cases described in the first section then usually proceed with the phrase: 'You shall then make for her ...', followed by a variety of prescriptions, some to be taken by mouth and others to be introduced into the vagina or applied externally. In three cases, it is recommended that the vagina be fumigated.

The second section starts on the third and last page, and comprises eight paragraphs which are unfortunately so badly deficient that little sense can be made of some of them. However, paragraph 19 is concerned with recognition of who will give birth and 20 with a fumigation procedure to cause conception to occur. Paragraphs 21–2 describe pessaries to prevent conception, the first made of crocodile excrement, the second 454 ml of honey and the third sour milk. One can hardly doubt the likely effectiveness of these contraceptives!

The third section (paragraphs 26–32) is concerned with pregnancy testing and starts with observing that the vessels of the breasts are distended. Other methods are more fanciful and paragraph 28 recommends placing an onion bulb deep in her flesh, with a positive outcome being determined by the odour of the onion appearing at her nose. Paragraph 30 provides the fragmentary indication of an incantation, apparently to help the test described in the previous paragraph. This is the only incantation in the Kahun gynaecological papyrus.

Section four comprises two paragraphs which do not fall into any of the previous categories. One prescribes treatment for toothache during pregnancy (33) and the other describes what appears to be a fistula between bladder and vagina with incontinence of urine 'in an irksome place' (34).

In view of the damaged state of the Kahun papyrus, it is fortunate that there are substantial gynaecological components in the Berlin, Carlsberg, Ebers, London and Ramesseum papyri (q.v.). There are no exact parallel passages between the Kahun and other papyri but there is considerable similarity between Kahun 26 and Berlin 196 and between Kahun 28 and Carlsberg iv (1,x + 4–x + 6).

The Kahun papyrus is, in many respects, disappointing to the medical reader. It contains very little which relates to present concepts of gynaecology, and nothing at all about obstetrics.

The Hearst papyrus

In the spring of 1901, a roll of papyrus was brought to the camp of the Hearst Egyptian Expedition near Deir el-Ballas by a peasant of the village, as a token of thanks for being allowed to take *sebakh* from the waste-heaps of the excavations to be used as fertilizer (Reisner, 1905). The papyrus was named in honour of Phoebe Hearst, the mother of William Randolph Hearst, the American millionaire newspaper proprietor. She financed much of the work of the University of California in Egypt, and in particular the Hearst Expedition under Reisner, who published the hieratic text and a brief guide to the contents in 1905. Wreszinski published the hieroglyphic transcription and translation into German in 1912. The latest translation into German is in the *Grundriss* (Table 2.2) and it does not appear to have been translated into English. The papyrus, which is believed to date from the reign of the Eighteenth Dynasty pharaoh Tuthmosis iii, is kept in the University of California.

Contents

The Hearst papyrus comprises eighteen pages, conveniently divided into 260 paragraphs. The contents include sections on the alimentary and urinary systems, teeth, bones, hair, blood, bites, the *metu* and remedies for unidentified conditions. There are also a number of incantations. Almost 100 paragraphs have parallels in the Ebers papyrus, some being identical. There are no other parallels, apart from one with the Berlin papyrus and two with Ramesseum v. No part is concerned with gynaecology.

The Chester Beatty papyri

Sir Alfred Chester Beatty was a multi-millionaire industrialist, collector of books and art, and a philanthropist who presented nineteen papyri to the British Museum, where some are on exhibition. They are part of a larger find during excavations in Deir el-Medina (the village of the necropolis workers at Thebes), which is now dispersed, with the legal texts in the Ashmolean Museum, Oxford, the letters in the French Institute, Cairo, and the largest literary manuscript in the Chester Beatty Library and Gallery, Dublin. The manuscripts in the British Museum include literary texts, rituals, incantations and the medical texts.

These papyri appear to have belonged to a private family archive, begun by the scribe Qen-her-khepeshef in the Nineteenth Dynasty, and passed through his wife Niut-nakht to the children of her second marriage (Pestman, 1982). One child was named after Niut-nakht's first husband (fig. 2.3). The collection seems to have remained within this family for over a century, increasing in scope with new owners until it was deposited in a tomb chapel, where it remained until discovery in 1928 (Parkinson and Quirke, 1995). Some of the contents of the archive were purely medical, but there is no suggestion that any of the owners held the title *swnw*, which we translate as physician or doctor (see Chapter 6).

2.3 Stela of Qen-her-khepeshef adoring Hathor, from the necropolis workers' village at Deir el-Medina, 19th Dynasty. Qen-her-khepeshef and his family are the only persons known to have possessed a medical papyrus, although none was a doctor. (British Museum, EA 278)

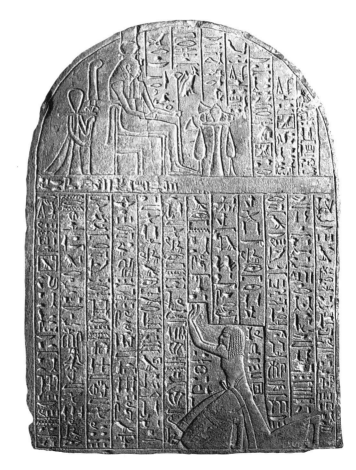

The condition of these papyri was generally poor and, even after extensive reconstruction, they still contain many lacunae. They were first published, with translation into English, by Gardiner in 1935 but he wrote of number VI, the most important from the medical point of view, 'The subject of the recto is too technical to be profitably dealt with here, and Mr W. R. Dawson ... will discuss it in detail elsewhere.' This did not seem to happen but Jonckheere translated it (into French) in 1947. The whole of number VI, together with most of the undermentioned sections, are translated (into German) in the *Grundriss*.

Contents

The third section of Chester Beatty v (BM 10685) comprises magical incantations for use against headaches, including *ges-tep* (literally 'half head'). This corresponds to the Greek 'hemi-krania', from which our word 'migraine' is derived. There are prescriptions but they seem to be of a predominantly magical nature.

The recto of Chester Beatty papyrus VI (BM 10686) comprises eight pages conveniently divided into forty-one paragraphs, almost entirely concerned with diseases of the anus. A range of symptoms are considered, and we may be reasonably certain of the nature of some of the underlying pathology (see Chapter 4). However, some words and phrases still defy translation and most paragraphs simply list 'Another prescription'. Some of these were to be taken by mouth, some were for local application to the anus, and at least twelve were to be 'poured into the anus' as an enema, a form of medication which drew comment from Herodotus. The only parallels are four in the Berlin papyrus. They are all prescriptions for enemas and there is no mention of disease. One of the parallels is similar to Ebers 157 in the section dealing with anal diseases. The very short verso contains a few remedies, together with many incantations against unidentifiable illnesses.

Chester Beatty VII (BM 10687) contains many spells on both recto and verso, the former being concerned with stings by scorpions and considered in Chapter 5. This is the only section here mentioned which does not appear in translation in the *Grundriss*.

Gardiner said of Chester Beatty VIII (BM 10688) 'This, the least interesting papyrus of the collection, has cost uncommonly much trouble to put in order' and he considered it to have been deliberately mutilated in antiquity. Among many magicoreligious texts there is a prescription (5,1–3), although it is unclear what disease it is intended to cure.

Chester Beatty XV (BM 10695) is only one page but the best preserved. Lines 5–9 contain two prescriptions for destroying 'thirst in the mouth'.

The Berlin Papyrus

This important papyrus was acquired by Giuseppe Passalacqua in Saqqara, and was sold in 1827 as a part of a large collection of antiquities to Friedrich Wilhelm IV of Prussia for the Berlin Museum, where it is still preserved (number 3038). Passalacqua became the first curator of the Egyptian collection until succeeded by Lepsius in 1865. Nothing is known of the provenance but the style and writing are typical of the Nineteenth Dynasty. It was initially studied by Brugsch and sometimes known as the Papyrus Brugsch, but the first full publication with translation into German was by Wreszinski in 1909. The definitive translation (into German) is in the *Grundriss* and I am unaware of any translation into English. The Berlin Museum also contains a fragment of another medical papyrus (number 3027) dating from the Eighteenth Dynasty.

The Berlin shares with the Ebers papyrus the distinction of a declared ancient and magico-religious origin. Paragraph 163a states that the original was 'found amongst writings of ancient times in chests of writing materials under the feet of Anubis, in Letopolis, in the time of the majesty of the king of Upper and Lower Egypt Den' (First Dynasty). In three places there is a reference to the author, who is mentioned in no other medical papyrus. There is a division of opinion concerning his name.

> Sealed by the scribe of the god's words, chief of the skilful *swnw* Netjer-hetepu. (Berlin 163a)
>
> made . . . by skilfulness of the *swnw*, of the excellent ones, Netjer-hetepu. (Berlin 163h)
>
> A spell ending: . . . Isis the great, it is she who makes the art of Ra, the *swnw*(s) Netjer-hetep. (Berlin 190)

The first passage makes it clear that a scribe and doctor was the author or compiler. This is supported by the second passage, while the third passage, the penultimate paragraph of the recto, looks like the scribe's colophon. The problem comes in deciding whether Netjer-hetepu is his name or whether it simply means 'who propitiates the god' (a disease-demon in this case). The latter was the view of the authors of the *Grundriss*, and their view was supported by a parallel phrase in Chester Beatty VII (1,4–2,5), 'Behold I am Horus the physician, soothing the god' (Gardiner, 1935). Furthermore there is no seated man determinative after Netjer-hetepu, which would be expected at the end of a man's name. The third passage is more difficult: *swnw* is plural and there is a god determinative after *netjer-hetep*. It has been accepted that Netjer-hetep was the name of the physician by both Jonckheere (1958) and Leca (1988), but Ghaliounghui (1983) adhered to the view stated in the *Grundriss*. It seems unlikely that we shall ever know for certain.

Contents

This papyrus comprises twenty-four pages (twenty-one recto and three verso). Paragraphs are numbered 1–191 (on the recto) and 192–204 (on the verso). Much of the Berlin papyrus is parallel to parts of the Ebers papyrus, and the very long paragraph 163 provides a most important duplication of Ebers 856, which is concerned with the *metu*. This provided important confirmation of the scribal error in Ebers 856b for the total number of *metu* (see Table 3.2).

Paragraphs 13–18 contain a section on diseases of the breast which is paralleled only by Ebers 810 (= Berlin 17). There is no useful indication of underlying pathology other than reference to a swelling (*besy*) in 14. Paragraph 192 appears to be a bizarre form of contraception. Paragraphs 193–9 are concerned with fertility tests, with some parallels in Kahun and Carlsberg. Paragraph 199 is the celebrated (but invalid) test for distinguishing between a male and a female child (p. 191).

The London medical papyrus

Nothing is known of the provenance or early history of this papyrus which was owned by the Royal Institution of London until it was transferred to the British Museum in 1860 (accession number 10059). It was first translated into German by Wreszinski in 1912 in the same publication which presented the Hearst papyrus. Translation (into German) is included in the *Grundriss* (Table 2.2).

This papyrus is in poor condition and is a palimpsest written over an earlier work at a date close to the reign of Tutankhamun. It comprises nineteen pages with sixty-one paragraphs, of which only twenty-five are medical, the rest being magical. There is a small section on gynaecology (40–5), and seventeen other paragraphs have parallels in the Ebers papyrus. There are no other parallels.

Papyrus Carlsberg VIII

The origin of this papyrus is unknown. It has been dated to the Nineteenth or Twentieth Dynasty but the style suggests an original from the Twelfth Dynasty or only shortly after the Kahun papyrus. It is written on recto and verso in two different hands. The recto is concerned with diseases of the eyes, but is badly damaged. However, it appears to be an exact copy of the corresponding sections of the Ebers papyrus. It has been possible to read much of the verso after painstaking reconstruction. The papyrus is owned by the Carlsberg Foundation, but housed in the Egyptological Institute of the University of Copenhagen. It was first published with translation into English by Iversen in 1939, and later in the *Grundriss* (Table 2.2).

Contents

The verso of Carlsberg VIII appears to cover two pages and it is possible to identify seven paragraphs which are confusingly designated by Roman numerals. Both Iversen and the *Grundriss* employ paragraph, page and line numbers thus 'Carlsberg III (1,6–x+3)'. In this example, III is the paragraph, 1 is the page, 6 is the line on which III commences and x+3 is the line on which it ends, x being the first line after a lacuna of undetermined length. All the surviving parts of the papyrus are concerned with the detection of pregnancy, the sex of the unborn child and the ability to conceive. Paragraphs III, V and VI appear to be substantially the same as Berlin 199, 195 and 198; IV is parallel to Kahun 28 (see above). There is some similarity between VII and Berlin 193 and 194.

The Ramesseum papyri III, IV and V

In 1896, Quibell found seventeen papyri in a wooden box at the bottom of a shaft under the brick magazines behind the great temple of the Ramesseum (Thebes). Gardiner (1955) remarked that other goods in the tomb shaft suggested the professional outfit of a magician and medical practitioner. However, the owner of the tomb is unknown. Reference to Amenemhat III (Twelfth Dynasty) in papyrus VI indicates that the date must be later than about 1854 BC, and Gardiner suggests Thirteenth Dynasty (early Second Intermediate Period). Three of the papyri have some medical content. All were badly damaged and Gardiner explained the vicissitudes of the conservation, reconstruction and translation. The hieratic text was published by Gardiner in 1955, and the hieroglyphic transcription and English commentary by Barns in 1956. The *Grundriss* contains the latest translation (into German) (Table 2.2).

Contents

The medical interest in the Ramesseum papyri is confined to III, IV and V, all of which are written in vertical columns. Ramesseum V is unique among the medical papyri in being written in cursive hieroglyphs like the Kahun veterinary papyrus.

The recto of Ramesseum III comprises thirty-one paragraphs in section A, and thirty-four in section B. These range over a wide field of medicine and include sections on the eyes, gynaecology and diseases of children. There are a few parallels with the

Ebers papyrus. Ramesseum IV is divided into five sections (A–E) with a total of forty-five paragraphs, again including diseases of women and children. Several sections relate to parturition: 'To separate [him] from his mother ... who is giving birth' (IV, C, 28–30), but they are predominantly magical and give no indication of obstetric practice.

Ramesseum V is the best conserved and its hieroglyphic script suggests that it may be the earliest. In accord with the general trend from pragmatic medicine to magic, it contains more practical medicine than Ramesseum III or IV. There is a horizontal title above the columns of prescriptions written vertically. These are arranged in two registers. The upper contains prescriptions I–X and the lower XI–XX. The content is largely confined to remedies for the *metu*, in this case referring to muscles and tendons. There are a few parallels with the corresponding section of the Ebers papyrus (Ebers 627–96).

The Brooklyn papyrus on snake bites

This remarkable papyrus (Brooklyn Museum 47.218.48 and 47.218.85) is concerned exclusively with snake bites. The two numbers refer to the upper and lower halves of the roll, which had been cut in half. It has been dated to the Thirtieth Dynasty or perhaps the early Ptolemaic Period, but written in Middle Egyptian. This was either because it was a copy of a much earlier document or because an author in the Late Period chose the idiom of the classical period of Egyptian literature for his text. A very full account of this work has been published posthumously, with translation (into French) by Sauneron (1989). The beginning and end of the papyrus are missing but the middle parts are generally in good condition with few lacunae.

Contents

The text proceeds page by page, alternating between the two parts of the papyrus. Thus each complete page starts with 47.218.48 and finishes with 47.218.85. The title and start of the work are missing, and the extant part of the first section commences at line 15 of the lower part (designated page 1) and continues on to pages 2 of both upper and lower parts, terminating at line 16 of the latter. The first section comprises a systematic description of snakes and their bites. The last line states that there have been descriptions of thirty-eight snakes and their bites, of which the first thirteen are lost.

The second section starts on line 17, page 2 of the lower part (47.218.85), and continues almost complete up to the fifth pair of pages. Only the right-hand halves of the sixth pair of pages remain. The second section commences at paragraph 39 with an important introduction:

> Beginning of the collection of remedies to ... drive out the poison of all ...
> snakes, all scorpions, all tarantulas (?) and all serpents, in the hand of the *kherep* priests of Serqet and to drive away all snakes and to seal their mouths.

The second section then continues with many remedies and a few spells for those bitten by snakes. The format for the remedies is strictly pragmatic, and most are based on the species of snake responsible for the bite, or the symptoms suffered by the victim. The remedies are in the typical format of prescriptions that appear in the Ebers and other medical papyri which were apparently intended for lay doctors. This papyrus provides the most striking evidence for the closely parallel roles of the physician (*swnw*) and the various priests concerned with healing (see Chapter 6). The contents are considered in Chapter 8.

Demotic medical writings

There are several late medical and magico-medical texts written in the demotic script. Though written in the ancient Egyptian language, they were undoubtedly influenced by Greek thought, and can clarify and confirm some uncertain words and phrases found in the texts from the classical pharaonic period. Most are predominantly magical, like the London and Leiden papyrus dated to the third century AD, transliterated and translated into English by Griffith and Thompson (1904). The papyrus was sold by Anastasi (the Swedish consul in Alexandria) in two parts because it was not realised that they were continuous. The Leiden text was acquired by the Dutch government in 1828, and the London text by the British Museum in 1857 (BM 10070). It is predominantly Egyptian but contains many very useful Greek glosses. On the other hand, a papyrus from Crocodilopolis (P. Vindob, D.6257), dated to the second half of the second century AD, is entirely free of magic and incantations of any sort. It lists many remedies for a variety of ailments, combining classical Egyptian drugs with new remedies from the Mediterranean area that were never mentioned in the extant pharaonic medical texts (Reymond, 1976).

Medical ostraca

There are many examples of remedies written on potsherds or flakes of white limestone. These range from the Amarna Period (Eighteenth Dynasty) to the time of the Roman occupation (Jonckheere, 1954).

CHAPTER THREE

Concepts of anatomy, physiology and pathology

Anatomy

Africanus, quoting the lost works of the Egyptian historian Manetho, wrote about the third pharaoh of the First Dynasty:

> Athothis [or Djer], his [i.e. Menes'] son, for fifty-seven years. He built the palace at Memphis, and his anatomical works are extant, for he was a physician.

Eusebius, quoting the same source, wrote:

> Athothis, his son, ruled for twenty-seven years. He built the palace at Memphis; he practised medicine and wrote anatomical books.

Although the citation of Manetho is consistent, no systematic Egyptian work on anatomy has survived, and it is very difficult to believe that there was any serious study of anatomy at the beginning of the third millennium BC. It is almost certain that no appropriate climate of enquiry existed at that time. Nevertheless, the anatomical insight shown for certain parts of the body in some of the medical papyri, the Edwin Smith in particular, strongly supports the view that there had been quite detailed study of anatomy at an early date and it is possible that a treatise on anatomy might have existed.

There is no evidence that human dissection was undertaken in Egypt until Herophilus, the Greek physician from Chalcedon, worked at the Alexandrian medical school in the early Ptolemaic Period (see Chapter 10). His works have not survived but there is ample reference by Celsus, Galen and others to show that he enjoyed unrestricted access to human cadavers for dissection, and even the possibility of vivisection on condemned but living criminals (Jackson, 1988; von Staden, 1989). Respect for the dead would have prevented this under the Egyptian pharaohs and also in Greece itself. After Herophilus, human dissection ceased.

Possible sources of anatomical knowledge

In spite of the obstacles placed in the way of human dissection, the Egyptian doctor must nevertheless have had the opportunity to observe the human skeleton. Although there was a rich Egyptian vocabulary for external parts of the body, we know relatively few names of bones with the exception of the skull, lower jaw, vertebrae, ribs and clavicles (collar-bones). Battle casualties and serious industrial accidents would provide an opportunity to gain further anatomical insight. Sections of the Edwin

Table 3.1 Canopic jars with their contents and protectors

CONTENTS	SON OF HORUS	HEAD AFTER 18TH DYNASTY	PROTECTIVE GODDESS
liver	Imsety	human	Isis
lungs	Hapy	baboon	Nephthys
stomach	Duamutef	jackal	Neith
intestines	Qebhsenuef	hawk	Serqet

Smith papyrus, considered below, suggest that these opportunities were not wasted. However, Celsus (Prooemium 40–2) rightly stressed the difficulties of observing internal anatomical relationships in the living subject.

The embalmers showed great technical expertise, whether or not they understood the details of the underlying anatomy. They were able to remove those internal organs most likely to putrefy through a relatively small incision (fig. 3.1) and transfer them, after preservation, to canopic jars under the protection of the four sons of Horus and the corresponding protective goddesses (Table 3.1). However, their most remarkable achievement was the removal of the brain through the nose. This required a perforation through the ethmoid bone, seldom exceeding 2 cm in diameter (fig. 3.2).

It is by no means clear to what extent the anatomical skills of the embalmers were passed to the doctors. Herodotus made it very clear that, in his time, the embalmers were regarded as unclean, which might have precluded dialogue with the doctors

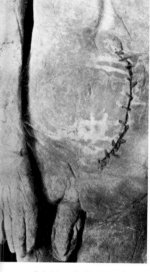

3.1 (above) Embalmer's incision of the 21st Dynasty which, contrary to the usual practice, had been sutured. The mummy was one of a cache of forty-four priests of Amum which also included the subject shown in fig. 4.4. (Cairo Museum; from Smith and Dawson, 1924)

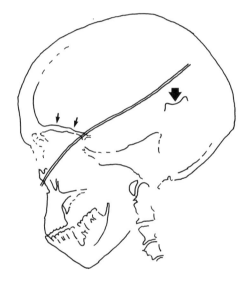

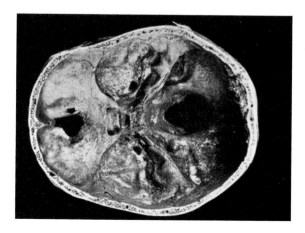

3.2 (left) The route for removal of the brain during embalming. The diagram is drawn from the lateral radiograph of a Ptolemaic head, with a modern radio-opaque catheter inserted through the nose, to show the route of brain removal through a hole created in the cribriform plate of the ethmoid bone. The large arrow indicates a detached part of the fossa for the pituitary gland which would have lain in the path of the removal of the brain. The two small arrows show the cribriform plate of the ethmoid bone which is broken through posteriorly (from Isherwood, Jarvis and Fawcitt, 1979). The photograph shows, from above, the base of another Ptolemaic skull after removal of the vault of the skull by horizontal saw cuts (cemetery 14, Khor Ambukol, Nubia). The ethmoidal aperture made by the embalmers on the left side is shown by an arrow. (From Smith and Jones, 1910)

(*swnw*). However, attitudes were different in earlier periods and there are occasional references to contacts between doctors and embalmers. Gloss A for Case 9 of the Edwin Smith papyrus states:

> As for 'a *hayt* bandage for the use of the *swnw*', it is a bandage (*seshed*) which is under the hand of the embalmer . . .

Gloss A for Case 19 seems to indicate that the *swnw* might be familiar with standard reference works available to the embalmers:

> As for 'his two eyes are blood-shot', it means that the colour of his two eyes is red like the colour of the *shas*-flowers. The 'Treatise on what pertains to the embalmer' says concerning it: 'His two eyes are red [with] disease like an eye at the end of its weakness'.

The 'Treatise on what pertains to the embalmer' is lost, but this extract suggests more than a trivial concern with the state of their subjects before their demise. It is thus conceivable that they were consulted before death and in that case they would inevitably have come into contact with the *swnw*.

Perhaps more cogent is the fact that the grandfather of the Middle Kingdom *wer swnw* (chief physician) Minemsehenet (Appendix B, no. 70) was an embalmer, Nebneb by name (van de Walle and de Meulenaere, 1973). Thus relationships between doctors and embalmers cannot always have been distant, and it seems likely that Nebneb would have passed useful information to his grandson, had he lived long enough. Finally, we may note that *swnw* (the usual word for 'doctor') could also mean 'embalmer' in the Ptolemaic Period.

Evidence from the medical papyri

Clement of Alexandria, born about AD 150, was a convert to Christianity but displayed an extensive knowledge of pagan religion. He reported that the Egyptians possessed a book concerning the structure of the body (Chapter 2). It might conceivably have been the book which Manetho improbably attributed to Djer. No such book has been found, although fragments may have survived in the Ebers and the Berlin papyri. It may also have been cited in some of the glosses of the Edwin Smith papyrus. In all, we have tantalisingly little from which to build a picture of the ancient Egyptian knowledge of anatomy. There is, nevertheless, a rich vocabulary for both internal and external parts of the body, some of which are shown in fig. 3.3.

The vessel (*metu*) book. This refers to parts of paragraphs 854 and 856 of the Ebers papyrus, and paragraph 163 of the Berlin papyrus which parallels paragraph 856 of the Ebers. Each is divided into a number of sub-paragraphs designated by letters. They describe the connections of the *metu*, which is the plural of *met*, a word having no direct equivalent in English. Its meanings include blood vessels, various ducts and also tendons and muscles, particularly those which are long and thin. It may also include nerves but it is unclear whether the ancient Egyptians had any concept of the nervous system. What is transported by the *metu* is often specified and this may be blood (in two instances), air, mucus, urine, semen, disease-bearing entities and also malign or benign spirits (Table 3.2).

It is hardly surprising that those *metu* which would appear to be arteries were thought to contain air. This was the general belief until the time of Galen who, in the latter part of the second century AD, opened a dog's artery between ligatures under water and showed conclusively that it contained blood and not air. The misconception arose because arteries usually contract after death and contain little if any blood when opened at postmortem or dissection. Once pierced, their natural elasticity causes them to open, giving the impression that they originally contained air. The Latin word *arteria* means windpipe as well as artery. Gloss A of Case 34 in the Edwin Smith papyrus mentions two *metu* beneath the clavicles (collar-bones), one on the right and one on the left of the throat, which lead to the lung. It is just possible that these refer to the trachea dividing into the two bronchi (Breasted, 1930).

There would appear to be two separate systematic descriptions of the *metu*, with some overlap for the ears, arms and legs. The first listing is Ebers 854 and the second Ebers 856, with its parallel text Berlin 163. The introduction to the latter in Ebers 856b is as follows:

> As to a man, there are 12 *metu* in him, to his heart. It is they which give to all his members/limbs.

Table 3.2 The distribution of the *metu* as described in the vessel book

ANATOMICAL DESTINATION	EBERS PAPYRUS 854	856	BERLIN 163	CONTENTS / FUNCTION
to his heart	–	12 b[1]	22 b	not specified (Ebers) air (Berlin)
to his heart, unite at anus	–	–	all h	
to his heart, unite at anus	–	all h	–	
to the anus	4 o	–	–	water and air
to the back of his head	–	2 g	2 g	not specified
to his forehead	–	2 g	2 g	not specified
in his neck/throat[2]	–	–	2 g	not specified
to his eye	–	2 g	–	not specified
to his eyebrow[3]	–	2 g	2 g	not specified
to his nose	–	2 g	2 g	not specified
to his right ear	2 f	2 g	2 g	breath of life enters
to his left ear	2 f	2 g	2 g	breath of death enters
in his two temples	4 c	–	–	blood and water (to the eyes)
to the head	4 d	–	–	create disease of hair
to his right shoulder	2 f	–	–	breath of life enters
to his left shoulder	2 f	–	–	breath of death enters
in his two nostrils	4 b	–	–	two give mucus; two give blood
to his [sic] breast(s)	–	2 c	2 c	heat to the anus
to the two arms	6 g	–	–	not specified
to his ? upper arm	–	2 f	2 f	? mucus
to the buttocks	2 k	–	–	not specified
to his two legs	6 h	–	–	not specified
to his thigh(s)	–	2 d	2 d	may cause disease
to the bladder	2 n	–	–	urine
to his two testicles	4 i	–	–	semen
to the liver	4 l	–	–	water and air
to the lung and spleen	4 m	–	–	water and air

Figures indicate the number of *metu*.

Letters refer to the sub-paragraphs of Ebers 854, 856 and Berlin 163.

1 It is believed that 12 is a scribal error for 22.

2 Alternatively, read as 'in his two eyes'.

3 One eyebrow in Ebers; two eyebrows in Berlin.

a

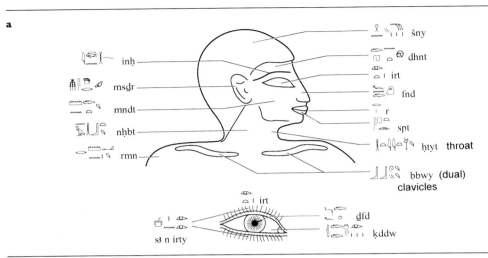

3.3 Some examples of Egyptian anatomical terms. Few of the writings are unique and I have tended to show the more complete forms. (a) Head and neck. (b) Some internal organs. (c) Female reproductive organs and the fetus. (d) Male genito-urinary tract.

b

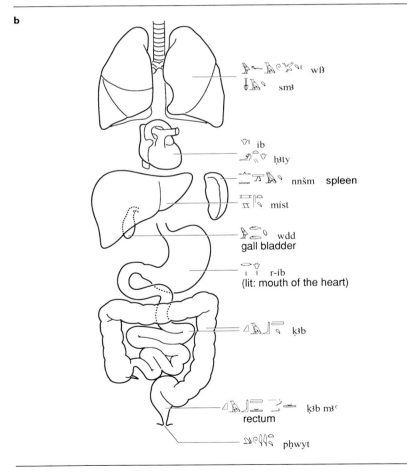

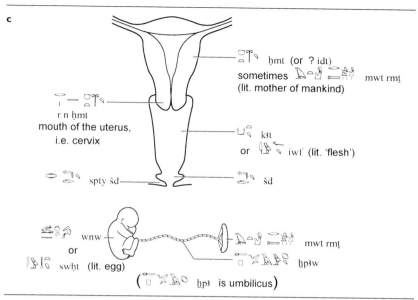

c

ḥmt (or ? idt)
sometimes mwt rmt
(lit. mother of mankind)

r n ḥmt
mouth of the uterus,
i.e. cervix

k3t

or iwf (lit. 'flesh')

spty šd

šd

wnw

or

swḥt (lit. egg)

mwt rmt

ḥp3w

(ḥp3 is umbilicus)

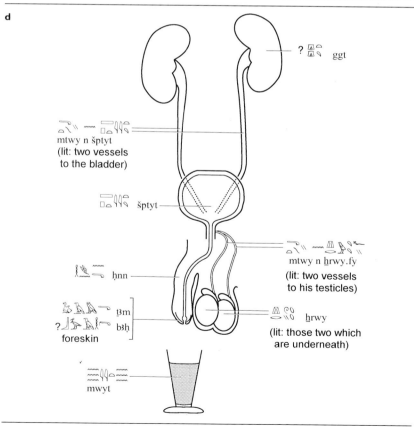

d

? ggt

mtwy n šptyt
(lit: two vessels
to the bladder)

šptyt

mtwy n ẖrwy.fy
(lit: two vessels
to his testicles)

ḥnn

3m
b3ḥ
foreskin

ẖrwy
(lit: those two which
are underneath)

mwyt

However, the parallel passage in Berlin 163b reads:

> . . . 22 *metu* in him. They lead/?draw off air to his heart. It is they which give wind/air to each of his two arms.

It is generally believed that the number twelve in the Ebers is a scribal error for the figure of twenty-two in the Berlin which is, in fact, the exact total for the *metu* in Ebers 856 and Berlin 163 combined (Table 3.2). Ebers 856h (with a close parallel in Berlin 163h) contains the enigmatic statement that 'All come to his heart. They distribute to his nose and all unite at his anus.' This would seem to apply to all of twenty-two *metu* listed in Ebers 856 and Berlin 163. Such a scheme would accord very well with Egyptian concepts of the circulation of noxious substances from the bowels through the *metu* to the rest of the body (p. 61). Nevertheless, it remains extremely difficult to see how the *metu* could lead to the heart, to a specified organ or region and still unite at the anus. Clearly they cannot correspond to any anatomical structures recognised at present. However, it is conceivable that there was word play between the words for 'anus' (*pehuyt*) and 'end' (*pehuy*). Preparation of a circulation diagram is fraught with difficulty but has been attempted by Majno (1975). Blood is not mentioned in Ebers 856.

Ebers 854 is an independent description listing the distribution of fifty-two *metu* to individual parts of the body. Since this number of *metu* far exceeds the totals for Ebers 854 and Berlin 163, it may represent an independent tradition, in which case we cannot assume that these *metu* 'all come to the heart, distribute to the nose and all unite at the anus', although four are specifically distributed to the anus and are 'flooded with faeces' (Ebers 854o).

Ebers 854 comprises a variety of *metu*. Some could relate to the vascular system while others appear to relate to certain structures and duct systems, which we may be tempted to identify. Blood is mentioned twice: two of the *metu* to the nostrils (Ebers 854b) are described as giving blood, and two mucus; four *metu* to the temples (Ebers 854c) are stated to give blood to the two eyes. (The two *metu* which are listed separately in Ebers 856g as being directed specifically to the eyes might be the very conspicuous optic nerves, since the small blood vessels which enter the eye could easily have escaped notice.)

The identification of the six *metu* to the two arms (Ebers 854g) is open to considerable uncertainty if they refer to the vascular system. In the upper arm there is only one major artery, the brachial artery, which divides into the radial and ulnar arteries at the elbow. Pulsations of all three may be detected and this would give the *swnw* a total of three *metu* per arm. This view is supported by the separate statement that there are two *metu* to the two upper arms (Ebers 856f and Berlin 163f). However, one cannot exclude the possibility that veins were also brought into the count. Alternatively, if the *metu* here refer to nerves, they might be the radial, ulnar and median, the three major branches of the brachial plexus which supply the arm. Unfortunately, the contents or function of these *metu* is not specified. Similar uncertainty clouds the identification of the six *metu* to the two legs (Ebers 854h). In the thigh they would probably have been aware of only the femoral artery with its obvious pulsation in the groin. At the knee it divides into the large peroneal and posterior tibial arteries, again giving a total of three large arteries to a limb. This view is supported by the statement that there are two *metu* to the two thighs (Ebers 856d; Berlin 163d). If, on the other hand, the *metu* referred to nerves, it would be difficult in the case of the leg to say which these might be.

Anatomical identification is much easier in the case of the *metu* to the bladder and testicles. Ebers 854n states quite clearly that 'there are two *metu* to the bladder: it is they which give urine'. Lefebvre (1956) took the view that, since the *metu* were thought to come from the heart, these could not be the ureters. This view may be contested on the grounds of independent traditions for Ebers 854 and Ebers 856/Berlin 163, as outlined above. The *metu* to the bladder are not included in the tally of twenty-two *metu* connected to the heart; therefore there seems nothing to preclude their being ureters. A similar argument applies to Ebers 854i which states 'there are two *metu* to his two testicles: it is they which give semen'. It therefore seems reasonable to identify them with the vas deferens in the spermatic cord, which can easily be felt through the skin in the living man.

In the case of the liver (Ebers 854l), it is specified that the four *metu* give air and water. It is tempting to believe that these might represent the hepatic artery, the hepatic and portal veins and the bile duct. Similarly one would like to believe that the *metu* to the lung and spleen (Ebers 854m) would include bronchi and pulmonary blood vessels. However, this can only be conjecture.

In the case of the ears and shoulders (Ebers 854f), the scientific tenor is abruptly interrupted by magical passages relating to the entry of the breath of life on the right and the breath of death on the left. Probably because of the prevalence of right-handedness, most cultures exhibit a bias against the left side with the word for 'left' having an alternative unfavourable meaning (e.g. *gauche* in French and *sinister* in Latin). Nevertheless, the Egyptian word for right is closely related to their word for west, and the word for left relates to east. The east bank of the Nile was associated with life and the west bank with death. It is thus interesting that the right (i.e. west) side of the body should be associated with life, and the left (i.e. east) side with death.

It will be clear that the vessel book, while containing glimpses of anatomical reality, does not provide any basis for believing that the ancient Egyptians had any clear concept of the circulatory system, distributing blood to all parts of the body. Nevertheless, they were clear that the heart could 'speak' through the *metu* in all the limbs of a patient (see pp. 55 and 113). This was very well known to the Greeks, particularly Herophilus, but the circulation of the blood was not discovered until the work of Harvey in the seventeenth century AD.

The Edwin Smith papyrus. There are passages in the Edwin Smith papyrus which offer quite remarkable insight into knowledge of anatomy. These are mostly in the glosses that must have been added subsequently to the original composition, which Breasted (1930) believed to have been written during the Old Kingdom (see p. 27). Since the only extant copy of the papyrus works systematically downwards from the head and stops at the chest, these glimpses of anatomical knowledge are unfortunately confined to certain sections of the upper part of the body. The best anatomical detail relates to the skull and merits consideration in detail.

As a starting point for the skull, there can be little doubt that this is represented by the Egyptian word *djennet*. Glosses in Cases 4 and 7 make it clear that the paired parietal bones (forming the vault of the skull) were known as *paqyt* (fig. 3.4), a word also used for the shell of a turtle to which the similarity is evident. In one instance the word is used to mean the frontal bone of the skull (Case 9). There is a separate word for the back of the head or occiput (*ha*), and a region of the skull called the *gema* is defined in Gloss B of Case 18:

As for '*gema*', it is what is in between the corner of his eye and the orifice of his ear, to the back of his lower jaw.

This would appear to describe the temporal bone and, more particularly, the zygomatic process of that bone.

There is further evidence that the bones of vault of the skull were recognised as separate entities. Gloss A of Case 7 defines the term *tepau*:

As for 'perforating the *tepau* [of his skull]', it is what is between shell and shell (*paqyt*) of his skull. The *tepau* are of leather (or hide).

There are three possible interpretations for *tepau*. The most obvious suggestion is that it refers to the falx cerebri (Westendorf, 1992), a strong fibrous membrane in the midline which separates the cerebral hemispheres and could have been seen in a major head injury exposing the brain. It must also have been known to the embalmers. However, Breasted (1930) favoured *tepau* meaning the sutures, which join the individual bones of the cranium. These are broad and conspicuous in infancy, but less

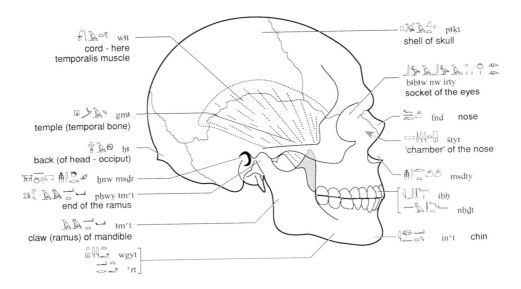

w3t
cord - here
temporalis muscle

gm3
temple (temporal bone)

h3
back (of head - occiput)

ḫnw msḏr

pḥwy 3mꜥt
end of the ramus

3mꜥt
claw (ramus) of mandible

wgyt

ꜥrt

p3ḳt
shell of skull

b3b3w nw irty
socket of the eyes

fnd   nose

štyt
'chamber' of the nose

msḏty

ibḥ

nḥḏt

inꜥt   chin

3.4 The lateral aspect of the skull. This has special relevance to the Edwin Smith papyrus, cases 1–27, some of which are cited in the text.

obvious in the adult. The ancient Egyptians were certainly aware of the existence of the fontanelle, a fibrous plate filling the gap between the parietal and frontal bones in very young children. Cases 6 and 8 both refer to '. . . the weakness of the crown of the head of a child, before it becomes whole'. A new approach is by Chapman (1992), who made the interesting suggestion that the two *paqyt* referred to the inner and outer tables of the skull. These separate to form the frontal sinus, and he proposed that *tepau* might refer to this structure. The word *tepau* also appears as an unknown disease of the head in Ebers 712.

The contents of the skull were known not only to the embalmer but also as a result of observation of head injuries. It seems from Case 6 of the Edwin Smith papyrus that the appearance of the brain was recognised:

If you examine a man [having] a gaping wound in his head, reaching the bone, smashing his skull and breaking open his brain (lit. the viscera (*ais*) of his skull), you should feel (palpate) his wound. You find that smash which is in his skull [like] the corrugations which appear on [molten] copper in the crucible, and something therein throbs and flutters under your fingers like the weak place in the crown of the head of a child when it has not become whole.

This remarkable passage (duplicated in the second examination of Case 8) is the earliest known description of the brain. Gloss B in Case 6 leaves no room for doubt that the corrugations refer to the slag which forms on molten copper and bears some resemblance to the surface of the brain. The weak place in the crown of the head of a child must refer to the anterior fontanelle which usually remains open until the second year of life.

Iversen (1947), the *Grundriss* and Faulkner (1962) take the word *ais* to mean viscera, and therefore the viscera of the skull would be the brain. However, Breasted takes *ais* to mean brain and translates the phrase as 'the brain of his skull'. The difference is largely academic and does not alter our general conclusion that the presence of the brain within the skull was recognised. There is another word '*amem*' which means brain (Iversen, 1947; the *Grundriss*; Faulkner, 1962), but it only appears in the medical papyri as a remedy in the form of the brain of various animals.

Finally in this section, we note that the Egyptians recognised that the brain was covered by a fibrous membrane (*netnet*), probably the dura mater, and was surrounded by fluid. We are left in no doubt by Gloss A of Case 6:

> As for 'a smash of his skull exposing the brain', the smash is large, opening to the interior of his skull, [to] the membrane (*netnet*) enclosing the brain. It breaks into his fluid in the interior of his head.

The word *netnet* is very rare but its determinative (Gardiner sign-list F 27) is the skin of a cow and the meaning seems certain. The fluid in the interior of the head would appear to be the cerebrospinal fluid, but it would surely be difficult, if not impossible, to recognise in the presence of the bleeding which accompanies a head injury.

There are two words for the lower jaw, *wegyt* and *aret*, which are used interchangeably and sometimes in the same sentence. The determinative (Gardiner sign-list F 19) is an excellent anatomical drawing of the mandible. The vertical part of the mandible (the ramus; fig. 3.4) has its own name, *amat*, and the articulation with the temporal bone is well described in Gloss A of Case 22.

> As for 'the end of his ramus', it means the end of his mandible. The ramus, the end of it (is) in his temple (*gema*) like the claw of the *ama* bird (when it) grasps an object.

The articular process of the mandible does vaguely resemble one claw of a two-clawed bird, although unfortunately the *ama* bird has never been identified. Insight into this area is enhanced by a clear description of the temporalis muscle in a case of lock-jaw (Gloss B of Case 7). This gloss sets out to explain the unfamiliar anatomical use of the Old Kingdom word for cord.

> As for 'the cord of his mandible is contracted', it means a stiffening of the *metu* at the back of his rami, fastened into his temple (*gema*), that is at the back of his jaw (*wegyt*), without moving to and fro. It is not easy for him to open his mouth because of the pain.

Figure 3.4 clearly shows that the *metu* in this case must refer to the powerful temporalis muscles which, together with the masseters, are mainly responsible for closure of the jaws. The origin and insertion of the temporalis muscle is described with a precision which makes its identification quite definite.

An understanding of the nasal cavity is revealed in Gloss A of Case 12, which sets out to explain the anatomical use of the word *shetyt*, which normally refers to the chamber of a building:

As for 'a fracture of the chamber (*shetyt*) of his nose', it means the middle of his nose [from] the bottom to the back, extending to between the eyebrows.

This gives a clear indication of the conformation of the nasal cavity, information which must have been familiar to the embalmers for removal of the brain through the nose.

These few examples are sufficient to show that, where we have documentary evidence, the anatomical knowledge of the *swnw* was remarkably good for the second and third millennium BC. If this level of knowledge was attained for the skull, lower jaw and nose, we can surmise that it would probably have reached a similar level for other parts which are not covered by the Edwin Smith papyrus. What we can infer certainly accords with the statement of Clement that an anatomical book was in existence, and it highlights the tragedy of its loss.

Hieroglyphs of medical relevance

Hieroglyphs provide us with several hundred miniature portraits of man, woman, animals, plants, inanimate objects and many of their component parts. Some of these portray items of anatomical or pathological interest (fig. 3.5). Gardiner's sign-list

3.5 Some anatomical structures used as the subject for hieroglyphs. External structures (except for the ear) tended to be human, whereas internal organs were generally those of animals. The well full of water (N 41) is used as a biliteral *h+m* in words meaning woman and uterus: it thence acquired some of the properties of a determinative, as the female equivalent of the phallus (D 52). Aa 1, F 36, F 39, S 24, D 52 and N 41 have extensive use as phonetics in many words unrelated to anatomical structures or their function. The numbers refer to the Gardiner sign-list.

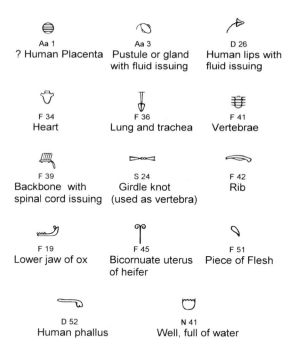

Aa 1	Aa 3	D 26
? Human Placenta	Pustule or gland with fluid issuing	Human lips with fluid issuing
F 34	F 36	F 41
Heart	Lung and trachea	Vertebrae
F 39	S 24	F 42
Backbone with spinal cord issuing	Girdle knot (used as vertebra)	Rib
F 19	F 45	F 51
Lower jaw of ox	Bicornuate uterus of heifer	Piece of Flesh
D 52	N 41	
Human phallus	Well, full of water	

contains sixty-three parts of the human body. It is striking that every one of these shows only external features, and thus provides no insight into knowledge of internal anatomy. This may be seen as confirmation of the belief that human dissection did not take place in the Old Kingdom when most of the hieroglyphs became formalised. Alternatively, it might have seemed improper to show internal parts of the human body. However, Aa 1 in Gardiner's unclassified group is thought to be a human placenta, and is very widely used as the phonetic sign for '*kh*'. Gardiner (1957) states that it may be used as a one-hieroglyph word for the placenta itself, although no such word appears in the *Wörterbuch der medizinischen Texte* of the *Grundriss*. Aa 2 is described by Gardiner as 'pustule or gland', while Aa 3 is the same with fluid issuing from it. These hieroglyphs have extensive use as determinatives for a range of words with unclean implications, such as 'embalm' (*wet*), 'wound', probably infected (*webenu*), 'pus' (*ryt*) and 'disease' (*khayt*). Steuer (1948) advanced the view that Aa 3 was derived from an embalmer's pot being poured, which would explain the lugs on the side, while conforming to the concept of infection as the counterpart of post-mortem decomposition (see below in relation to *wekhedu*). In its non-medical use it tends to be used without the liquid issuing from it (Aa 2). In D 26 is shown a fluid issuing between lips, and this appears as a determinative in words such as 'spit' (*peseg*). Its use is, however, extended to become the determinative for many important medical words, including 'vomit' (*besh*), 'blood' (*senef*) and 'menstruation' (*hesmen*).

In contrast to the reticence in showing human internal organs, nineteen of the fifty-one hieroglyphs showing parts of mammals display many internal structures, some of which are shown in fig. 3.5. Gardiner sign-list F 34 shows a not unreasonable diagram of the heart, and F 36 the lungs and trachea; F 36 acts as a triliteral in the Egyptian word *sma* meaning 'unite' and is elaborately shown in representations of the unification of the two kingdoms as, for example, at Abu Simbel. In some instances, it is possible to see what appear to be the cartilaginous rings of the trachea and the depressions on the lungs caused by the ribs. Vertebrae are seen in F 41, and F 39 shows a length of the vertebral column with spinal cord issuing from one end. Gardiner lists S 24 as a girdle knot but it would certainly pass for a fish vertebra in longitudinal section. This may be relevant to the fact that S 24 is also used in *tjes* meaning vertebra or spine. A reasonable representation of a rib is given in F 42, and F 19 is an unmistakable picture of the lower jaw-bone of an ox; F 45 is the bicornuate uterus of a heifer and F 51 is 'a piece of flesh', a very widely used determinative in, for example, 'liver' (*miset*), 'lung' (*sma*) and 'anus' (*pehwyt*). The flesh determinative is used freely in words for internal parts of the human body, and is very valuable for distinguishing anatomical terms from homophones with entirely different meanings.

There are two hieroglyphs with important, though by no means exclusively, sexual implications. The human phallus (D 52) has clear overtones of masculinity as a determinative in such words as 'husband' (*hy*). It is also the determinative in words such as 'phallus' (*henen*), 'urine' (*mwyt*) and 'copulate' (*nehep, nek, rekh* or *da*). In its excretory role, it may be embellished by liquid issuing from the tip (D 53). However, D 52 also functions as a biliteral phonetic for '*m+t*' in a wide range of words with no implications whatsoever of masculinity, sex or excretions. These include such innocuous words as 'discuss', 'precise', 'instruct' and 'midday'. It functions as a biliteral phonetic in the important word *metu* discussed at length above. The phallus appears twice in the word *metut* meaning both 'semen' and 'poison'. Its first appearance (D 52) is as a biliteral phonetic (*m+t*) and the second (D 53) as a determinative. In the meaning of 'poison' this relates to the poisonous semen of the god Seth who made a homosexual assault on Horus. The link between semen and poison is also implicit in the fear that the ghost of a dead person could have sexual relations with a sleeping person. Spells to avoid this danger include the phrase 'let your seed be ineffective'.

There is no corresponding hieroglyph to represent femininity, but Gardiner (1957) said that N 41, representing 'a well full of water', could act as a determinative for the female organs. However, this is complicated by the fact that it is a biliteral phonetic for *h+m* and features as a determinative only in words where it also functions as a biliteral phonetic (e.g. *hemet* – uterus). As in the case of D 52, it is also a biliteral phonetic in words which are nothing to do with femininity, such as 'assuredly', 'steering oar' and 'guest'.

Names of the internal organs

It may be useful at this stage to summarise the names of the main internal organs which were recognised by the ancient Egyptians. In some cases, the names throw light on their understanding of the structure, location and function of these organs. At least it is an indication of awareness of their existence.

The heart was known by two words *ib* and *haty*, used interchangeably in the medical papyri. The former was written simply as the hieroglyph F 34 (fig. 3.5), while the latter contains phonetic hieroglyphs with F 34 as a determinative. The word *ib* but never *haty* was also used to describe the seat of the emotions as in English. Many compound words included *ib*; for example *aw-ib*, literally 'long of heart', is usually translated as 'joyful'.

The stomach was known as *r-ib*, literally 'the mouth of the heart', and the two organs were not always clearly distinguished. This reminds us that the word 'stomach' is derived from the Greek *stoma*, meaning mouth, and the entrance to the stomach is still known as the cardia. The word *khet* has a much broader meaning of 'belly', 'body' or even 'uterus'.

'Liver' was *miset*, 'lung' *sma*, 'spleen' *nenshem*, 'bladder' *sheptyt* and 'brain' *amem* or alternatively *ais* or *ais n djennet* – the viscera of the skull (see p. 50). Lungs, liver, stomach, intestines and brain were removed during mummification, but the heart was carefully retained in position. Therefore the existence of all these organs must have been known at least to the embalmers. The kidneys, however, were a different matter. Outside the abdominal cavity and buried deeply in perinephric fat, it is entirely possible that they escaped detection. They were usually left behind in the embalming process and this resulted in the first detection of the ova of schistosoma in mummy tissue (p. 69). Faulkner (1962) and Lesko (1982–90) give *ggt* as kidney, but this word does not appear in the medical papyri and so is not listed in the *Wörterbuch* of the *Grundriss*.

Physiology

We have no information that any book of physiology was available in ancient Egypt. The evidence of the medical papyri indicates that concepts of physiology were simple and often erroneous.

The nervous system

There is no evidence that the ancient Egyptians associated the brain with thought or control of the body. At embalmment, the brain was the only major organ to be removed and discarded, unequivocal evidence of their failure to recognise its function. Emotion was related to *ib*, one of the two words for heart (see above). This identification of the heart as the seat of the emotions was widely held throughout the ancient and classical world and survives in current English usage. Before the work of Herophilus (see Chapter 10), Alcmaeon of Croton, Diogenes of Apollonia and Plato were exceptions in believing that the brain had a controlling function. However, the Hippocratic corpus (430–330 BC) does give an indication of its true role which seems unequivocal:

> It ought to be generally known that the source of our pleasure, merriment, laughter and amusement, as of our grief, pain, anxiety and tears, is none other

than the brain. It is specially the organ which enables us to think, see and hear.
. . . I therefore assert that the brain is the interpreter of comprehension.

The Edwin Smith papyrus gives valuable insight into the role of the spinal cord in transmission of information from the brain to the lower part of the body. Case 31 is concerned with a dislocation of the neck and describes how 'you find him not knowing his two arms and his two legs because of it'. It continues 'his phallus is erect and urine drips from his member'. This is a very apt description of quadriplegia (motor and sensory paralysis of all four limbs), erection and incontinence; all are consequences of a high spinal injury. The meaning of all the phrases cannot be in doubt and is made doubly clear from a series of glosses.

The circulatory system

The entire pharaonic period lay nearly two millennia before discovery of the circulation of the blood by Harvey in the seventeenth century AD. There is ample evidence that they believed the arteries contained air and that the whole concept of a circulatory system was unknown. However, the ancient Egyptians seemed to appreciate that the peripheral pulses reflected the beating of the heart, implicit in the quotation from the Ebers papyrus (854a) at the beginning of Chapter 6. Nevertheless, they believed that this resulted from the air which the *metu* were thought to contain. This is made clear in a misplaced gloss in the Ebers papyrus (855e). The passage to which it refers is unknown:

As to 'the heart weakens', it means the heart does not speak, or it means the *metu* are dumb. There is no remedy for them or information under your two hands, which normally appears because of the air with which they are filled.

There is constant stress on a *swnw* placing his hand upon the patient (see Chapter 6) and it seems likely that feeling the pulse was an important part of the examination.

The respiratory system

Outside the medical papyri, there is frequent reference to the breath of life (*tjaw n ankh*) received from the king or one of the gods. It cannot be doubted that they appreciated the life-giving importance of breathing. Their concept of what happened to the air which was breathed is less clear, but the following misplaced gloss from the Ebers papyrus (855a) provides an interesting overall view of the function of the respiratory system:

As for 'the breath which enters into the nose', it enters into the heart and the lungs. It is they which give to the entire body.

The overall scheme of cardio-respiratory function would seem to be that air was drawn in through the nose into the lungs. It was then transmitted to the heart and thence circulated to all parts of the body, giving rise to the peripheral pulses. It is interesting that, if for 'air' we substitute 'oxygen' (in solution and chemical combination in blood), the whole concept is remarkably close to the truth. What became of the air is not defined but it may be of significance that the vessel book says that all the *metu* unite at the anus.

Other systems

The medical papyri do not give any clear account of other physiological systems. The stomach book of the Ebers papyrus (188–208) appears to accept that food and drink pass into the stomach (*r-ib*) and their residue eventually 'goes down' (*ha*) to the anus.

It makes clear that the process can go wrong in various ways (see below), but there is no evidence of any understanding of the processes of digestion and absorption of nutriment. Vomiting was known by several words (e.g. *qa*, *qis*, *qas*, *besh*) and defecation by *fegen*, embellished with an unmistakable determinative.

There is very little mention of the physiology of the urinary system in the medical papyri. Ebers 854n states: 'There are two *metu* to the bladder (*sheptyt*). It is they which give urine (*muyt*).' Thus it was known that the bladder contained urine, and it is tempting to believe that these *metu* were the ureters (see fig. 3.3d and pp. 48–9). However, the kidneys are never mentioned in the medical papyri and it remains unclear why they were left in the body at embalmment (p. 54). Furthermore, they do not feature in the lists of organs which might be placed under divine protection. The commonest word for micturition was *wesesh* but is better translated as 'elimination' and may include defecation, loss of blood, passage of worms, etc. (*Grundriss*).

The essentials of reproduction were clearly understood and the relationship of sexual intercourse to procreation was well known. However, the ovaries were probably not recognised and no Egyptian word is known for them. The uterus was sometimes known as *mut remetj* (the mother of mankind), and its role may have been perceived purely as the environment for maturation of the male seed, without recognition of the genetic contribution of the mother. Nevertheless, inheritance through the female line was important to the ancient Egyptians. The testicles were known as *kherwy* (those two which are underneath) and Ebers 854i states: 'There are two *metu* to his testicles. It is they which give semen (*metut*).' There seems little doubt that their function was clearly understood.

Concepts of pathology

The ancient Egyptian concepts of the causation and nature of disease processes varied widely from the pragmatic to the magical. It is possible to draw a sharp contrast between trauma and internal medical disorders. In the case of the former, the causation was all too obvious and the experienced *swnw* would often be able to predict the outcome. Treatment was usually logical, having regard to the facilities which were available at the time, and resort to magic was unusual. Internal medical disorders presented an entirely different picture. In such conditions as infections, tumours and heart failure, they could not be aware of the cause, and the outcome would often be extremely difficult to predict. Furthermore, they had very few drugs which could have a decisive influence on the course of the disease and their surgical repertoire was limited. Thus it is hardly surprising that the causation of medical disorders was frequently attributed to supernatural causes and magic was an important factor in treatment (see Chapter 5).

Trauma

The *swnw* would have encountered trauma in many forms, including warfare, bites of dangerous animals and industrial accidents arising from mining, quarrying and the erection of large buildings. A wall painting in the tomb of Ipwy at Deir el-Medina (fig. 3.6) displays a variety of minor industrial injuries in satirical vein. Our main source of information is the Edwin Smith papyrus (see above and Chapter 2). The text and particularly the glosses give clear insight into an advanced understanding of the nature of injuries, at least a millennium before the Hippocratic era of medicine. It is particularly tragic that the only existing copy of the papyrus stops before consideration of the lower part of the body.   .

Gloss A of Cases 5 and 41 (see below) refer to an additional book on the treatment

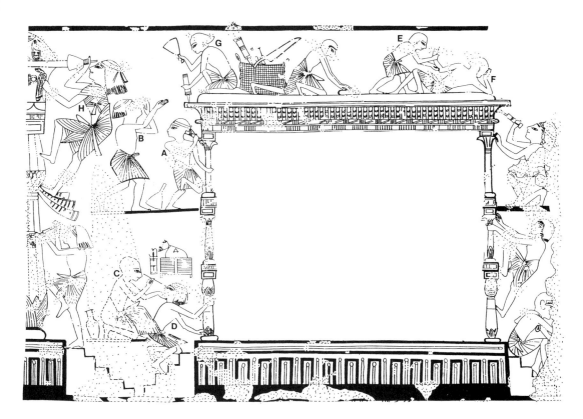

3.6 A unique relief from the tomb of the necropolis worker Ipwy in Deir el-Medina (Tomb 217), 20th Dynasty. This shows a remarkable series of occupational injuries and their treatment. A appears to have dropped his mallet on the foot of B. C seems to be removing a foreign body from the eye of D who continues working. E looks as though he is reducing a dislocated shoulder of F (see fig. 8.9). G may have been responsible for a foreign body in the eye of the unfortunate B, on whom H might well fall. This new drawing by Richard Parkinson is based on the painting by Nina Davies in Davies (1927).

of wounds. No copy of any part of this book has been found and it is not mentioned by Clement of Alexandria. Therefore it may have been lost in antiquity, although the Edwin Smith papyrus could well have relied upon it to a far greater extent than is indicated by these two references.

There is a rich vocabulary to describe injuries, and fortunately the glosses often define their meaning with precision. Some of the words are well known outside the medical field, but their medical use is found only in the Edwin Smith papyrus. Other words are quite unknown except for their use in the papyrus. All the references in the following section relate to the Edwin Smith papyrus (Breasted, 1930), except where specifically mentioned. Management of trauma is considered in Chapter 8.

Soft tissue injury. The general term for a flesh wound is *webenu*, with various determinatives including the pustule and fluid issuing between lips. Majno (1975) drew attention to the possibility that these two determinatives were used to distinguish between an infected and a clean, though bleeding, wound. The word *kefet* also means flesh wound and the two terms may be used interchangeably. Used together these words are translated as a gash. The usual word for lips (*sepet*) is used to describe the edges of wound. Gloss B of Case 1 (restored) says that when a wound does not have two lips it means that the wound is narrow and not gaping.

Fractures. The Edwin Smith papyrus has an impressive vocabulary to describe different types of fractures. The usual word for fracture is *heseb* with a cross for the determinative, implying a discontinuity; it is unknown outside the Edwin Smith papyrus.

A simple closed fracture is described with great clarity as one in which the flesh is healthy (*wedja*) without a wound (*webenu*) (Edwin Smith, Case 8).

A special form of fracture is specified by the word *sed*, which appears twenty-three times in the Edwin Smith papyrus and is translated by Breasted as 'smash'. It appears to be a more severe type of injury and is defined in Gloss A of Case 5:

> As for 'a *sed* of his skull', it means a *sed* of his skull, bones appearing in that smash, sinking into the interior of his skull. The book (*tjaw*) pertaining to wounds states: 'It means a *sed* of his skull into many fragments which sink into the interior of his skull'.

The word *sed* is well known outside the medical papyri to mean 'break into', 'break open', etc. (as, for example, a pottery jar). In the context of Case 5, *sed* seems to include at least three special aspects of a fracture. First, there are multiple fragments of bone (comminuted fracture). Secondly, there is involvement of another organ (complicated fracture), the brain in this case and also in Cases 6 and 8. Thirdly, in the context of the skull, this is a depressed fracture. However, the pattern of usage of the word *sed* in relation to fractures elsewhere is not sufficiently consistent to say that it has the specific meanings of comminuted, complicated, compound or depressed fractures. The word *sed* is also used to describe soft-tissue injuries and, in the Ebers papyrus, to indicate the therapeutic opening of an abscess.

The next special word for bony injury is *peshen*, an ancient word which has the general meaning of 'split' outside the medical papyri. Its medical meaning is made explicit in Gloss A of Case 4:

> As for 'splitting his skull', it means separating shell (*paqyt*) from shell of his skull, while fragments remain in the flesh of his head and do not fall to the ground.

This presents a clear picture of the skull cleft with a sword or battle axe. However, it is conceivable that it refers to separation of the inner and outer tables of the skull (p. 50).

The ancient Egyptians seem to have understood the principle of an impacted fracture in which the fragments of bone are driven into one another so that they cannot move in relation to one another. This they described as a crush (*sehem* with the pestle determinative, Gardiner sign-list U 33), a state of affairs clearly described in Gloss A of Case 33:

> As for 'a crush of the vertebrae in his neck', he is speaking of a falling of a vertebra of his neck into another of his, one entering into another, without moving to and fro.

It would be difficult to improve on this simple and explicit definition of an impacted fracture. An alternative description of the same phenomenon is in Case 32 which describes 'a vertebra sinking as a foot settles into cultivated ground'.

A special type of fracture was *tehem*, a well known word interpreted in the context of the Edwin Smith papyrus to mean perforation of a flat bone to damage an underlying organ (Breasted, 1930; the *Grundriss*; Faulkner, 1962). This type of injury is described for the skull (Case 3), maxilla (Case 15), temporal bone (Cases 18, 19 and 20), chin (Case 27), cervical vertebra (Case 29) and manubrium sterni (upper part of the breast bone – Case 40).

Injuries to joints. These are separated into dislocations and sprains. Dislocations (*wenekh*) are described for the lower jaw (Edwin Smith, Case 25), the vertebrae

CONCEPTS OF ANATOMY, PHYSIOLOGY AND PATHOLOGY

(Case 31), the clavicle (Case 34) and the articulation between the ribs and the sternum (Case 43). The meaning of *wenekh* is formally defined in Gloss A of Case 31:

> As for 'a dislocation (*wenekh*) in a vertebra of his neck', he is speaking of separation of one vertebra of his neck from another, the flesh which is over it being uninjured (*wedja*). As one says 'a dislocation is things which were joined together and one is severed (*pehedj*) from another'.

Although the meaning of *pehedj* is debatable, the account of the dislocated jaw in Case 25 (p. 178) leaves no doubt as to the meaning of *wenekh*.

Breasted translated *nerut* as 'sprain' largely on the basis of Gloss A in Case 30, which describes a *nerut* of the cervical vertebrae.

> As for 'a sprain', he is speaking of a breaking open (*neg*) of two members [although] it is still in its place.

Edwin Smith Case 42 describes a *nerut* of the ribs and states specifically that there is no dislocation (*wenekh*). Case 48 describes a *nerut* of the vertebral column with pain on extending the legs. When the hips are flexed, this is a diagnostic sign of a prolapsed lumbar intervertebral disc pressing on a nerve, and in Case 30 it is recorded that flexion of the neck (looking at the shoulders and breast) is painful. Thus it may be concluded that *nerut* does indeed involve a loosening of a joint but without an actual dislocation and the word 'sprain' is a reasonable translation.

Snake bite and scorpion sting. The magical aspects of the treatment of snake bite and scorpion sting, particularly as outlined in the Metternich stela (Chapter 5), leave no doubt that the ancient Egyptians realised that a toxic substance (*metut*) was injected by the animal, and this was the cause of the pain, difficulty in breathing and other effects. There is repeated mention of the desirability of casting the poison on to the ground by magical means and occasionally of applying 'the knife treatment' to the wound (p. 188). A pragmatic approach to the treatment of snake bite, relatively free of magic, is revealed in the Brooklyn papyrus no. 47.218.48 and 47.218.85 (see Chapters 2 and 8).

Medical disorders

When we leave the field of trauma, ancient Egyptian medicine loses much of its pragmatism and there is increased evidence of empiricism, speculation, unproven remedies and magic. This may be explained by their lack of understanding of the cause of most internal disorders. Such knowledge lay far in the future.

Infection. Bacterial infection was regarded as a normal consequence of open wounds until the advent of asepsis, antisepsis and antibiotics. The cause must have been quite unknown in ancient Egypt. The classic signs of superficial infection are pain, swelling, redness and heat. There is an explicit description of an infected wound in Gloss A of Case 41 of the Edwin Smith papyrus:

> As for 'a diseased (*sma*) wound (*webenu*) in his breast, inflamed (*neser*)', it means that the wound which is in his breast is sluggish(?) and it does not cover itself (i.e. close up). High fever (lit. heat – *shemmet*) comes forth from it. Its two lips (*sepety*) are red (*desher*) and its mouth is open. The book pertaining to wounds states concerning it 'It means there is very great swelling (*sheu*). One says it is high inflammation (*neser*).'

The common word for flame is *neser* and, used in its medical sense of inflammation, still carries the flame determinative (Gardiner sign-list Q 7). This remarkable passage specifies all the essential characteristics of an infected wound except for pain, but elsewhere it is stated that 'the flesh cannot receive a bandage', perhaps because of the pain. In addition, it is made clear that the wound cannot close itself.

It is tempting but unjustified to believe that the ancient Egyptians realised that bacteria entered the wound from outside the body and thereby caused infection. They were very familiar with the concept of something evil entering the body from outside. Gloss D of Case 8 states:

> As for 'something entering from outside', it means the breath of an outside-god or death. It is not an entering of what is created by his flesh.

Reference has been made above (p. 49) to the breath of death entering through the left ear, and below there is reference to the heart showing disordered function (*neba*) as a result of 'something entering from outside', the whole phrase with an unidentifiable god determinative. Things which enter from the outside are described by Westendorf (1992) as sickness-demons (see Chapter 5) and indeed they do appear to belong to the realm of magic rather than an anticipated recognition of infection.

Abscess formation. It would be expected that the ancient Egyptians must have been familiar with the formation of an abscess. As there is no convincing evidence in mummies or representations, we must rely on accounts in the medical papyri. These are discussed in Chapter 4, and the surgical treatment in Chapter 8. There are clear accounts of rounded swellings with liquid contents which are treated with the knife. However, without mention of heat, redness and pain, it is difficult to exclude the possibility that they were describing a cyst, perhaps the very common sebaceous cyst.

The common word for pus is *ryt*, which carries the so-called pus determinative. However, Ebers 871 uses the word *wekhedu*, in relation to a condition which very strongly suggests an abscess in the axilla (p. 76). *Wekhedu* is a very difficult word of uncertain and possibly multiple meanings, which are considered below.

The role of the *metu* in the causation of disease. There can be no doubt that the *metu* were considered essential to life and health, and a substantial section of the Ebers papyrus is devoted to remedies for strengthening or softening them (Ebers 627–94). However, the situation is greatly complicated by the multiple meanings of the word *metu* which, in the latter context, presumably refers to muscles. Ebbell (1937) sometimes interpreted *metu* as the male member, weakness of which he equated with impotence (Ebers 663). This ingenious interpretation is not acceptable, and the hieroglyph representing the phallus (Gardiner sign-list D 52) in *metu* is here a biliteral for '*m+t*' rather than a determinative. A more specific disease of the *metu* is a 'swelling of the *metu*'. In Ebers 872 this is described as rounded and solid, arising from an injury to the vessel, possibly suggesting a post-traumatic aneurysm (a localised ballooning of an artery). In Ebers 873 the 'swelling of the *metu*' is as though it contained air and had formed knots. It is not clear what this might be.

Disease of the heart (see Chapter 4) is attributed to the *metu* in Ebers 855c, which describes the causation of an unknown pathological condition of the heart (*shes*) thus:

> It is the *met* (singular of *metu*) whose name is the 'receiver' which causes it. It is this which gives water to the heart.

Similarly, Ebers 854l says that the four *metu* to the liver are 'those which cause all illness to appear because of overflooding with blood'. Both Ebers 856h and Berlin 163h say that disease of the anus happens because of the *metu*.

Of special interest is the suggestion that the *metu* might carry infected material to the body. Ebers 855g comprises a most important gloss to a passage which is lost:

> As to 'the heart spreads itself out', it means that the *metu* of the heart contain faeces.

This suggests the possibility of septicaemia arising from infected bowel contents. Ebers 856h and Berlin 163h state that 'all [*metu*] come to his heart ... and unite at his anus' which, as a meeting point of *metu*, seemed to enjoy a position second only to the heart. The ancient Egyptian concept of the network of *metu* would therefore be well disposed to permit the spread of toxic substances from the bowel. The nature of such a substance is crucial to an understanding of Egyptian medicine and in this connection we now return to consideration of the extended meanings of *wekhedu*.

Some pathological terms of uncertain meaning

Our understanding of ancient Egyptian medicine is gravely handicapped by a number of pathological terms of which the meaning is either unknown or else is the subject of debate and disagreement. In general, these are left untranslated in this book (see Appendix D), but the following section discusses some of the possible interpretations which have been advanced.

Wekhedu – pain matter or morbid principle? Few aspects of ancient Egyptian medicine are more difficult to comprehend than the nature of *wekhedu*, a word used on many occasions in most of the medical papyri, but unfortunately never defined in a gloss. The implication is that it was well understood by contemporary readers, while we are forced to determine its meaning by implication from the contexts in which it is used. The subject has been extensively considered in the *Grundriss* and also by Steuer (1948) and Steuer and Saunders (1959). *Wekhedu* is almost certainly related to the well attested verb *wekhed* meaning 'to suffer'. In four paragraphs of the Ebers papyrus *wekhedu* appears with the feminine termination as *wekhedut*, always along-side *wekhedu* as though it had a separate identity, as in the following example (Ebers 246) in which one god prepares a remedy for another:

> A fifth remedy that Nut prepared for Ra himself ... every ailing part is bandaged therewith, whether it is for *wekhedu* or *wekhedut* ...

A person suffering from *wekhedu* is referred to as a *wekhedy*, following the normal Egyptian termination '*y*' to indicate a person in relation to a noun or adjective. *Wekhedu*, and sometimes *wekhedut* as well, was said to afflict many organs, including the belly, skin, mouth, chest, back, heart, head, eyes and teeth. Many remedies are 'to drive out or to ward off *wekhedu*', which had the capacity to move about the body (Ebers 856a):

> Beginning of the *Book of Wanderings* (*hebheb*) of *wekhedu* in all the limbs of a man, as was found in writings under the two feet of Anubis in Letopolis ...

The word *hebheb* has been alternatively translated as 'traverse' or 'pull through' but the general concept is clear that *wekhedu* may pass from one part of the body to another. This citation is the opening sub-paragraph of the list of *metu* in Ebers 856 (see Table 3.2) and it seems clear that these *metu* (see above) would be the channels through which *wekhedu* was expected to spread; this hypothesis was proposed in the *Grundriss* and propounded in detail by Steuer (1948) and Steuer and Saunders (1959) and imaginatively illustrated by Majno (1975). The theory runs as follows. It was well known that, after death, putrefaction commenced in the bowels and then spread to the whole body. This was, no doubt, the basis of the early removal of the bowels in the process of mummification (Andrews, 1984). It was not difficult to extrapolate from death to believe that putrefaction in the bowel could spread to other parts of the body during life, the 'morbid principle' being *wekhedu* and the *metu* the means of its transmission. The *metu* had the right connections, linking the heart and the anus, as cited above. The association between *wekhedu* and decomposition after death is strengthened by the claim in the quotation from Ebers 856a above that the original papyrus was found under the feet of Anubis, the god of mummification. There is, however, no specific statement in the medical papyri which describes this process by which *wekhedu* passes from the anus to the rest of the body through the *metu*, but what is written accords with this approach. The inference is also strongly supported by the Egyptians' concentration on purgatives and enemas (Herodotus II, 77) which would be logical to remove *wekhedu* and prevent its spread:

> Every month for three successive days they purge themselves, for their health's sake, with emetics and enemas, in the belief that diseases come from the food a man eats.

A very similar concept was taught by the Greek school of medicine which flourished in Cnidos immediately before the Hippocratic school in Cos. This school held the view that *perittoma* was formed under abnormal conditions in the bowels and this 'morbid principle' then spread to the rest of the body to cause disease in other organs (Steuer and Saunders, 1959). *Perittoma* was the pathological counterpart of *kopros* which was the normal state of the faeces. The Egyptian parallel would be that *wekhedu* was the pathological state of the bowel contents, in contrast to *hes* which means normal faeces. However, *perittoma* does not feature explicitly in the Hippocratic corpus although the idea of disease originating in the bowels was never lost. The concepts of *wekhedu* and *perittoma* accord well with modern ideas of toxaemia arising from abnormal growth of commensal aerobic organisms in the small bowel.

How then should we translate the word *wekhedu* in terms of modern concepts of medicine? There is no agreement. One school of thought uses words based on 'pain'. Lefebvre (1956) used 'les douleurs de toute sorte', von Deines and Westendorf (1961) in the *Grundriss* 'Schmerzstoffe' and Ghaliounghui (1987) follows the *Grundriss* with 'pain matter'. Faulkner (1962) simply gave 'pain' for both *wekhedu* and *wekhedut*. This seems too restrictive and would not accord with the complete absence of the word in the Edwin Smith papyrus dealing with trauma. Furthermore, there are at least five other Egyptian words for 'pain'. Ebbell (1937) used 'purulency' which seems appropriate in certain cases, particularly the account of axillary abscess (Ebers 871) mentioned above and cited in Chapter 4. However, this is also too restrictive, particularly in relation to the heart, an organ in which purulency is hardly a major problem. Ghaliounghui (1987), in recognition of the multiple aspects of *wekhedu* as infection (sepsis, septicaemia, pyaemia, toxaemia) and perhaps the spread of malignant disease, suggests it might be better to use '*wekhedu* – morbid principle'. Perhaps the wisest course is to follow Leca (1988) who avoids a direct translation.

Setet. This word starts with the hieroglyph representing an animal skin pierced by an arrow (Gardiner sign-list F 29) and ends with the so-called pustule determinative (fig. 3.5). The former appears in the verb *set* (shoot, thrust, pierce, etc.) and derived nouns with the same determinative mean arrow, target, etc. It thus appeared very reasonable for Dawson (1934b) to suggest that the meaning of *setet* in the medical texts should be 'shooting pains'.

However, Gardiner makes it clear that F 29 may also be a biliteral phonetic for *s+t*, and it does appear in a few words which are quite unrelated to shooting, such as 'ground'. In at least two instances (Ebers 102 and 206) *setet* carries the liquid determinative, and the authors of the *Grundriss* translate *setet* as 'Schleimstoffe' (slime, mucus or 'mucosities'). Ebbell (1937) favoured 'phlegm'. Unfortunately, no gloss defines *setet*, nor do its contexts in the medical papyri resolve its true meaning.

The *aaa*-disease. This condition is mentioned by name twenty-two times in the medical papyri, and these citations are accompanied by another twenty-eight 'other remedies'. Phonetically, the word is *aaa*, and the determinative is the discharging phallus. It is unknown as a noun outside the medical papyri and no gloss explains its meaning. As early as 1853, Brugsch suggested it meant a 'maladie divine mortifère'. However, Ebbell (1937) translated it as 'haematuria' (blood in the urine), with a footnote to say 'by this *Bilharzia haematobia* (sic) must no doubt be meant'. Jonckheere (1944) expanded the meaning to 'hématurie parasitaire', caused by schistosomiasis, the commonest cause of haematuria in Egypt (see Chapter 4). Lefebvre (1956) supported this interpretation.

In 1961, the *Wörterbuch* of the *Grundriss* proposed a radically different meaning of 'Samen' or 'Giftstoffe'. Their concept was essentially that of an evil spirit in the form of an incubus who impregnated its victims with its poisonous semen while they were asleep, a concept further considered in Chapter 5. This is supported by the fact that there is a rare verb *aaa*, with the same determinative, which means 'to discharge semen'. Furthermore, many of the remedies against *aaa* are to be taken at night when an incubus would be most active. Therefore, *aaa* appears to be a poisonous and toxic substance introduced into the body by magical means, and was considered to be the cause of a variety of diseases to be treated with remedies as well as incantations.

The *Grundriss* interpretation is supported by the majority of texts in which *aaa* is mentioned. Berlin 58 refers to 'driving out the *aaa* of a god or goddess', and six other paragraphs to 'driving out the *aaa* of a god or dead man', while two refer to the *aaa* of a dead man or woman, one of these being a spell. There is, furthermore, nothing to link *aaa* directly with the bladder (see p. 91). Six citations refer to '*aaa* of the belly and heart' while three refer only to '*aaa* of the heart', in each case heart being written as *haty*, which cannot be confused with any other organ. It is inconceivable that the Egyptians would have believed the heart to be involved in schistosomiasis. It should also be noted that none of these passages mentions haematuria.

Ebers 62 is the critical passage for identifying *aaa* as schistosomiasis:

Another remedy, useful as something prepared for the belly: reeds (? sedge), 1; *shames*-plant, 1; grind fine, cook with honey, and eaten by a man in whose belly [there are] *hereret*-worms. It is the *aaa* which created them. Not killed by any [other] remedy.

The identity of the *hereret*-worm is unknown, but it has been suggested that they are the adult parasitic worms of schistosomiasis. However, it is explained on pp. 68–9 that their recognition in antiquity would have been extremely unlikely. Furthermore, Ebers paragraphs 56–61 all start 'Another [remedy]', following paragraph 55 which is a 'Remedy to kill the *hefat*-worm'. Therefore, assuming that the paragraphs have remained in their original order, paragraph 62 should also be intended to kill the *hefat*-worm, with which 'useful as something prepared for the belly' would not necessarily conflict. The identity of the *hefat*-worm (see Table 4.1) is unknown, although elsewhere Ebbell (1937) suggested roundworm (e.g. *Ascaris lumbricoides*). Evidence for the existence of schistosomiasis in ancient Egypt is considered in Chapter 4.

CHAPTER FOUR

The pattern of disease

It is often assumed that the ancient Egyptians must have suffered from much the same range of diseases that afflict the country today. This may well be true for degenerative diseases, such as osteoarthritis and arteriosclerosis. However, the assumption is not valid for many conditions where causative factors may have changed. For example, the incidence of cancer seems to have been much less, but how far this is due to the shorter expectation of life, genetic factors or absence of carcinogenic factors in the environment can only be conjectural at present. The greatest difficulties arise with infective conditions. Within recent times, certain parasites have changed their geographical boundaries, as environmental factors have altered the distribution of alternative hosts. There have also been major changes in the virulence of many bacteria and viruses. Certain bacteria were unknown in the Old World in pharaonic times, and there is, for example, no convincing case of syphilis from ancient Egypt (Buikstra, Baker and Cook, 1993).

Although the study of disease in ancient Egypt has been actively pursued for almost two hundred years, attention tends to have been concentrated on interesting cases, almost always belonging to a privileged minority. The most favoured techniques have been unwrapping of mummies, followed by dissection, histological examination of tissues (since 1889) and radiography (since 1898). Armelagos and Mills (1993) presented a compelling argument to adopt a population perspective, involving large numbers rather than concentrating on individuals. This approach is now realistic, with new analytical techniques which are relatively non-destructive and require only small samples of tissue. Important examples are recovery of deoxyribonucleic acid (DNA) and detection of antibodies, considered below.

Evidence of disease in pharaonic times

Study of the pattern of disease in pharaonic times depends on three main sources – human remains, representations of persons and accounts of disease in the papyri. These three sources do not greatly overlap in the details which they provide, and it may be helpful to review their scope and limitations before considering individual diseases.

Human remains

The dry hot climate of Egypt is better suited to the preservation of human remains than that of any other country in the world. A simple burial in hot sand often results in desiccation proceeding faster than putrefaction. The end result is a dehydrated body, often with remarkably good preservation of detail (fig. 4.1). Unfortunately, bodies simply buried in the sand were often scavenged by wild animals, particularly jackals. Coffins of basketwork were then used to prevent this, but so impeded the process of desiccation that putrefaction often occurred with loss of the body. This dilemma was ultimately resolved by artificial mummification, practised first for the royal family from at least the early Fourth Dynasty (Andrews, 1984). Soon afterwards it became available for members of the court as the gift of the king.

All royal mummies from the Old Kingdom are lost but three mummies of members of the court have survived, a fourth being lost in the air raid on the Royal College of

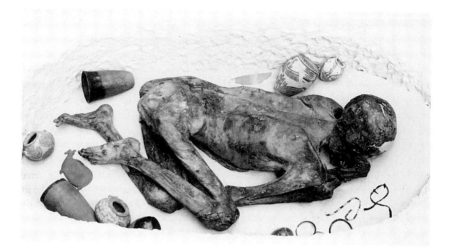

4.1 A late Predynastic burial from Gebelein, Naqada II Period, showing excellent preservation resulting from desiccation caused by burial in dry sand with no coffin. (British Museum, EA 32751)

Surgeons of England (see below). In the Middle and New Kingdoms, mummification became more generally available and reached its technical peak in the Twenty-first Dynasty. A large number of royal mummies of the Eighteenth and Nineteenth Dynasties were found in caches in Thebes and are preserved in Cairo Museum. The mummy of Tutankhamun remains in his tomb in the Valley of the Kings.

The pathological information available from mummies is severely restricted by certain technical aspects of the embalming procedure, which was described during the Twenty-seventh Dynasty by Herodotus (II, 86). As much as possible of the brain was removed through the nose and discarded. The lungs and the abdominal contents were removed and, after an elaborate preservation procedure, were placed in the four canopic jars as listed in Table 3.1. However, their state of preservation is often too poor to reveal the presence of disease. Heart and kidneys usually remained in the body and may be available for study, along with parts of other organs accidentally left behind.

The skeleton, muscles and skin remained in place and, under ideal conditions, were well preserved as, for example, in the case of Seti I (Nineteenth Dynasty). The head of the pharaoh Seqenenra was so well preserved that his injuries may still be clearly seen (see fig. 8.6). Nevertheless, over-enthusiastic use of resin, pitch and cosmetic packing often caused severe damage to soft tissue. Another cause of damage was the attempts of tomb robbers to remove valuable items from the body.

During the last century, public unwrapping of mummies became a popular event (Granville, 1825; Pettigrew, 1834) but yielded comparatively little useful pathological information. The pioneer of systematic palaeopathology was Sir Marc Armand Ruffer, Professor of Bacteriology in the Cairo Medical School (1896–1917); his studies were collected in a volume (1921) published after his death. More recently there has been a long-running multi-disciplinary study at Manchester University under the leadership of Rosalie David (1979). The Granville mummy (Itry-senu) was re-examined in 1994 (Harer and Taylor, in preparation).

The current emphasis is on the extraction of maximal information with minimal destruction of the material. Simple radiography has given way to the far more informative computed tomography, which can be undertaken without opening the mummy cartonnage (Isherwood and Hart, 1992; Baldock *et al.*, 1994). Images of cross-sections can be prepared at any level, together with sections in other planes (fig. 4.2). Different ranges of densities can be selectively amplified to show bone, soft tissue or artificial implants. Body cavities can be explored by fibre-optic endoscopy which requires only a small hole for the introduction of the instrument. Samples of tissues can then be removed and, after rehydration, can be stained and examined by light microscopy and by electron microscopy in both the transmission and scanning modes. Studies of antibodies (see below) can be undertaken on very small samples of skin, and have enormous potential for population-based studies.

A particularly exciting development was the recovery and replication of DNA from ancient human remains (Pääbo, 1985). This opened the possibility of determining individual genetic profiles, with important future applications. These include sex determination, kinship studies, genetic diseases and perhaps identification of ethnic groups (Hedges and Sykes, 1993). Bacterial, viral and parasitic DNA may also be sampled from infected individuals. It is important to distinguish between nuclear DNA (about 3,000,000,000 base pairs) and maternally transmitted mitochondrial DNA (about 16,000 base pairs). (Three base pairs are required to code for each amino acid, of which there may be many hundreds in a protein.) Mitochondrial DNA is easier to recover, especially from the osteocytes in bone, which is the commonest available tissue to study. As might be expected, the technical problems are formidable and the DNA is usually damaged. The best recoveries to date, using the polymerase chain reaction, are of the order of 100–200 base pairs. Fortunately, such short sequences can often yield valuable information. A major problem is contamination with foreign DNA from insects, moulds and those who have handled specimens.

Skeletal remains are a very important resource, particularly for population-based studies. A large group of cemeteries just south of Aswan was flooded after the old Aswan dam was raised by seven metres from 1908. A rescue dig was undertaken in 1907 by George Reisner; Elliot Smith, Professor of Anatomy in the Cairo Medical School (1900–9), assisted by Wood Jones, examined *in situ* some 6000 bodies and skeletons from fifty-seven cemeteries, ranging from pre-historic to Roman times (Smith and Jones, 1910). A collection of 360 pathological specimens was deposited in the Hunterian Museum of the Royal College of Surgeons of England in 1908. Unfortunately, many were lost, together with their records, during an air-raid in 1941. Wood Jones was appointed Professor of Human and Comparative Anatomy at the Royal College of Surgeons in 1945, soon after the loss of the specimens which he had collected thirty-eight years before. Most of the surviving specimens of the Nubian Pathological Collection were transferred (1948–68) to the Natural History Museum of London (Molleson, 1993), and have featured prominently in many studies.

Major limitations in the study of human remains from ancient Egypt have been reviewed by Buikstra, Baker and Cook (1993). There have been too many examples of poor documentation at excavation, and loss or destruction of specimens. Newly developed diagnostic techniques frequently demand re-examination of material. This is, of course, impossible if the specimen or its identification has been lost. Then there is often confusion between disease processes and *post-mortem* damage due, for example, to attack by natron, mould or insects. Differential diagnostic criteria have become much more rigorous in recent years, as is so evident when material is re-examined and original diagnoses cannot be sustained.

Representations of the body

Much of ancient Egyptian art followed strict iconographic conventions, with individual peculiarities subordinated to the portrayal of idealised features. Thus pharaohs and others tend to be portrayed in the full vigour of youth with perfectly proportioned limbs, well developed muscles and the minimum of fat. Likewise, the

4.2 Computed tomography of the 22nd Dynasty mummy Tjent-mut-en-gebtiu (British Museum, EA 22939) still within the cartonnage. On the left is the composite image produced from combined topogram views. Top right is a lateral topogram, showing a winged goddess on the anterior surface of the neck. Bottom right is a transverse section of the torso with the cartonnage clearly visible, showing the vertebral column and ribs with the two upper arms to the sides. Internal structures are wrapped organs replaced in the thorax, each containing a small object (Baldock *et al.*, 1994). The wealth of detail may be compared with conventional radiographs of the same mummy by Dawson and Gray (1968).

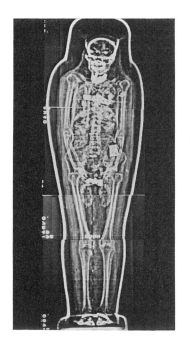
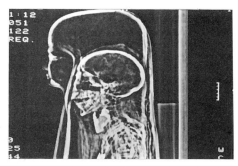
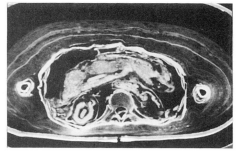

women are usually shown as tall, slender and beautiful, with graceful poise. However, under certain circumstances the canon of proportions was set aside and we have what appears to be a degree of realistic portrayal.

Realistic portrayal of the deceased was often employed in funerary statues and stelae. The Egyptian concept of life in the afterworld was based on life as it had been enjoyed while alive. Central to this was the preservation of the body of the deceased and hence mummification. However, it was well known that tomb robbing was prevalent and the mummy was often destroyed. Therefore, a portrayal of the body was required as a contingency substitute for the mummy. This took the form of serdab statues, *ka* statues, conventional 'husband and wife' statues (see fig. 4.6), and also reliefs and paintings on the walls of the tomb chapel. Depiction of physical abnormalities ensured that the representation was a valid substitute for the real body, should it be required. Similar considerations applied to the portrayal of servants, so that they should be immediately identifiable by their infirmities when summoned by magic to serve the deceased in the hereafter.

There are, however, important caveats in the literal interpretation of deformities in these representations. It is possible that certain disabilities were conventionally shown to illustrate a particular state or those who undertook a particular job. Thus it is conceivable that obesity might be used to imply prosperity, that all dwarfs were shown with short limbs (whether or not they were achondroplasiac) and that blindness might be no more than a convention when a harpist is shown. A special problem arises in the case of the highly atypical artistic style of the Amarna Period when Amenhotep IV (Akhenaten, *c.* 1352–1336 BC) was displayed in an apparently naturalistic style, although with highly abnormal physical features. Did his appearance indicate disease or had he introduced a new iconographic convention to break with that of previous pharaohs? These difficult problems are considered later in this chapter in relation to the diseases which are portrayed.

Disease in the medical papyri

It might be thought that the medical papyri would be the obvious sources of information on disease in ancient Egypt. It is true that injuries are very well described and it is not difficult to visualise the clinical condition. However, it is much more difficult to identify medical as opposed to surgical conditions from the papyri. The Edwin Smith surgical papyrus is almost unique in its excellent descriptions of the conditions before proceeding to treatment. In contrast, the main medical (as opposed to surgical) papyri tend to assume that the diagnosis has already been made and merely identify it by a name which is often difficult or impossible to translate. So many sections of the Ebers, Hearst and Berlin papyri follow the general format 'as for a man suffering from ABC, you shall prepare for him XYZ ...' leaving us none the wiser as to the meaning of ABC.

Certain sections of these papyri do approach the style of the Edwin Smith papyrus in providing a brief description of the history and clinical findings. This is particularly true of the section devoted to the stomach in the Ebers papyrus (188–207). However, even here there are great difficulties in understanding the words used to describe signs and symptoms, so it is often impossible to be certain of the diagnosis. The words are frequently unknown outside the medical papyri and the medical texts may provide no firm evidence of their meaning. Alternatively, their meaning may be well established in the non-medical sense, but it appears that they must have a special meaning when used in the medical sense. This is true today, when doctors have hijacked many English words and given them a special meaning when used in medicine – as, for example, the term 'flail chest' used for multiple rib fractures.

Parasitic diseases

Parasitic diseases have been a major health problem in Egypt until the present day. Numerous disease terms carry a worm determinative and many case descriptions in the medical papyri are strongly suggestive of the worm infestations which might be expected. However, it is very difficult to make a positive identification of specific parasites from the Egyptian texts. The alternative source of information is from examination of human remains. There was a historic positive identification of calcified Bilharzia (Schistosoma) ova in the kidneys of two mummies of the Twentieth Dynasty by Ruffer (1910a). Since then, histology, radiography and, more recently, immunological techniques have yielded positive results on a wider scale (see below).

Schistosomiasis (bilharziasis)

This is still a major cause of chronic ill health in Egypt; recent figures on the control of schistosomiasis from the World Health Organization (1993) show that about 12 per cent of the population are infected. There are three main species of the platyhelminth worm *Schistosoma* but the most important for Egypt are *S. mansoni* and *S. haematobium*, first described by Bilharz in 1852. There is a complex life cycle alternating between two hosts, humans and fresh water snails of the genus *Bulinus* which live on the banks of rivers. If the snail can be eradicated, the cycle is disrupted and the disease can be brought under control.

The infection is acquired from immersion in water containing cercariae, the free-swimming form of the worm released by the snail. The cercariae penetrate the intact skin and enter the veins of the human host. The adult male is about 1 cm in length and the female about double this but much thinner. It would not be easy to see the worms in antiquity. It would be necessary to examine blood which was diluted with water before it had clotted, and the worms disappear by autolysis within twenty-four hours of the death of the host (Ghaliounghui, 1987). Although magnifying glasses had not been invented in pharaonic times, persons with gross short sight (myopia) would be able to see objects too small to be seen by those with normal eyesight. The detail of miniature engravings on jewellery suggests that such people were employed for their close vision.

The adult worms are believed to pair in the portal vein (leading from the bowels to the liver) and then migrate to the veins of the bladder and rectum, where the eggs are deposited. The eggs of *S. haematobium* are oval, about 0.14×0.05 mm, and invisible to the naked eye. They can be found in most of the internal organs of the human host but especially in the urinary tract. The eggs ulcerate through the bladder, with blood and eggs being passed in the urine. The condition is self-limiting provided re-infection does not take place. However, once the eggs reach fresh water, they rupture, releasing the miracidia which swim away to seek their intermediate host. Within the snail, the miracidia develop into sporocysts, producing large numbers of cercariae which then escape into the water to seek a human host and so to start another cycle.

The main symptom is haematuria (blood in the urine), and Napoleon's troops reported that Egypt was the land of menstruating men. This may result in serious anaemia, with lassitude, loss of appetite, urinary infection and loss of resistance to other infections. There may be interference with liver function and this is said to be one cause of gynaecomastia (breast development in the male) which is so frequently illustrated in statues and reliefs (see fig. 4.11). Ghaliounghui (1973) raised this as a possible explanation for the portrayed physique of the heretic pharaoh Akhenaten (Amenhotep IV). There is an association between schistosomiasis and bladder cancer, perhaps due to liberation of nitrosamines which are known to be carcinogenic (Hicks, 1983). Schistosomiasis of the rectum can be painful and may explain the high percentage of ancient Egyptian remedies for 'cooling and refreshing' the anus (Majno, personal communication, 1995).

The first archaeological evidence for the existence of schistosomiasis in ancient Egypt was the finding of calcified ova by Ruffer (see above) and more recently confirmed by Millet *et al.* (1980) in Nakht, an unembalmed desiccated mummy of the New Kingdom. A technique which can be widely applied is the demonstration of schistosome circulating anodic antigen (Miller *et al.*, 1993). Deelder *et al.* (1990) reported positive results with extracts from skin and brain of unembalmed bodies from the Predynastic Period and New Kingdom (Nakht, see above). Miller *et al.* (1992) demonstrated the antigen in fifteen of twenty-three mummies from the Ballana Period (AD 350–550).

Two items from ancient Egypt may suggest measures for avoidance of contact with the cercariae. The negative confessions in Chapter 125 of the *Book of the Dead* include: 'I have not waded in the water' (papyrus of Ani; Faulkner, 1972). Secondly, it has been postulated that the penile sheaths (*karnatiw*) shown in some tomb murals were worn to prevent access of the parasite to the urinary tract, in the mistaken belief that access was by the same route as the most obvious symptom (haematuria) became apparent. Penile sheaths occur in other cultures with no such rationale for their use.

It has often been proposed that the Egyptian word *aaa* means haematuria and, in particular, that caused by schistosomiasis. Later in this chapter the difficulties of identification of haematuria in the medical papyri are discussed, and Chapter 3 explains the grounds for believing that *aaa* is unlikely to mean either haematuria or schistosomiasis.

Dracunculiasis (guinea-worm)

Although now eradicated from Egypt, guinea-worm (*Dracunculus medinensis*) infestation was a major health hazard in the past. A calcified male guinea-worm was found in the abdominal wall of a mummy (no. 1770 of the Manchester Museum Mummy Project) dated to approximately 1000 BC (Tapp, 1979).

As in the case of the schistosomes, the guinea-worm has a complex life cycle alternating between two hosts, humans and cyclops (a tiny crustacean). The infection is acquired by swallowing water containing infected cyclops, which then release larval guinea-worms in the intestines of the new host. The larvae wander through the body tissues, where they reach maturity and mating then takes place. The male is only 2 cm in length and dies after impregnating the female. The gravid female worms migrate to the subcutaneous tissue of the human host and attain a length of about a metre. The gravid female then perforates the skin of the ankle, forming an ulcer, before depositing the ova in water when the feet of the host are immersed. The ova hatch into larvae which infect a cyclops, wherein they develop to the infective stage, awaiting ingestion by the next human host.

When the female guinea-worm presents at the skin, it is possible to wind it out of the body on a stick. This is a long, slow and dangerous procedure, provoking a serious reaction if the worm breaks in the process. The mummy referred to above had the right leg amputated above the knee and the left leg below the knee. In view of the presence of the male calcified guinea-worm, it is conceivable that unsuccessful attempts at removal of female guinea-worms may have been the cause of the loss of the legs.

A possible reference to removal of a guinea-worm is found in Ebers 875, the latter part of which is cited in Chapter 8 in relation to surgical instruments:

Instructions for *aat* swelling in any limbs of a man.
a) If you examine the protuberance of the *aat* swellings in any limbs of a man, you must place a bandage on it. You find it goes and comes and *deqer.ti* to/against the flesh which is under it.
b) You shall then say concerning it: [it is] *aq* of *aat* swellings.
c) You should then undertake for it the knife treatment. You should cut open with the *des*-knife, and you should grasp with a *henu*-instrument, grasping what is inside it with the *henu*-instrument. You should cut it out with the *des*-knife. There is inside something which is in it like the *mendjer* of a mouse. Then you should cut it out . . . at its sides, touching the flesh with a *shas*-knife, grasped with a *henuyt*-instrument of carob of any kind (*djaret*). That which is like a head is likewise.

'Going and coming' would be compatible with the appearance of the guinea-worm, although this phrase is quite common in the medical papyri in contexts which have no relation to the appearance of worms. The 'knife treatment' as detailed could describe an attempt to remove a worm, particularly if *mendjer* is interpreted as the intestines of a mouse. The *Grundriss* gives 'internal organ' for *mendjer* and Miller (personal communication, 1994) has suggested 'intestines' which, for a mouse, would look not unlike a female guinea-worm. The untranslated word *aq* (under b) would mean 'enter' were it not for the determinative of lips spitting out fluid. Parant (1982) suggested that *aq* might be a metathesis for *qa(a)* meaning 'to spit out or vomit', for which the determinative would be entirely correct. This interpretation would be consistent with a guinea-worm presenting at an ulcer in the leg and discharging ova. The next problem is the meaning of the word *deqer*. This is a very rare word which seems to have several meanings (Parant, 1982). These include 'to cling' or 'to press', which is the preferred rendering by the *Grundriss* and Ghaliounghui (1987) in this context. However, an alternative meaning is 'to spin' and it has been proposed that, in Ebers 875, it refers to winding out the worm on a piece of wood (Miller, 1989). The verb is in the old perfective form and could be used as a passive.

Filariasis

There are several genera of the order Filarioidea which infect humans, the carrier being the mosquito. Adult worms of some species can block the lymphatics, causing swelling and thickening of the skin (elephantiasis). This could be difficult to detect in a mummy, but might be expected to be shown in some tomb pictures of servants. In fact, there are many representations of enlarged male external genitalia (Weeks, 1970), but the typical swollen legs of elephantiasis are almost never seen. Ghaliounghui (1949) favoured schistosomiasis as the cause of the enlargement of the genitalia. Tapp and Wildsmith (1992) examined skin thought to be scrotum of the Leeds mummy Natsef-Amun and reported filarial worms. The Filaria *Onchocerca volvulus* affects the eyes and is a potent cause of blindness.

Strongyloidiasis

The parasitic worm *Strongyloides* also invades the body through the feet, but then passes through the vascular system to reach the lungs, and ascends the tracheo-bronchial tree to reach the alimentary system via the larynx and the oesophagus. Eggs are laid which pass out with the faeces. These hatch in water and the cycle is continued without an intermediate host. Tapp (1979) found larval forms of Strongyloides worms in the intestinal wall of the mummy Asru (probably Twenty-fifth Dynasty) of the Manchester Museum Mummy Project: the intestines had been removed and placed between the legs, not in a canopic jar.

It is highly unlikely that the ancient Egyptians would have been aware of the existence of Strongyloides worms, and there is no obvious link with any passage in the medical papyri.

Roundworms (*Ascaris lumbricoides*)

This very common intestinal parasite undergoes an internal cycle within the human host, in whom eggs laid in the intestine hatch into larvae which migrate to the lungs, regaining the alimentary tract by the same route as the Strongyloides worm (above). Adult worms are quite large and may be passed with the stools, where they can be conspicuous and distressing. It is likely that this would have been known to the ancient Egyptians, and Ebbell (1937) suggested, on no firm basis, that they were the still unidentified *hefat*-worm (see below). Cockburn and his colleagues (1975) found evidence of Ascaris infection in the mummy PUM II, unwrapped in the United States.

Tapeworms (*Taenia saginata* and *Taenia solium*)

Eggs of tapeworms are ingested in undercooked meat and hatch into long flat intestinal worms, firmly attached by the head which is upstream, but discarding caudal segments which contain the eggs. As with roundworms, the segments would have been noticed in the stools, and Ebbell again suggested, on no firm basis, that they were the unidentified *pened*-worm (see below).

The only firm evidence for tapeworm infestation in ancient Egypt is the finding of eggs of *Taenia* species in the mummy ROM I (Nakht), cited above in relation to schistosomiasis, and examined in Toronto (Hart *et al.*, 1977). Nakht was also infested with Trichinella, most commonly acquired from eating undercooked pork.

Unidentified Egyptian worms

The medical papyri contain unequivocal references to intestinal infestation by para-

phonetics

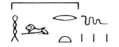

ḥrrwt:
hereret-worms

phonetics

pnd:
pened-worm

phonetics

ḥȝt:
hefat-worm

4.3 Examples of Egyptian words for various types of worms. The determinative (Gardiner sign-list I 14) is also used for snakes.

sitic worms but their identification is fraught with difficulty. The worm determinative is the same as one of those used for snakes (Gardiner sign-list I 14; fig. 4.3) but, fortunately, the context usually makes the distinction clear. *Hereret* and perhaps *djedfet* are general terms for intestinal worms. Ebbell's interpretation of *hereret* as the schistosome parasite (Chapter 3) has not been generally accepted in more recent studies.

There are a number of words carrying the worm determinative, which the *Grundriss* and Westendorf (1992) believe to have only metaphorical meaning in the sense that worms seem to appear by spontaneous generation in certain disease states, an erroneous belief perhaps based on the appearance of maggots in infected wounds. These words include *hesbet* (Ebers 102 = 296), *betju* (Ebers 205), *sa* and *sep* (Ebers 617) and *fenet* (Hearst 196, Berlin 20 and Ramesseum III, B,3). No specific remedies are proposed for these.

Many intestinal parasites, such as roundworms, threadworms and segments of tapeworms, have a very distinctive appearance in the stools, and would surely have been recognised and given specific names. Unfortunately, the papyri do not provide any guide on recognition of the worms, and simply assume that the identification has already been made. Only two Egyptian names appear to relate to specific worms: these are the *hefat*-worm and the *pened*-worm. There are no clear grounds for their identification, and there is currently no confirmation for Ebbell's suggestions of

Table 4.1 Identifiable remedies for specific intestinal parasitic worms

HERBAL REMEDIES		MINERAL REMEDIES	
H P	acacia leaves	H P	salt of Lower Egypt
H	barley	P	natron
P	bread	P	red ochre
H P	carob (*djaret*)	H	malachite
P	conyza (*innek*)	P	desert oil
P	cumin		
H P	cyperus grass		ANIMAL REMEDIES
H P	dates	H P	honey
P	earth almonds (*sheny-ta*)	P	white oil
P	juniper berries	P	ox fat
P	pine oil	P	goose fat
H P	sedge		
H	*kaa* part of sycomore		VEHICLES
H	*kaw* sycomore figs	H P	beer
H	roots of pomegranate	P	milk
H P	wormwood/absinthe	P	wine

The *hefat*-worm (H) features in Ebers 50–61, 64–6, 68, 70–1; Berlin 2–7; Ramesseum III (A,29).
The *pened*-worm (P) features in Ebers 66–7, 69, 72–85.
Egyptian names in parentheses indicate that the meaning is less certain or that alternative meanings have been attributed to the word (see Table 7.5).

roundworm (*Ascaris*) for *hefat* and tapeworm (*Taenia*) for *pened*. Many remedies are listed for each of these worms (Table 4.1). Some ingredients would support the nutrition of the host, while others were believed to kill the worms. Pomegranate and wormwood are known vermifuges. There is considerable overlap of the many ingredients of the remedies recommended for each of the worms. The following are typical of the genre:

> Another [remedy] to drive out the *hefat*-worm: *afa* (probably wild lettuce; see Table 7.5), 1; wormwood/absinthe (*sam*), 1; vegetable mucus (*hesa*), 1; mix as one thing and eat. He will then evacuate (*wesesh*) all worms (*djedfet*) which are in his belly. (Ebers 64)

> Another remedy to kill the *pened*-worm: *khet*-part of the *kesbet*-tree, 5 *ro*; strong beer, 20 *ro*; cooked, strained and drunk immediately. (Ebers 72)

Neither the headings nor the ingredients of the remedies offer any help in identification of the worms.

Malaria

The epidemiology of infection with protozoal parasites of the genus *Plasmodium* strongly suggests that malaria must have existed in pharaonic times when conditions for the mosquito carrier must have been more favourable than today. There would be no gross pathological changes to be found in mummies, and the medical papyri (unlike the Hippocratic corpus) are silent on the characteristic recurrent fever at three- or four-day intervals, which surely could not have escaped notice. Miller *et al.* (1994) applied the *Para*Sight™-F test to a series of naturally desiccated bodies from the Predynastic Period and embalmed mummies of the New Kingdom, Twenty-fifth Dynasty and Nubian Ballana Period (AD 350–550). This test detects antigen produced by *Plasmodium falciparum* (causing tertian fever), and it was found in mummies from all the periods investigated. The authors concluded that this suggests all were suffering from malaria at the time of their deaths.

Bacterial and viral infections

There are great difficulties in the demonstration of bacterial or viral diseases in mummies or skeletons. Furthermore, there are few clues in the medical papyri or in illustrations in tombs. However, advances in the demonstration of bacterial DNA or detection of antigens by new technology may cast more light on the subject in the future.

Tuberculosis (*Mycobacterium tuberculosis*)

Ruffer (1910b) reported tuberculosis of the spine in Nesparehan, a priest of Amun of the Twenty-first Dynasty (fig. 4.4). This shows the typical features of Pott's disease with collapse of a thoracic vertebra, producing an angular kyphosis (hump-back) well seen in the lateral view. An unpleasant but well known complication of Pott's disease is the tuberculous suppuration which had tracked downwards under the sheath of the psoas major muscle (filet steak), towards the right iliac fossa, forming a very large psoas abscess.

Ruffer's case has remained the best authenticated case of spinal tuberculosis from ancient Egypt. All known possible cases, ranging from Predynastic to Twenty-first Dynasty, were reviewed by Morse, Brothwell and Ucko (1964) and later, with additional material, by Buikstra, Baker and Cook (1993). These included nine cases reported by Derry (1938), the Nubian collection of the Royal College of Surgeons of England (see above), and thirteen specimens, mainly Predynastic, collected by Flinders Petrie and Quibell in 1895 from 2000 graves in Naqada. Both groups of reviewers were in agreement that there was very little doubt that tuberculosis was the cause of the pathology in most but not all cases. In some cases it was not possible to

4.4 The best example of spinal tuberculosis (Pott's disease) is in Nesparehan, from the cache of forty-four priests of Amun from the 21st Dynasty. The lateral view shows the acute angulation of the spine (kyphosis) due to collapse of the vertebral body, and the anterior view shows a psoas abscess in the lower part of the right abdomen. This drawing by Mrs Cecil M. Firth is from Ruffer (1910b).

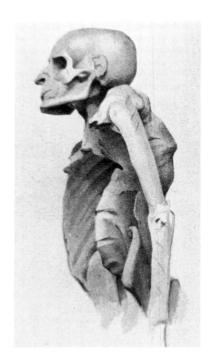
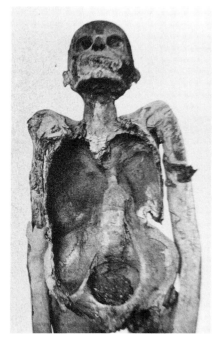

exclude compression fractures, osteomyelitis and bone cysts. Morse's review included a single case of collapsed lung with pleural adhesions, which might have been pulmonary tuberculosis (see also Sandison, 1972).

There are many representations of hump-backed servants in tomb chapels but it is difficult to distinguish between Pott's disease, porter's hump, ankylosing spondylitis (Zorab, 1961) and simply poor posture. The problem of hump-back has been reviewed by Leca (1988) and Miller (1991b). Although there can be no doubt of the existence of tuberculosis in ancient Egypt, nothing in the medical papyri can be directly related to the disease and the bacillus has yet to be demonstrated in a mummy.

Leprosy

Leprosy is a chronic progressive infection due to *Mycobacterium leprae*, now treatable with antibiotics but formerly incurable. It is acquired by close personal contact over a long period, often among members of the same family. Leprosy results in deformity by two entirely different processes. The first is the formation of hard nodules in the skin: without treatment, these enlarge and coalesce, resulting in the characteristic leonine facial appearance. The second process results from loss of sensation due to the involvement of nerves: loss of peripheral sensation ultimately results in loss of fingers and toes.

Møller-Christensen (1967) and Sandison (1980) were unaware of any mummy from the pharaonic period which presented the appearance of nodular leprosy, but it is possible that mummification would have been denied to victims of a disease if it was known to be infectious and requiring isolation from the community during life. However, a Coptic Christian burial at El Bigha in Nubia (sixth century AD) was strongly suggestive of leprosy (Smith and Derry, 1910), although it was not possible to demonstrate the organism.

Evidence for leprosy in the medical papyri is tenuous. Ebbell (1937) translated Khonsu's tumour (*aat net Khonsu*) as tubercular (i.e. nodular) leprosy, and this view was supported by Lefebvre (1956). This is based on the following extracts of Ebers 874:

> Instructions for a tumour of Khonsu (*aat net Khonsu*). If you examine a large tumour of Khonsu in any part of a man and it is terrible and it has made many swellings. Something has appeared in it like that in which there is air. ... Then you shall say concerning it: It is a swelling of Khonsu. You should not do anything against it.

Perhaps a somewhat different type of Khonsu's tumour (*anut*) features in Ebers 877:

> Instructions for an *anut*-tumour of the slaughter of Khonsu. If you examine an *anut*-tumour of the slaughter of Khonsu in any part of a man and you find its head pointed and its base (?) is straight; his two eyes are green (*wadj*) and burning; his flesh is hot under it ... If you find them on his two arms, his pelvis and his thighs, pus [being] in them, you should not do anything against it.

Ebbell considered this to be 'lepra mutilans' and Leca (1988) said it would appear difficult to refute the diagnosis of leprosy. However, much depends on the translation of difficult words which are not well known, and these passages could equally well relate to cancer, bubonic plague or even neurofibromatosis.

Tetanus (*Clostridium tetani*)

Evidence of tetanus could not be expected in human remains. However, Case 7 of the Edwin Smith papyrus gives a graphic description of lock-jaw and distortion of the face, which makes tetanus a very likely diagnosis. This case is considered in Chapter 8.

Plague (*Pasteurella pestis*)

History has been punctuated with catastrophic epidemics of plague caused by the organism *Pasteurella pestis*, normally carried by rats and transferred to humans by the fleas with which the rats are usually infested. Pneumonic plague was rapidly fatal and one would hardly expect evidence in mummies. Bubonic plague was characterised by inflammation and enlargement of lymph glands, draining the area where the rat flea had bitten the human host. Khonsu's tumours, considered above in relation to leprosy and listed in Table 8.1, might possibly refer to the buboes of bubonic plague. However, no mummy has been reported as bearing signs of such an infection, and the medical papyri are otherwise silent on the subject. There is some evidence that bubonic plague did not reach Egypt until after the Moslem conquest (Dols, 1974).

Sepsis and abscesses

We can be reasonably certain that abscesses must have been of common occurrence in ancient Egypt. In the absence of convincing evidence in mummies and representations, we must rely on passages in the medical papyri.

Interposed among the forty-eight cases of trauma in the Edwin Smith papyrus is an account of a *seher* of the breast in a man, as judged by the male possessive pronoun (Case 46, which is the only occasion where this word is used). It is translated as 'abscess' by Breasted, while the *Grundriss* tentatively suggests only 'swelling'. The treatment section says that there is 'heat in the mouth of the wound' and refers to fluid exuding from the head of the *seher*. Gloss A continues thus:

As for 'an abscess (*seher*) with prominent head in his (sic) breast', it means that there is a large swelling due to injury in his breast, soft like a fluid under the hand.

There is no recommendation that an incision be made to drain the contents of the abscess, perhaps because fluid was already exuding.

The Ebers papyrus contains two descriptions of what are probably abscesses, both with recommendations for the knife treatment. The first is (Ebers 869):

Instructions for a swelling of pus (*ryt*). If you examine a swelling of pus in any limb of a man and you find it [with] its head raised and it is enclosed and it is rounded, you shall say concerning it: 'a swelling of pus, an illness which will be treated by me with the knife treatment'. There is something in it like mucus (?). Something comes forth like wax. It [i.e. the swelling] makes a pocket. If anything [remains] in its pocket, it recurs.

The word *ryt* carries the so-called pus determinative (see fig. 3.5) and its meaning seems secure. However, there is no mention of heat, redness and pain (the other cardinal signs of infection), and the possibility of recurrence if anything remains raises the possibility of sebaceous cyst.

The second case (Ebers 871) uses the word *wekhedu* instead of *ryt*; the precise meaning of *wekhedu* has never been resolved, but it must have had meanings other than solely 'pus' (see Chapter 3). Nevertheless, in this instance the context supports the meaning 'pus' more strongly than the previous passage does for *ryt*.

If you examine a swelling of *wekhedu* at the top of both your (sic) arms and you find that it is producing water. It is hard under your fingers and it is firm/unyielding. It is soft but not very. You shall say concerning it: 'A swelling of *wekhedu* at the top of both your arms, an illness which I will treat.' You shall perform for it the knife treatment but beware of the *metu*. Something comes forth from it [like] water of gum/resin. It forms a pocket. You should not allow anything in it [to remain], in order that it may not recur. Treat it like the treatment of a wound in any member/limb of a man. Allow it to close itself. Ease the *metu*. [If] it swells after [the contents] are driven out, it is a characteristic of the sickness which it makes against a man.

This immediately suggests abscesses of the axillary lymph glands (in the armpit), caused by infection ascending the arms. This interpretation is strongly supported by the exhortation to beware of the *metu* when wielding the knife. This probably refers to the axillary artery which lies in perilously close proximity to the axillary lymph glands. However, in view of the diverse meanings of *metu*, it might also refer to the brachial plexus, which surrounds the axillary artery and provides the nerve supply to the arm. The recommendation that the wound be left to close itself is very strong support for an abscess. If it were a sebaceous cyst, there would be no objection to suturing the lips of the wound, whereas this would be very bad practice for an abscess. It is perhaps a rather common scribal error that the reference is to 'your' rather than the usual 'his' two arms.

Case 41 in the Edwin Smith papyrus gives a graphic and unmistakable account of an infected wound and is cited on p. 173. A variety of other swellings, some of uncertain nature, are considered in Chapter 8 in relation to their surgical treatment.

Osteomyelitis

A wide variety of organisms may infect bone, apart from *Mycobacterium tuberculo-*

sis, which is considered above. Sandison (1972) agreed with earlier observations that pyogenic osteomyelitis is surprisingly rare in skeletal remains, and there are many cases of healed compound fracture in which the bone shows no signs of infection.

Poliomyelitis

Roma was a doorkeeper of the Eighteenth or Nineteenth Dynasty and was portrayed on his funerary stela with a grossly wasted and shortened leg accompanied by an equinus deformity of the foot (fig. 4.5). Medical opinion is divided on the diagnosis. Some favour the view that this is poliomyelitis contracted in childhood, before completion of growth of the leg bones. The equinus deformity would then be a

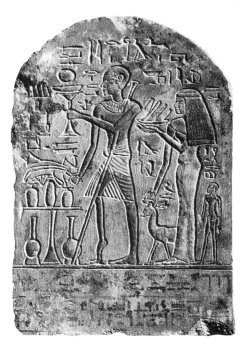

4.5 The grossly wasted and shortened leg belonged to Roma, a doorkeeper of the 18th or 19th Dynasty. The differential diagnosis includes club foot (talipes equinus) and poliomyelitis, considered further in the text. Roma does not appear to be using his staff as a crutch, as in the case of Intef (fig. 4.10). (Carlsberg Glyptotek Museum, Copenhagen, AIN 134)

compensation for walking on the shortened leg. Alternatively, it has often been suggested that this was primarily an equinus variety of club foot (see below), with secondary wasting and shortening of the leg. Much depends on the accuracy with which the artist portrayed the condition. However, on the available evidence, poliomyelitis seems the more likely diagnosis, since club foot does not usually cause such extreme shortening of the leg. It is interesting that Roma appears with a stick which could be used as a crutch, and that his disability had clearly not prevented his attaining high office, marrying and having at least one child. A still more convincing crutch is considered below (see fig. 4.10) in relation to hydrocephalus.

Smallpox (variola)

Ruffer and Ferguson (1911) reported a skin lesion resembling smallpox in a mummy of the Twentieth Dynasty. Sandison (1972, 1980) reviewed the rather tenuous evidence for smallpox in human remains. If the diagnoses are correct, the most distinguished case would be Ramses V, described by Elliot Smith (1912). Nothing in the extant medical papyri can be related to smallpox.

Deformities

We are better informed on deformities in ancient Egypt because of their persistence in mummified and skeletal remains and also representations in tomb chapels and on ostraca. However, the medical papyri say nothing on the subject, presumably because they had no means of treating deformities.

Dwarfism

There is copious evidence for the existence of dwarfs in ancient Egypt, comprehensively reviewed by Dawson (1938), Weeks (1970) and Dasen (1993), who cite skeletal remains of dwarfs ranging from the Predynastic Period to the Twenty-first Dynasty. Egyptian words for dwarf and pygmy are *nem* and *deneg*, the latter dating from the Sixth Dynasty of the Old Kingdom and appearing in the letter of King Pepy II to Harkhuf, the nomarch of Aswan:

> You said that you sent a dwarf (*deneg*) of the god's dances ... Please bring this dwarf with you ... to do the god's dances to gladden the heart of ... the king Neferkara (Pepy II). If he comes with you in the boat, arrange trustworthy people to be around him on the two sides of the boat, who shall guard him lest he falls into the water ... For [my] majesty wishes to see him more than the gifts of Sinai and Punt ... etc.

This extraordinary passage leaves little doubt of the value placed on dwarfs, who were employed as personal attendants, overseers of linen, animal tenders, jewellers and entertainers. Some achieved high rank and received a privileged burial, particularly Seneb who held important priesthoods in addition to being overseer of weaving in the palace (fig. 4.6). A dwarf is shown steering a calcite model boat in the tomb of Tutankhamun in the Cairo Museum (JdE 535).

Dasen listed 207 representations of dwarfs in ancient Egypt. Most representations show achondroplasia, a type of dwarfism in which the head and trunk are normal but the limbs are short. Seneb is a classic example, who shows all the characteristics of the condition in the superb statue found in his tomb in Giza and now in the Cairo Museum (JdE 51281). The preservation of Seneb's dignity is impressive, with the tender embrace of his wife, and two of his three children occupying the space where his lower legs should be. Reliefs on his false door include a further variety of artistic devices to preserve his dignity, though in no way concealing his deformity (see Dasen, 1993). The hieroglyph in 'dwarf' at Harkhuf's tomb also shows achondroplasia.

It is unclear whether the representation of achondroplasia was always factual, or merely an iconographic convention for the display of any dwarf, whether achondroplasiac or not. The pituitary type of dwarf, for example, has normal adult proportions and differs only in overall size. The large collection of illustrations of Dasen shows hardly a single dwarf with normal proportions of limbs. The problem must be set against established conventions in Egyptian two-dimensional art, one of which was that the size of a person denoted his status. Thus husbands were usually shown on a larger scale than their wives, and servants smaller than either. This convention was even observed in the case of Seneb who is shown in reliefs as taller than, or at least no smaller than, his servants (Cairo Museum, JdE 51297; in Dasen, 1993). The problem was therefore how to indicate that someone was a dwarf without reducing his size, which could be misinterpreted as denoting inferior status. The use of achondroplasiac proportions would seem to be a convenient way out of this dilemma. It is particularly effective as the Egyptian canon of proportions of the human figure was so strictly maintained that short limbs were immediately apparent. A similar problem was the portrayal of children. Size denoted their position in the family hierarchy, and childhood was indicated by such devices as the side lock of youth and the finger in the mouth (fig. 4.6).

The medical papyri are totally silent on dwarfism. It is unlikely that dwarfism was regarded as a disease and no treatment would have been of any avail. Dwarfism would probably have been regarded as a divine manifestation, and it is noteworthy that Bes, a very popular benign protector-god (see Chapter 5), showed many of the features of achondroplasia.

4.6 (right) Seneb, a classic example of an achondroplasiac dwarf, with two children replacing the normal position of his legs. This example is from his tomb in Giza, Old Kingdom, 4th or early 5th Dynasty. (Cairo Museum, JdE 51281)

4.7 (far right) The most illustrious known sufferer from club foot was the pharaoh Saptah of the 19th Dynasty, whose mummy is now in the Cairo Museum (CG 61080). (From Smith, 1912)

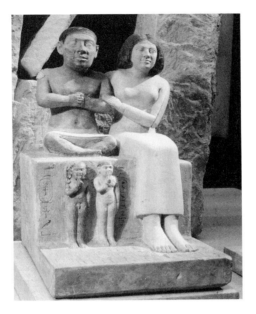

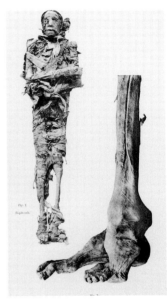

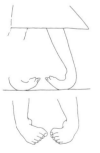

4.8 The top diagram shows a representation of bilaterally deformed feet in the Middle Kingdom tomb of Baqt I in Beni Hassan. Above the subject's head is the word *djeneb* meaning 'crooked'. Below, for comparison, is a modern representation of talipes equino-varus, the commonest form of club foot.

Club foot (talipes)

There was apparently no effective treatment for this condition in ancient Egypt and there is evidence of some gross instances of the condition. The most impressive is the pharaoh Saptah who reigned for six years at the end of the Nineteenth Dynasty (*c.* 1194 BC). However, his mummy shows shortening of the left leg and such a gross deformity of the ankle that the diagnosis is not entirely certain (fig. 4.7). It was originally considered to be club foot (Elliot Smith, 1912) but the possibility of poliomyelitis has also been raised (Forbes, 1993). Other skeletal abnormalities in Saptah's body support this diagnosis. There are several representations of inward-turned feet (Dasen, 1993) which correspond very closely to talipes equino-varus as seen today (fig. 4.8). Like dwarfs, such people seemed to hold responsible positions in the household of the tomb owner.

Hydrocephalus

This condition results from a rise in pressure of cerebrospinal fluid in infants before the skull is fully ossified. The skull enlarges, and this is in striking contrast to the facial bones which remain normal. Derry (1912–13) described such a case in a skeleton of a man estimated to be at least thirty years of age, found in a cemetery of Roman date at Shurafa. The facial bones are not enlarged but the circumference of the skull is 66 cm, compared with a normal value of about 55 cm (fig. 4.9). The long bones show

4.9 Hydrocephalus in a skull of the Roman Period from Shurafa (Petrie and MacKay, 1915). Note the enlargement of the cranial vault contrasting with the normal size of the facial bones. See fig. 4.10 for use of a staff as a crutch, exactly as Derry (1912–13) suggested from an examination of the skeleton belonging to this skull. (Natural History Museum, London)

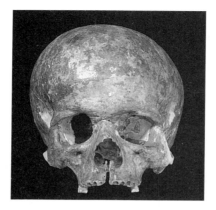
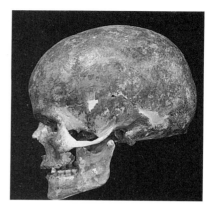

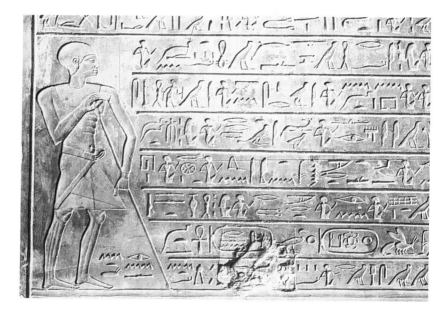

4.10 The stela of Intef (12th Dynasty) showing his use of a staff as a crutch, exactly as suggested by Derry (1912–13) from an examination of the skeleton belonging to the skull shown in fig. 4.9. (British Museum, EA 562).

evidence of a left-sided weakness and over-development of the right arm, perhaps from use of a long staff as a crutch. On the basis of excessive size of the bony ridges for insertion of certain muscles, Derry proposed the use of a crutch as follows:

> ... it is suggested that this man supported himself by the use of a long staff placed across the body so as to reach the ground on the left side, and grasped high up by the right hand, the left perhaps giving slight assistance. In this manner he could support his body momentarily while bringing the right foot forward.

The stela of Intef (Twelfth Dynasty; BM 562) shows the use of a staff exactly as Derry proposed (fig. 4.10), with some signs of malfunction of the left leg. The staff is similar to that of Roma (see fig. 4.5) but, in the case of Intef, it is being used as a crutch, whereas Roma has rested his staff against his shoulder to use his hands for other purposes.

Cancer and other tumours

The incidence of cancer increases with age, and it is therefore less common in populations with low expectations of life, as must have been the case in ancient Egypt. Furthermore, carcinogens produced by human activity would be far less before the beginning of industrialisation. Nevertheless, untreated cancer often produces large tumours before death, and it is therefore surprising that cancers are very rare, as in many ancient populations, in both mummies and skeletal remains. The latter are very informative in this respect because they can show either tumours arising from the bone itself (either primary or secondary), or else destruction of bone from a tumour growing nearby and destroying the bone by pressure.

Surprisingly, no bony tumours were reported in the skeletons examined by Elliot Smith and Wood Jones at Aswan before the building of the first Aswan dam (see above). Indeed, Elliot Smith and Dawson (1924) were unable to report from their extensive experience any true case of cancer from the pharaonic period. More recently there are a very few isolated reports of tumours reviewed by Ghaliounghui in a symposium on palaeo-oncology edited by Retsas (1986). Hussein (1949–50) found the usual skeletal reaction to meningiomata (benign tumours arising from the membrane covering the brain) in two skulls of the Twentieth and Twenty-first Dynasties. Rowling (1961a, b) and Sandison (1980), among others, reported an osteochondroma in a femur of the Fifth Dynasty found in Giza. Leca (1988) showed the same lesion in his much clearer figure 55. Wells (1963) attributed multiple erosions of a skull from the Old Kingdom to carcinoma of the naso-pharynx with widely scattered secondaries. There were twenty-six lesions in all. The cystadenoma of the ovary in the Granville mummy (Irty-senu) in the British Museum, originally thought to have been malignant, is now believed to have been benign (Harer and Taylor, in preparation). These few examples illustrate what Ghaliounghui called a meagre harvest.

Evidence of cancer in the medical papyri is very uncertain. Khonsu's tumours were considered above in relation to leprosy, and there is the following passage from Ebers 813:

> Another [remedy] for one in whom there is eating (*wenemet*) of the uterus (*hemet*), and ulcers appear in her vulva. Fresh dates, 1; *hekenu*, 1; stone from the shore, broken with water, left overnight in the dew and poured into her vagina.

Ebbell (1937) suggested that the well attested word for 'eating' here means cancer, but the *Grundriss* and Ghaliounghui (1987) remained more cautious. Nevertheless, one could hardly deny that 'eating' is a very graphic description of advanced malignancy. Kahun 2 has also been thought to indicate cancer of the uterus:

> Instructions for a woman suffering in her uterus by wandering (sic). You shall say concerning it: What is the smell? If she says to you: I smell roast meat, then you shall say concerning it: it is the *nemsu*-disorder of the uterus. You shall then do for it: her fumigation over everything which she smells as roast meat.

The diagnosis here hinges on the smell of roast meat and is tenuous in the extreme. The word *nemsu* does not appear elsewhere in the medical papyri.

Nutritional, endocrine and metabolic disorders

Obesity

Obesity is difficult to detect after the processes of mummification; the most important evidence is in statues, stelae, reliefs and paintings. However, the problems of interpretation are considerable and were reviewed by Weeks (1970). As with dwarfism (above) the major problem is distinguishing between accurate portrayal and stylistic convention. Thus, pharaohs are not usually shown in a state of obesity, but generally as young men with a physique corresponding to the classical canon of proportions. Many tomb owners, on the other hand, are shown displaying rolls of fat and often

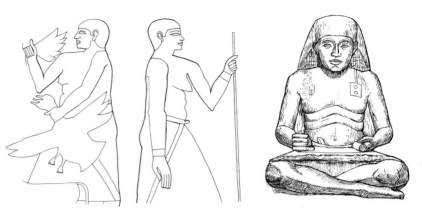

4.11 Formal representations of obesity in the case of important men. In the centre is a relief of Ankh-ma-hor in his 6th Dynasty tomb at Saqqara (see p. 126). His obesity has features of frank gynaecomastia. On the left is Hepi, an offering bearer in the same tomb. On the right is the statue (Cairo Museum, JdE 44861) of the legendary healer Amenhotep-son-of-Hapu (see fig. 6.3).

pendulous breasts which raise the question of gynaecomastia (enlargement of the male breasts) (fig. 4.11). Weeks contrasts this with a different pattern of obesity in representations of servants and labourers. The latter tend to show relatively normal limbs and a paunchy belly, sometimes embellished with an umbilical hernia. Weeks draws the parallel of the modern 'beer-belly', perhaps related to hard work and an unbalanced diet. It seems quite likely that there was a well established convention for displaying an important and prosperous man, in maturity, as one who had enjoyed the best available food over many years, without the necessity to undertake un-welcome exertion. Harpists are often shown with a third and distinctive pattern of obesity (see fig. 9.3). Wives of tomb owners are usually portrayed tall, slender and beautiful, in stark contrast to some of their mummies. Some women have more plausible figures in husband and wife statues but frank obesity is quite unusual.

Liver disease simulating obesity

Certain aspects of obesity may be simulated by an effusion of fluid into the abdominal cavity (ascites), resulting from obstruction of the blood draining the alimentary tract as it passes through the liver. This may occur in schistosomiasis. Walter Loebl (personal communication, 1995) has drawn attention to the stela of Bak, Akhenaten's chief sculptor (fig. 4.12). He points out that the pattern of obesity is not that seen conventionally in tombs but is typical of Symmers' fibrosis, caused by chronic hepato-splenic schistosomiasis. This results in obstruction of the portal venous system in the liver causing portal hypertension, and thereby effusion of fluid into the peritoneal cavity (ascites). This causes distension of the abdomen, with disappearance of the umbilicus, which is highly unusual in Egyptian art. The statue of Bak shows no umbilicus (possibly due to clothing) and no rolls of fat, but he has swollen ankles, all features contrary to normal Egyptian representation of obesity. He also shows gynaecomastia, which is a known complication of liver disease secondary to schistosomiasis. Loebl's diagnosis depends, of course, on Bak's portrayal being naturalistic and accurate but, because the stela dates from the highly unconventional Amarna Period, this is uncertain.

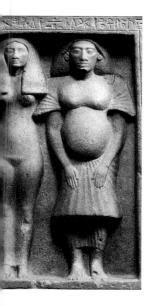

A second diagnostic problem is the Queen of Punt, shown in relief in Hatshepsut's temple at Deir el-Bahri (fig. 4.13). Suggestions have included Dercum's disease, steatopygy, elephantiasis, achondroplasia and pseudo-hypertrophic progressive muscular dystrophy (Weeks, 1970).

Malnutrition

It is difficult to diagnose malnutrition in the bodily remains of ancient Egyptians, but gross malnutrition must have occurred in famine years when the Nile failed to rise (see fig. 1.6). Bones give some indication, partly through Harris' lines which indicate arrested growth, and partly through osteoporosis (Armelagos and Mills, 1993). Studies of isotopic ratios in bone, skin and hair can indicate major dietary components, and thus predict deficiencies which are to be expected (White, 1991). Dietary toxins include lead (Harer, 1993).

Akhenaten

The ultimate diagnostic problem is Akhenaten, the heretic monotheistic pharaoh of the Eighteenth Dynasty who began his reign as Amenhotep IV but changed his name after rejecting the worship of Amun and other gods, substituting the Aten (the solar disc). During his reign as Akhenaten (the Amarna Period), the traditional canon of proportions for the royal family was totally changed. In the middle of his reign,

4.12 (above) Stela of Bak, Akhenaten's chief sculptor (18th Dynasty), a possible case of Symmers' fibrosis of the liver or perhaps simply an example of the artistic trends of the Amarna Period. (Ägyptisches Museum, Papyrussammlung, Berlin, 1/63, photo M. Büsing)

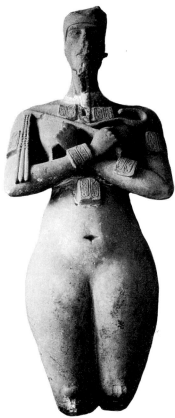

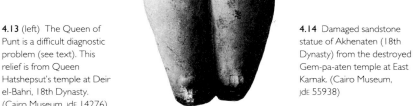

4.13 (left) The Queen of Punt is a difficult diagnostic problem (see text). This relief is from Queen Hatshepsut's temple at Deir el-Bahri, 18th Dynasty. (Cairo Museum, JdE 14276)

4.14 Damaged sandstone statue of Akhenaten (18th Dynasty) from the destroyed Gem-pa-aten temple at East Karnak. (Cairo Museum, JdE 55938)

Akhenaten is represented as tall and languid, with a massive lower jaw, well developed breasts and feminine hips, but spindly lower legs (fig. 4.14). His abdomen is full but his umbilicus is preserved. He was married to the beautiful Nefertiti and was often shown with six daughters, one of whom married Tutankhamun. The fundamental question is whether Akhenaten really looked like this, or whether he chose his gynaecoid portrayal for other reasons, perhaps to indicate his role as the mother of his people. Nefertiti is usually portrayed in the same style as Akhenaten in reliefs of the Amarna Period.

On the basis of the Amarna portrayals, Elliot Smith proposed the diagnosis of Frölich's syndrome (dystrophia adiposo-genitalis), now known to include a variety of different entities. I am indebted to Dr Charles Edmonds, the endocrinologist, for his opinion that the likeliest diagnosis from the artistic representations is Klinefelter's syndrome. This is a congenital chromosomal abnormality with doubling of the female x strand normally present in the male XY chromosome, which then becomes XXY (the normal configurations are XY for male and XX for female). There is often mild obesity but the subjects are usually quite tall with long legs. Muscularity tends to be underdeveloped, with small testes and gynaecomastia. Although sexual drive may be normal, infertility is the rule. Akhenaten's six daughters, if they are his own, are hardly compatible with this or indeed any likely diagnosis of endocrine dysfunction, other than simple adolescent gynaecomastia.

All might be resolved if Akhenaten's mummy were available for examination. Unfortunately, there are major problems of identification which may never be resolved. Tomb 55 in the Valley of the Kings (KV 55) was opened in 1907, but with less than adequate recording (Aldred, 1988). Inside was a golden shrine dedicated to Akhenaten's mother, Queen Tiye, and a damaged coffin now thought to have been made for Kiya, the 'wife and great beloved' of Akhenaten (but not his principal queen). This contained the remains of a body, originally thought to be Queen Tiye although, according to Elliot Smith (1912), the coffin and gold bands encircling the mummy bore the name of Akhenaten. Elliot Smith (1912) and Reeves (1990) believed the evidence to favour Akhenaten, whereas Harrison (1966), Aldred (1988) and Allen (1994) favoured Smenkh-ka-ra, a pharaoh who appeared to reign for at most a year after Akhenaten but whose male identity is now debated.

Elliot Smith (1912) undertook the first autopsy, when the gold bands were unfortunately stolen and never recovered. A much more detailed examination was undertaken by Harrison (1966), who found a complete disarticulated skeleton lacking only the manubrium sterni. He concluded that the remains were undoubtedly those of a male, 1.7 m (5 ft 7 in) in height, and less than twenty-five years of age, an estimate hardly compatible with Akhenaten's reign of sixteen years. He found no evidence of hydrocephalus (reported by Elliot Smith) and 'no possible resemblance to Akhenaten as depicted in his monuments'. Skeletal measurements were, however, very close to those of Tutankhamun. Furthermore, both Tutankhamun and the body in question were blood group A_2, with the serum antigen MN, all suggesting close consanguinity. It is proposed, therefore, that Akhenaten might have been the father of Tutankhamun and even the mysterious Smenkh-ka-ra.

It is not entirely certain that the bones examined by Elliot Smith and Harrison were indeed those found in Tomb 55. At the time of excavation, the remains were pronounced by two medical men, one an unknown but 'prominent American obstetrician', to be those of a woman. Even if they are the same remains, there can be no certainty that they are those of Akhenaten. However, if they are Akhenaten's remains, there can be no justification for making a diagnosis based on the king's portraiture alone.

Diseases of internal organs

The cardio-vascular system

Although the heart was left in the body during mummification, it would be difficult to find evidence of cardiac pathology. However, atherosclerosis and calcification of large arteries have often been found, and are well shown in figures 17 and 23 of Isherwood, Jarvis and Fawcitt (1979). There is little to be learned about cardio-vascular disease in statues, reliefs and paintings, and the main sources of information are in the medical papyri, which are difficult to interpret in terms of modern concepts of cardiology.

In Chapter 3 it was explained that the ancient Egyptians had no understanding of the circulation of the blood, although it was known that the heart 'spoke' through the peripheral vessels (*metu*), which we can interpret as feeling the pulse (Ebers 854a, cited at the beginning of Chapter 6). It was explained in Chapter 3 that the original word for heart was *ib*, later supplemented by *haty* which had a far more precise anatomical meaning. Westendorf (1992) pointed out how the later term often replaced the earlier term in glosses, as for example in Ebers 855e:

> As to: 'the heart (*ib*) weakens', it means the heart (*haty*) does not speak, or it means the vessels of the heart (*haty*) are dumb.

Paragraph 855 of the Ebers papyrus is largely composed of a series of glosses explaining terms used to describe pathological states of the heart (Table 4.2). In most cases we have lost the original material to which the glosses refer, although there are glosses that appear to explain the underlined passages in the following difficult paragraph 154 of the Berlin papyrus. It is likely that glosses would have been welcomed, even in the New Kingdom!

> Another [remedy for] a nest of wandering of heat. His abdomen is heavy laden: his stomach (*r-ib*) is diseased: his heart (*ib*) is <u>hot</u> (*tau*) <u>and stinging</u> (*khensu*): his clothes are a burden to him: he cannot endure many clothes: his heart (*ibb*)* is <u>shrouded in darkness</u> (*wekh*): his heart (*haty*) is <u>powerless</u> (*depet*) and <u>flooded</u> (*igep*), like a man who has eaten the *kau*-fruit of sycomore.

> * The word for heart (*ibb*), as written here, means 'thirst', but is presumed to be a homophone for heart (*ib*), as reconstructed from the gloss.

The glosses for *wekh*, *depet* (Ebers 855w) and *igep* (Ebers 855t) are shown in Table 4.2. The rather unhelpful glosses for *tau* and *khensu* appear in Ebers 855s, where the affected organ is written as mouth (*r*), but this is clearly a scribal error for *ib* (as in Berlin 154):

> As to: 'the mouth (*r*) is hot (*tau*) and stinging (*khensu*)'; as to: 'the heart (*ib*) stings', it means spreading of heat over his heart (*haty*). It means that the heart (*ib*) is hot because of heat like a man whom torture is stinging.

The glosses in Group I of Table 4.2 appear to relate to the failing heart. The word *wegeg* is well attested to mean 'weakness' or 'feebleness'. Ebers 855f explains that *fet*, meaning 'disgust' in its non-medical context, is here a synonym for *wegeg* (weakness). *Wered* is well known to mean weary and it is reasonable to believe that kneeling must have a similar interpretation. The word *amed* is not known outside the medical papyri but the explanation eloquently describes a state of gross cardiac failure with absent pulses (see above). In two cases the condition is ascribed to *wekhedu* and this is a most cogent reason for believing that the meaning of *wekhedu* can extend beyond 'purulence'.

Table 4.2 The cardiac glosses of the Ebers papyrus

PARA.	TERM	MEANING	'THE EXPLANATION'
Group I – the failing heart			
855m	*wegeg n wiauyt*	weakness of old age	there is *wekhedu* on his heart*
855f	*fet*	turn aside	weakness (*wegeg*) of the heart*
855x	*wered*	weary	as through travelling far
855k	*maset*	kneeling	heart* constricted, small and heated
855l₂	*mas*	kneeling	it is weak (*iar*) because of *wekhedu*
855e	*amed*	? weakness	heart* does not speak; *metu* are dumb
855c	*shes*	? weakness	caused by the *met* called receiver
855d	*ad*	decay/debility*	it is a *khasef* (meaning unclear)
Group II – possible congestive heart failure			
855t	*igep*	flooded	the heart is covered up
855b	*bah*	flooded	a liquid of the mouth
855z	*meh*	drowned	heart is forgetful
855v	*sewesh*	? compression*	filling of heart* with blood
Group III – displacement or enlargement of the heart			
855p	*her set.f*	in its place*	mass of heart* on his left side
855o	*deher*	bitter	heart sinking below its place
855n	*rut*	dancing*	heart moves away from left breast
855q	*nepa*	? fluttering*	movement of the heart downwards
Group IV – miscellaneous			
855g	*sesh*	spreads itself out	*metu* of the heart* holding faeces
855l	*wesher*	drying up	? blood coagulates in the heart*
855u	*aq*	perish	caused by breath of lector priest
855u	*meht*	forgetful	caused by breath of lector priest
855x	*djednu*	hot	weariness through travelling far
855w	*wekh*	shrouded in darkness	narrow
855w	*depet*	? powerless	dark because of anger
855y	*neba*	unclear	something entering from outside

Columns 2 and 3 refer to the phrase 'as to xxx of the heart'. Column 4 gives the 'explanation'.

*Heart is written *haty*, otherwise *ib*.

Group II evokes the picture of congestive cardiac failure in which the pressure of the blood entering the heart is raised beyond the pumping capacity of the heart. The ancient Egyptians could hardly have known that the heart was dilated with blood in congestive cardiac failure, but they might well have observed the distended veins and the accumulation of fluid in the legs and abdomen. The clinical picture certainly suggests 'flooding'. Ebers 855b speaks of a liquid in the mouth, which raises the possibilities of pulmonary oedema with exudation of fluid into the lungs as a result of left ventricular failure. In extreme cases this may present as froth in the mouth.

Group III starts with a clear statement that the heart 'in its place' is on the left side. They were presumably speaking of the apex beat which is normally some 10 cm to the left of the midline, although the bulk of the heart is only slightly to the left of the midline. It would be pleasing to believe that 'dancing' of the heart referred to an abnormal rhythm, but the explanation does not support this interpretation.

Group IV comprises a miscellaneous group of terms, some of which have well established meanings in a non-medical context. Perhaps the main interest of this group is the attribution of 'perishing of the heart' to the breath of the lector priest (see Chapter 5). The unfamiliar condition of *neba* is attributed to 'something entering from outside'. This probably refers to 'disease-demons' (see Chapter 5) but the question of infection is considered in Chapter 3.

There is a possible reference to ischaemic heart disease in Ebers 191 (= 194), in spite of this being within the *Book of the Stomach*. However, there are many examples of confusion between heart (*ib*) and stomach (*r-ib*) in the medical papyri.

> If you examine a man because of suffering in his stomach, and he suffers in his arm, his breast and the side of his stomach. One says concerning him/it: It is the *wadj*-disease. Then you shall say concerning it: Something has entered his mouth. Death is approaching.

In both angina and myocardial infarction, pain is concentrated in the left of the chest and may radiate down the left arm. Unfortunately, this passage does not specify which side, but the suggestion of coronary ischaemia is supported by the bad prognosis. *Wadj* has a pustule determinative and, as such, it does not appear elsewhere and its meaning is unknown. Without the pustule determinative, *wadj* can mean green, which could conceivably be an exaggerated reference to the colour of someone in cardiogenic shock. Something entering the mouth usually refers to a disease-demon (Chapter 5).

Ebers 207, although also within the *Book of the Stomach* and cited below, makes overt reference to the heart in relation to what appears to be food poisoning. The heart makes noises and 'thumps', for which the onomatopoeic Egyptian word is *deb-deb*, not so far from the 'lub-dup' used today to describe the normal heart sounds as heard through a stethoscope.

There are a number of remedies in the Chester Beatty and Ebers papyri for treating the heart, although with virtually no information on the pathology being treated. Chester Beatty (VI, 16–41) contains many recipes to 'cool or refresh (*seqebeb*) the heart (*haty*)' or to 'drive out heat'. These remedies are often indicated to have a similar effect on the anus. Remedies 'for the heart' in the Ebers papyrus are for an unspecified problem, for the relief of heat or to drive out *aaa*. None of these sheds light on disease processes in the present state of our knowledge.

The lungs

The lungs were often removed and placed in canopic jars, a process which was seldom favourable for pathological studies. However, Tapp (1979) obtained clear identification of lung tissue and was able to demonstrate sand pneumoconiosis. This still occurs in those living in the Sahara and Negev deserts, and is caused by the inhalation of blown sand. It is not unlike the silicosis of coal miners and stone workers, and could well have proceeded to pulmonary fibrosis. There is one possible case of pulmonary tuberculosis in a mummy (see above). Rowling (1961b) cited three cases of pneumonia, probably lobar.

In the papyri the key words are *seryt* (cough) and *wefa* and *sema* (lungs). Ebers 305 announces the 'Beginning of the remedies to drive out cough'. There follow twenty paragraphs simply headed 'another', which must be presumed to serve the same purpose. Ebers 321 does, in fact, say 'Another, an instant drink to drive out cough from/in the belly'. Further remedies for cough occur in Berlin 29–38, some of which are parallel to passages from the Ebers, cited above. Antitussives are considered in Chapter 7. Ebers 21 is a remedy very similar to many in Ebers 305–25 and is headed simply 'another to treat the lung'.

There is an interesting account of what appears to be a productive cough in Ebers 190:

> If you examine a man with a lifting (*fayt*, ? productive; lit. 'bearing') cough (*seryt*), and his disease is under his flanks, like lumps of faeces, it is liftings (*setjesu*) from his two flanks, and his stomach is constricted. Then you should prepare for him strong remedies for drinking: fresh (kind of) bread, cooked in oil and honey, wormwood/absinthe, 1/32; resin of the umbrella pine from Byblos, 1/16; ? valerian (*shasha*); add it together and cook as one thing. To be drunk on four days. If you examine him afterwards and you find him with his illness of the first time (i.e. as it was before), then he will get well.

This account would conform with unpleasant suppuration in the lungs such as might result from bronchiectasis, a saccular dilatation of the bronchial tree with sepsis in the pockets so formed. Alternatively, the *Grundriss* raised the possibility of this referring to faecal vomiting in advanced obstruction of the colon.

Ebers 192 probably relates to an upper respiratory tract infection with a streaming cold.

> If you examine a man suffering from his stomach and he is vomiting (*qas*) much: if you find it [as] catarrh (*khenet*) in front of him, his two eyes are blood-shot (*shesem*) and his nose is running (*takheb*), then you should say concerning it/him: it is a product of putrefaction of his mucus . . .

The section actually refers to the stomach (*r-ib*) and vomiting (*qas*), but the distinction between lung and stomach was often unclear and it is not impossible that the word for 'vomit' might also mean to 'bring up by coughing'. The *Grundriss* supports the meaning 'catarrh' for *khenet*, which is elsewhere related directly to the nose (see under 'Nose' below). The word *takheb* probably relates to the more common *tekheb* meaning 'bloated' or 'discharging fluid'.

The gastro-intestinal tract

The Book of the Stomach. Chapter 3 considered the reasons for believing that the Egyptian word for the stomach was *r-ib*, and this occurs in the titles of all paragraphs except four in the *Book of the Stomach* (Ebers 188–208). If fact, this book raises so many questions that the reader is forced back to question the real meaning of *r-ib*, as will be apparent below.

Eleven paragraphs have 'obstruction' (*shena*) in the title which takes various forms, the meaning being clear in the following examples:

> If you examine a man suffering from an obstruction in his stomach and you find it going and coming under your fingers like oil inside a skin . . . (Ebers 199)

> If you examine a man with obstruction of the stomach: he vomits and is very sick . . . (Ebers 202)

> If you examine a man with obstruction of his stomach: it is irksome for him to eat bread (i.e. food in general). His belly is constricted (Ebers 188)

The first example suggests vigorous peristaltic contraction in an attempt to overcome an obstruction, although admittedly more often seen as visible peristalsis than felt with the fingers. However, pyloric stenosis (obstruction of the outflow of the stomach) can be felt in infants to go and come under the fingers. The next two paragraphs suggest many possible diagnoses, including an obstruction at the lower end of the oesophagus, carcinoma of the stomach and pyloric stenosis secondary to peptic ulceration, to mention a few possibilities from modern practice. It is also unlikely that they could have distinguished obstruction in the stomach from obstruction lower down the alimentary tract, which also ultimately causes vomiting. Indeed, Ebers 202 continues:

> He suffers from it like *sekhet*-illness. You shall then say concerning it: It is a seizing up of faeces which is not yet 'knotted ?' . . . it is seizing up and making a clump.

This raises the possibility of faecal impaction, and Herodotus said that the Egyptians were obsessed with their bowels. Ebers 203 contains the phrase:

> You should then make for him a powerful remedy of oil in order that 'it comes down'.

Surprisingly, all remedies in this section are to be taken by mouth and they do not suggest enemas which lay well within their technical capabilities.

The start of Ebers 188, cited above, continues along lines which suggest that they thought the problem was not primarily in the stomach at all:

> You should examine him lying down. You find his belly is hot and [there is] obstruction in his stomach. You shall then say concerning it/him: It is a case involving the liver (*miset*). . . . <then follows a remedy to 'purge his belly'> . . . If after doing this, you find the two halves of his belly – the right side hot, the left side cold. Then you shall say concerning it/him: It is an illness that restricts his eating. Then you repeat your seeing him, and you find his belly is entirely cool. They you shall say: It is his liver which has been purged. He has received the treatment.

Ebers 207 may perhaps refer to some form of food poisoning:

> If you examine a man with an obstruction.
>
> a) His heart (literally, perhaps stomach was meant) makes noises. His face is pale and his heart makes thumps (*deb-deb*). If you examine him and find his heart is hot and his belly is prominent, it means it is a deep-seated swelling. He has eaten roast meat.
>
> b) You should then make something for washing out the roast meat, and for purging his intestine by a drink. Sweet beer left overnight with notched sycomore figs which have dried. Eat and drink for 4 days.
>
> c) You should rise early on account of it every day to see what has gone down from his anus. If it has gone down, *naadjet*, like black lumps, you shall say concerning it/him: It is this roast meat which has gone down to his stomach. His belly is in a bad state, blistered.
>
> d) If you examine him after doing this and something goes down from his anus like porridge of beans . . .

Although there are some difficult phrases and words, the overall picture seems fairly clear and this is surely the earliest record (1500 BC) of directions for the physician to examine the patient's stools.

Apart from the last instance, the cases with obstruction do not usually give the possibility of making a clear diagnosis, and the remedies offer few useful clues. We can do little more than guess what might have been the diagnoses. Nevertheless there is a clear picture of the practitioner trying his best to cure his patient, handicapped by a very limited understanding of anatomy, physiology and pathology.

The cases without obstruction are hardly any easier to diagnose:

> If you examine a man who suffers from his stomach. All his limbs are heavy [because of] the approach of weariness. You should then place your hand on his stomach. You find his stomach dragging. It goes and comes under your fingers. Then you shall say concerning him: this is a weariness of eating. It does not allow him to eat what is in front [of him]. You shall make for him his purge (totally): flour of dates, mashed in stale beer. Eating his bread (food) returns. ... (Ebers 189)

Perhaps this should be taken at face value to indicate general loss of appetite with a wonderful cure wrought by date flour.

In four cases in the stomach book, the trouble does not seem to lie primarily in the stomach at all. The case involving the liver (Ebers 188) is outlined above. Ebers 190 and 192 appear to relate to the respiratory system and were considered in that section. Ebers 191 (= 194) may well be ischaemic heart disease (see above).

In addition to Ebers 188, there is a small section of the Ebers papyrus (477–81) of 'remedies to treat the liver (*miset*)' but with no indication of diagnosis. Gallstones were extremely rare: Elliot Smith and Dawson (1924) reported only a single case in 30,000 bodies.

The large bowel, rectum and anus. We are on firmer ground further down the gastro-intestinal tract. There is no specific Egyptian word for constipation other than *shena*, which means obstruction, and its use is mainly confined to the upper gastro-intestinal tract (see above). Nevertheless, the *swnw* was clearly very familiar with constipation, as shown by the many remedies to clear the bowels (see Chapter 7). The phrase 'to open/purge the belly (*pekha khet*)' is not open to doubt and a typical remedy for this purpose is included in Ebers 7 (= Hearst 58):

> Remedy to open/purge the belly: Milk, 1/16 + 1/64 (25 ro); notched sycomore fig, 1/4; honey 1/4; boiled, strained and drunk on four days.

Other introductory phrases for aperients are:

> to drive out faeces (*hes*)
> to evacuate (*fegen*), with an explicit ideogram of defecation
> to void (*wesesh*)

The word *wesesh* (void or evacuate) often means 'to pass urine' (see below). However, there are many contexts where it must refer to the bowels, such as Ebers 64 which is quoted above in relation to elimination of the presumably intestinal *hefat*-worm. As is usually the case, *wesesh* here carries the determinative of a discharging phallus, which certainly suggests micturition. However, this determinative, especially when not discharging, has many possible meanings, and has misled people in the past.

It is hard to believe that ancient Egyptian healers were not often confronted with the problem of diarrhoea, but it is difficult to find an Egyptian word which covers the condition. Ebers 44–8 give remedies to stop evacuation (*wesesh*). Lefebvre (1956) interpreted this as 'to put an end to unduly frequent micturition' but the *Grundriss* left open the options with the interpretation 'remedy to stop elimination'. Ebers 251 describes the uses of the castor-oil plant (Chapter 7) and mentions its use for the *wehi*-disease, which could be constipation although the *Grundriss* has suggested the equally possible diarrhoea. Unfortunately, the word does not appear elsewhere.

The anus received detailed attention in ancient Egyptian medicine, especially in Ebers 138–64 and Chester Beatty VI. There are many remedies to 'cool or refresh (*seqebeb*) the anus (*pehuyt*)' and to 'drive out heat (*tau*)'. None of these words is open to misinterpretation, and they suggest an infection. The possibility of schistoso-miasis is considered above.

Ebers 161 specifically refers to the vessels (*metu*) of the anus and Ebbell's sugges-tion of haemorrhoids would seem definite, were it not for the many alternative mean-ings of *metu* (p. 44). The treatment in Ebers 161 is 'ox-fat, 1/64; acacia leaves, 1/64; bandaged thereon', which seems plausible for haemorrhoids. Chester Beatty VI, 6 refers to 'blood found running out behind him' among a series of remedies for the anus. Ebers 145 refers to a *wenekh* of the anus. The word *wenekh* is formally defined in Gloss A of Case 31 in the Edwin Smith papyrus (p. 59) where there can be little doubt that it means dislocation in relation to joint injuries. In the present context, the *Grundriss*, Ghaliounghui (1987) and Ebbell (1937) concur that prolapse is the likely meaning. Chester Beatty VI, 9 is headed 'a remedy to drive out a turning-back (*an*) of the anus' and the *Grundriss* proposed the special meaning of prolapse for *an* in this context. The remedy includes salt, oil and honey applied to the anus for four days. Other afflictions of the anus include swelling and ulceration (Chester Beatty VI, 2).

The urinary tract

The urinary tract has a special section of the Ebers papyrus (261–83) with isolated paragraphs elsewhere in the Ebers, and also in the Berlin and Hearst papyri. There are several parallels between the Ebers and Hearst papyri (see Table 7.8).

Many paragraphs use Egyptian words such as *wesesh*, *wekha* and *khaa*, which have the general meaning 'evacuation or voiding of waste products', and only in an appro-priate context is it possible to distinguish between defecation and micturition. This confusion is particularly unfortunate in the possible references to blood in the urine. Haematuria is such an important symptom in a country where schistosomiasis (see above) is endemic that it would be valuable to have a reference which unequivocally indicated that the Egyptians recognised this important symptom. The only possible references to haematuria are Ebers 49 (= Hearst 18) and Berlin 165 and 187. Ebers 49 commences with the words 'Another [remedy] for driving out the voiding (*wesesh*) of much blood'. Hearst 18 is similar but omits '*wesesh*'. The headings of Berlin 165 and 187 are essentially similar to Ebers 49 but the phonetic part of *wesesh* is lost in a lacuna in Berlin 187. All use the word *wesesh* without mention of urine, and it is not possible to exclude the possibility that they refer to the passage of blood with the stools as, for example, is very commonly caused by haemorrhoids. No text combines the unequivocal words urine and blood.

However, there can be no doubt that micturition is intended when the word for urine (*meuyt*) appears as, for example, in Ebers 262:

Another [remedy] to cause a child to void (*wesesh*) an accumulation of urine (*meuyt*) in his belly: an old book, boiled in oil; his belly is anointed [with it] to regulate (*maa*) his voiding (*weseshet*).

Ebers 274–5 and 277–80 are remedies 'to eliminate urine which is too plentiful (or too often)'. Unfortunately, the crucial word *asha* can mean both 'plentiful' and 'often', and it is unclear whether the condition described was polyuria (increased volume of urine) or increased frequency of micturition, very often due to cystitis. The latter condition is much more common and therefore the more likely interpretation. Rather similar is the remedy in Ebers 276 (= 281) which is 'to eliminate hurrying (*as*) of urine', which strongly suggests urgency of micturition, due to cystitis or an irri-table bladder. However, Ebers 264 refers to 'correcting (*aqa*) urine of excess (*haw*)' which sounds more like polyuria, perhaps due to diabetes. No less than nine reme-dies are 'to put the urine in order (*smaa*)' and it is difficult to say what that might mean, although easing of frequency of micturition is a possibility. Ebers 273 is a remedy 'made for a child who suffers wetness', still a familiar problem.

The rather enigmatic Ebers 265 is 'another [remedy] to eliminate heat (*tau*) in the bladder, when he suffers retention (*hedbu*) of urine'. The first part suggests cystitis, and the second outflow obstruction due perhaps to urethral stricture or an enlarged prostate. Both parts would certainly apply to a urethritis. Infection is also suggested by reference to what appears to be solid material in the urine: Ebers 261 is 'to drive out knots (*tjesu*) in the urine', and Ebers 267 for 'someone suffering from *henau* in his urine'. The word *henau* is otherwise unknown. It may derive from the very well known word *hena* meaning 'together with', but embellished with a plural and a pus determinative. The *Grundriss* translates as 'accumulations' and Ghaliounghui (1987) as 'agglomerations'. Over all one gains the impression of pus in the urine although it would be difficult to exclude the possibility of passage of stones or clots of blood. Stones in the kidney or bladder have very seldom been seen, either on direct examination of a mummy or by radiography (Sandison, 1972). Elliot Smith and Dawson (1924) reported only three cases of renal calculus and two of vesical calculus in 30,000 bodies of which they had accurate records.

The nervous system

The ancient Egyptians appeared to have little concept of the function of the nervous system and discarded the brain at mummification (Chapter 3). Nevertheless, there are some excellent descriptions of the neurological consequences of injuries, considered in Chapter 8. With the exception of trauma, the medical papyri have little to say about disorders of the nervous system, except for a possible reference to facial nerve paralysis (Bell's palsy) which usually affects only one side of the face. The relevant passage is Berlin 76 and the literal translation is:

> A fumigation (*kap*) for driving out a taking (*itj*) of one side (*ges*) of his face (*her*) [and] the bank (*idebu*) of his mouth (*r*).

The diagnosis of Bell's palsy depends on the acceptance of *itj* to indicate paralysis; although its usual meaning is 'take', it can also mean 'conquer'. The second problem is the word *idebu* (with a 'tusk' or 'tooth' determinative). The word *ideb* (with a 'tongue of land' determinative) means 'river bank' or 'shore' and it is likely that this was extended to mean 'corner' of the mouth and so shown by use of the 'tusk' or 'tooth' determinative. This may well be an example of special use of everyday words in the medical sense (p. 25). This interpretation follows that of Westendorf (1992).

Migraine is considered below.

Hernias and hydroceles

The more common types of hernia are protrusions, usually of bowel, through weaknesses in the abdominal wall, presenting intermittently as swellings under the skin in characteristic sites. Most hernias would be very difficult to see in a mummy, because they often disappear in the supine position, particularly after death when muscle tone is lost. Furthermore, the contents of the hernial sac might be removed from the inside by the embalmer, for placement of the intestines in the appropriate canopic jar. Elliot Smith (1912) found a bulky but empty scrotum in Ramses v (Twentieth Dynasty): he thought this suggested an inguinal hernia or possibly a hydrocele. The scrotum of the pharaoh Merenptah (Nineteenth Dynasty) had been removed.

Several tomb paintings and reliefs show servants and workmen with protuberances near or above the umbilicus (see fig. 8.3). Most of these have the characteristic appearance of an umbilical hernia. More difficult to diagnose is the scrotal swelling of the marsh fowler in the tomb of Ankh-ma-hor (fig. 4.15). This might well be a large inguinal hernia which had descended into the scrotum. However, if it is an accurate representation of the disorder, the appearance is closer to that of a hydrocele, which is an effusion of fluid into the tunica vaginalis which surrounds the testicle. Hydroceles do not communicate with the abdominal cavity and there is a distinct upper boundary to the swelling, as appears to be the case in fig. 4.15.

The most important reference to hernia in the medical papyri is Ebers 864, cited and considered in Chapter 8. The diagnosis is strongly suggested by reference to the swelling appearing on coughing, and the location 'above the umbilicus' suggests an umbilical or epigastric hernia (see fig. 8.3). Hernias in ancient Egypt were reviewed by Rowling (1967).

Bones and joints

The occurrence of tuberculosis of bone is very well established and has been considered above, together with non-tuberculous infection which was surprisingly rare. Gout has never been recognised in the pharaonic period although Elliot Smith and Dawson (1924) reported a single case from the Coptic (Christian) period. Rickets has not been seen, probably because of the intense sunlight resulting in the biosynthesis of vitamin D, which prevents rickets. Fractures were very common and are considered in Chapter 8.

The bony changes of wear and tear have been widely reported and include osteoarthritic 'lipping' of the vertebrae with loss of intervertebral discs. Ankylosing spondylitis (fusion of the spine) is well documented from Predynastic to Coptic times (Ruffer, 1921; Zorab, 1961).

Pains and aches

Migraine

One of the most celebrated passages in the medical papyri is Ebers 250:

> Another [remedy] for suffering (*meret*) in half the head (*ges-tep*). The skull of a cat-fish (*nar*), fried in oil. Anoint the head therewith.*
>
> *Another remedy for *ges-tep* is in Chester Beatty v, 4.

The headache of migraine is caused by excessive vasodilatation of blood vessels in the meningeal membranes which surround the brain. It normally occurs on one side only and the headache, often very severe, is therefore confined to one side. The Egyptian specification of *ges-tep* leaves very little doubt that migraine was intended. The Hippocratic corpus also refers to unilateral headache, using the word 'hemicrania', from which the English term 'migraine' is derived. This is one of the very few possible links between Egyptian and Greek medicine, but the name might well have arisen independently in the two countries.

Disorders of the *metu*

Chapter 3 explained how the word *metu* could refer to anything long and thin, including blood vessels, ducts, nerves, tendons and muscles. A compact section of the Ebers papyrus commences at Ebers 627 with 'Beginning of the ointments to strengthen the *metu*'. It is, as always, very difficult to know what is meant by the *metu* but, in this context, it seems likely that the whole section (Ebers 627–94) refers to the muscular system. Apart from remedies to strengthen the *metu*, there are others to soften, relieve

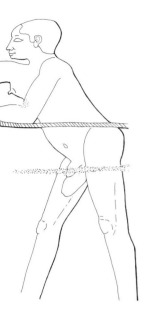

4.15 Relief showing a marsh fowler from the tomb of Ankh-ma-hor (6th Dynasty) at Saqqara (see p. 126). The differential diagnosis of the scrotal swelling is between a hydrocele and a scrotal extension of an inguinal hernia (see text).

pain and soothe. Most of the remedies are for surface application and were probably intended to relieve painful and aching muscles, to relieve cramps and perhaps in the hope of actually strengthening the muscles.

Disorders of the ears and nose

The ears

The ears comprised two of the seven openings in the head and were believed to be an important portal of entry for good and bad spirits, as for example in Ebers 856g:

> ... There are two *metu* in him to his right ear. The breath of life enters into them. There are two *metu* in him to his left ear. The breath of death enters into them.

Deafness was well understood and several words mean 'to be deaf'. Benitez (1988) reported a perforated ear-drum, suggesting a middle ear infection, in an exceptionally well preserved Ptolemaic mummy. Ebers 766 provides detailed instructions for an injury to the lobe of the ear (see Chapter 8). Diseases of the ears are covered in Ebers 764–70 and Berlin 70–1 and 200–3.

The nose

Injuries to the nose are well covered in the Edwin Smith papyrus (see Chapter 8), but medical disorders merit only four paragraphs in the Ebers papyrus. Ebers 761 is headed 'beginning of remedies for *resh*'. The word *resh* with a nose determinative seems to be related to *reshuet* (also with a nose determinative) meaning 'joy'. However, the *Grundriss* gives the more likely meaning of 'head cold or coryza'. For this condition, Ebers 761 recommends date juice, probably to be applied to the nostrils, while 763 gives an incantation directed against *resh* which 'makes ill the seven apertures of the head'. This is to be recited in association with the administration of milk of one who has borne a male child and fragrant gum. Ebers 418 is for the *khenet*-disease, considered to be catarrh (see under 'Lung' above), and now specifically related to the nose thus:

> Another [remedy] to drive out catarrh from the nose: galena, 1; *khet-awa*, 1; dry incense (*àntyu*), 1; honey, 1; paint therewith for four days. Do [it] and you will see [the result]! Behold it is true!

Ebers 762 provides a remedy for the unknown *nia*-disease of the nose.

Disorders of the skin

Mummies have shown a few examples of skin diseases (Sandison, 1967a) and there are remedies for the skin in sections 708–21 in the Ebers papyrus, 150–4 of the Hearst papyrus and also on the verso of the Edwin Smith papyrus (21, 3–8). Several of these are parallels. It is unfortunately not possible to identify specific skin diseases from the papyri and the remedies are more in the category of beauty care.

Ebers 708–11 are concerned with driving out *khenesh*, which the *Grundriss* translates as 'perspiration' and Faulkner (1962) as 'stink'. The remedies are for local application and include incense-resins, grains from the umbrella pine of Byblos, carob, ostrich egg and tortoise shell. Ebers 712 and 713 are probably misplaced and the section continues with 714, 'another to overturn or renew (*sepena*) the skin'. 'Overturn' is the usual meaning of *sepena* for which the determinative is a ship upside down. The remedy, for local application, is honey, red natron and salt. Ebers 715 is 'to beautify (*senefer*) the skin'; *inem* is a well attested word for skin. The remedy is powdered alabaster, natron, salt and honey. The remaining paragraphs of this section of the Ebers are concerned with wrinkles and stretching of the skin.

This section is remarkable for the omissions rather than for what is included. The conspicuous nature of skin diseases and their common occurrence must have driven countless patients to seek the help of *swnw*, priest and magician. One would have expected this branch of medicine to have generated a large corpus of remedies and spells.

Ageing

The ancient Egyptians were very conscious of the ageing process, and in the *Tale of Sinuhe* the hero gave the following account of himself at the time of his return to Egypt:

> So shall my limbs grow young again, for now old age has fallen on me: weakness has overtaken me, my eyes are heavy, and my arms weak; my legs fail to follow, and my heart is weary; I am near to death. May they conduct me to the cities of eternity!

The *Maxims of Ptahhotep* (Žába, 1956) begin as follows:

> The *Teaching of the Lord Vizier Ptahhotep*, under the majesty of King Isesi. May he live for all time and eternity! The Lord Vizier Ptahhotep said: 'Sovereign, my Lord! Old age has occurred, elderliness descended; woe is come and weakness is renewing itself; the heart passes the night in pain, every day; the eyes are dim, the ears deaf; strength is perishing for the heart's weariness; the mouth is silent and cannot speak; the heart is stopped and cannot recall yesterday; the bones suffer because of their length; goodness has become evil; all taste is gone. What age does to people is evil in every aspect; the nose is blocked and cannot breathe, because of the weakness due to standing and sitting. May One decree for this servant that a Staff of Old Age be made.' (Both translations after Richard Parkinson, personal communication, 1995)

It is interesting that deterioration which we would regard as cerebral is here attributed to the heart (see Chapter 3).

Several sections of the medical papyri are devoted to stemming the ravages of age. Ebers 451–63 comprises remedies to prevent the hair turning grey; Ebers 464–74 is devoted to remedies to cause the hair to grow on a bald head. In general the remedies are sympathetic and include various parts of black animals to be applied to grey hair, and the bristles of a hedgehog for baldness. The verso of the Edwin Smith papyrus ends with remedies to be applied for transforming an old man into a youth.

CHAPTER **FIVE**

Magic and religion in medicine

In pharaonic times there was little distinction between magic and religion, and supernatural influences were regarded as major controlling factors in the events of daily
life. This included not only such phenomena as the movement of celestial bodies and
the flooding of the Nile but also the causation of disease. Belief in the supernatural
origin of certain diseases continued and was prevalent in Europe for many centuries,
particularly in the case of the 'sacred disease' (epilepsy), 'king's evil' (scrofula) and
leprosy. Certainly in ancient Egypt, malign deities and disease-demons were believed
to bring many diseases, a process which could also be invoked by individuals to bring
misfortune to an adversary. If the cause of disease was thought to be supernatural, it
was also logical to look to the supernatural for its cure. This took many forms.
Certain deities were invoked to prevent or cure diseases and attacks by dangerous
animals. In addition, incantations were directly addressed to disease-demons, bidding
them leave the body.

Jackson (1988) has discussed the reasons why patients sought the help of the gods
in preference to that of doctors in the civilisations of Greece and Rome. These
included the cost, risk, uncertainty of outcome, discomfort and sheer physical pain
of ancient treatments. Similar though less well documented reasons probably applied
to Egypt, particularly in the Ptolemaic Period when Greek influence was paramount.
On all these counts, an appeal to the supernatural would seem an attractive option.
Furthermore, the deities were such an accepted part of daily life that invoking their
help would often have been the first rather than the last resort.

The cause of the illness would have been an important factor in the choice between
conventional treatment and magic. In the case of trauma in particular, the cause was
usually obvious, and it was often possible to predict the likely outcome. In contrast,
the aetiology of internal disorders was usually unknown and the outcome often uncertain. It is therefore not surprising that remedies for trauma only rarely contain
incantations, whereas they are very common in the treatment of medical conditions.

The contrast between trauma and medicine is, however, complicated by the times
when the surviving medical papyri were written (see Chapter 2). As dates advance,
there is a general trend for magical practice to increase at the expense of the practical approach to medicine, and there is a similar tendency in Babylonian medicine
(Kinnear Wilson, personal communication, 1994). However, the correlation between
date and the proportion of magical practice in medicine is much influenced by the Old
Kingdom date, proposed by Breasted (1930), for the original of the Edwin Smith
papyrus, which is a model of pragmatism and contains only one spell. Although the
early date of the Edwin Smith papyrus has now been challenged (p. 27), there is no
doubt that there is a great deal of magic in most of the later papyri.

There were a great many deities in ancient Egypt. Some were ambivalent towards
disease, being involved in both causation and cure. However, others were predominantly malevolent, believed to be capable of bringing misfortune and illness. The
practice of invoking malign deities has a direct continuity with demonic magic and
witchcraft, practices continuing to this day. Other Egyptian deities, Isis in particular,
were predominantly benign with special powers and inclination to ward off evil, and
to repair the damage caused by malign influences. Many Egyptian incantations concerned with healing invoke a benign deity, and the more powerful the better. The close

association between magic and religion continued throughout Greek and Roman times, eventually bringing magicians into conflict with the new Christian church.

Belief in the power of the supernatural is not to be confused with the deliberate deception practised by professional magicians and conjurors, whether in ancient or in modern times. There is a classic example of deception in the only account of Egyptian magic in the Bible. Pharaoh summoned his wise men and sorcerers, who turned their staffs into serpents, only to be swallowed by a serpent formed from Aaron's staff (Exodus 7: 8–13). Turning a staff into a serpent still remains in the repertoire of the snake charmer.

The therapeutic value of magic

It would be quite wrong to dismiss magic as irrelevant to the healing process. Suggestion and expectation of cure have a measurable curative value, particularly in the relief of pain, a phenomenon now known as the placebo effect (Chapter 7). Since, in pharaonic times, there may have been relatively few pharmacologically effective remedies, it was entirely reasonable to rely on the placebo effect which, for many conditions, would have been much better than nothing. One would expect the effect of a placebo to be greatly enhanced by the suggestion of magic and the pronouncement of an incantation.

In some instances it is possible to discern a rational basis for what appears at first sight to be purely magical practice. The clearest example of this concerns the circumstances under which certain herbs were gathered and prepared for medicinal use. There is a diurnal variation in the concentration of many alkaloids in various parts of plants, and where such alkaloids have therapeutic value – morphine is a good example – the efficacy of a preparation must therefore be related to the time of day when the plant is gathered. Even Galen (second century AD), who usually decried magic, recommended that a certain herb should be collected before sunrise. The basis for this cannot have been understood and the practice would appear to be magical. There must have been many such instances where the therapeutic efficiency of a herbal or indeed animal preparation could have been improved, apparently by magical means. On the other hand, many magical aspects of the preparation of herbs can have had no rational benefit other than to increase the expectation of cure.

Magic was also concerned in the practice of selecting a herbal remedy from a particular plant because of its resemblance to the organ requiring treatment, the principle of *similia similibus*. Alternatively, an animal preparation might be selected on the basis of a characteristic associated with that animal, such as keen eyesight. It could only be by chance if such a remedy had any therapeutic potential.

Gods and magicians concerned with healing

Myths related to healing practices

Certain myths of the Egyptian pantheon are fundamental to an understanding of some of the magical incantations, amulets and drugs used in healing. The most important myths of relevance to medicine concern the four children of the earth god Geb and his sister–wife Nut, the sky goddess – Osiris, Isis, Seth and Nephthys (Hart, 1986; Quirke, 1992). The Osiris legend was recounted, with Greek overtones, by the classical writer Plutarch (*de Iside et Osiride*), translated from the Greek by Griffiths (1970).

Osiris, first mentioned in the pyramid texts of Unas at the end of the Fifth Dynasty (*c.* 2345 BC), was a benign mythical ruler of Egypt in prehistoric times. He aroused the jealousy of his brother Seth, who attacked him and threw his dismembered body into the Nile. Isis, who had the reputation of being 'more clever than a million gods', exhibited supreme devotion to her brother and husband, undertaking a tireless search for the parts of his body. She then used her extensive magical skills to reassemble the body and, in the guise of a hawk, fluttered her wings to provide the breath of life. She revived him to the extent of enabling him to have sexual intercourse with her, still in the guise of a hawk. The product of conception was Horus-the-child. The impregnation of his sister–wife was the last earthly act of Osiris, who was thereafter ruler of the underworld, always depicted wrapped in mummy bandages, but with protruding hands holding the crook and flail, the emblems of kingship. His name became a part of the identity of each dead person, and countless inscriptions refer to the deceased as 'the Osiris, NN'.

Isis, the prototype single-parent mother, then devoted herself to care of her son, Horus-the-child, who is to be distinguished in this aspect from Horus the falcon god of the Old Kingdom and the symbol of divine kingship. Her exemplary care of her child, combined with her magical skills, made her the ideal deity to be invoked for protection and cure, the patient being identified with Horus-the-child. Isis brought about the victory of Horus over venomous animals, and this resulted in the concept of Horus-the-saviour, who had protective and curative powers in his own right (see below in relation to cippi). The Metternich stela (considered below) provides a very full collection of myths and incantations related to Isis and to the child Horus, who was stung by a scorpion and restored to health by Isis with the involvement of Ra and Thoth.

Horus then grew to maturity, acquiring the title of protector or avenger of his father. This pitted him against Seth who, in an independent tradition, appeared as his brother rather than his uncle. Horus and Seth contended for the throne of Egypt for many years, their antagonism culminating in Seth undertaking a homosexual assault on Horus, who later tore off Seth's testicles. The former unpleasant episode relates to the concept of poisonous semen, which was a recurring feature in the supernatural causation of disease in ancient Egypt (see Westendorf, 1992). The Egyptian word *metut* means both semen and poison, in each case with a phallus as biliteral phonetic for *m+t*, and a second (discharging) phallus as a determinative. This double meaning accords with the act of the malign incubus who could inseminate and thereby poison a sleeping victim.

In the course of their fighting, Seth pulled out Horus' eye, which was magically restored by Thoth (Djehuty). The restored or whole eye (the *wedjat* eye) became the most powerful of the protective amulets (Andrews, 1994). It also became the basis for the geometric progression of unitary fractions (1/2 to 1/64) used for the dosage of drugs (fig. 7.3). Horus eventually gained the ascendancy over Seth and thereby the throne of Egypt. However, Seth was retained, and even honoured, as a god who was the necessary personification of disorder and evil, parallel in certain respects to the devil in Christian theology.

Magicians

There is good evidence that various categories of magicians practised medicine independently of a conventional doctor or *swnw* (see Chapter 6), who was perhaps not available in the smaller communities. However, some magicians may have worked in association with a *swnw*. There are a few cases of double qualification, with a *swnw* carrying a magician's title in addition to his title as a doctor (see Table 6.4).

Khery-hebet, literally 'the one in charge of the festival rolls', is usually translated as 'lector priest', a role closely associated with religious performances, magic and, in particular, the reading of incantations and spells (see below). Two *swnw* are known to have held the title of lector priest: Mereru-ka, the illustrious vizier to Teti (Appendix B, no. 25) and Huy (App. B, no. 147), known only from Late Period graffiti in the temple of Sethos I at Abydos. The Westcar papyrus describes wonderful acts of magic undertaken by the chief lector priests Weba-iner and Djadja-em-ankh. Lector priests could also be malign, and a failing heart is ascribed to the breath and evil actions of a lector priest (Ebers 855u).

Sau means magician, and the word is closely related to *sa* meaning 'amulet' and 'protection'. All share the ideogram Gardiner sign-list v 17, which also appears in the word *sa* meaning 'phyle', 'company' or 'troop'. The quotation from the Ebers papyrus at the beginning of Chapter 6 is addressed to the *sau* as well as the *swnw* and the *wab* priest of Sekhmet, the presumption being that all three groups practised as healers. It seems likely that two of the three *swnw* listed on stelae in the temple of Serabit el-Khadim in a Sinai quarry may have held this title in addition to that of *swnw* (Gardiner, Peet and Cerny, 1952). The *swnw* whose name is lost (App. B, no. 82) clearly shows the ideogram (Gardiner sign-list v 17) for *sau*, with the phonogram for '*u*' (or '*w*') but without the seated man determinative. The ideogram is less clear in the case of Akmu (App. B, no. 67) but is likely to be the same. In both cases, Jonckheere (1958) made the suggestion that the reading was *sa* meaning 'phyle', 'troop' or 'gang', translating the whole phrase as 'physician to the troop', but that word is usually written with accompanying signs for a group of men.

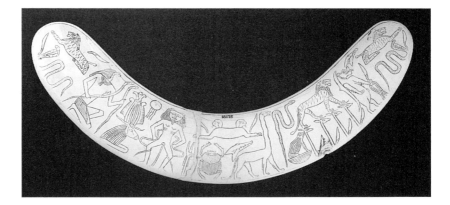

5.1 Ivory curved wand of 12th Dynasty, from Thebes, to provide magical protection for mother and child. (British Museum, EA 18175)

Hekay is a rare word for magician, confined to the Middle Kingdom, and related to Heka, the god of magic. It was sometimes qualified as *hekay n kap*, meaning magician of the (king's) private apartments (Ward, 1982). Magical protection of children of a local magnate is shown in a scene with nurses (*menat*) holding magic ivory wands (fig. 5.1) (Wildung, 1984). The role of the *hekay* in medicine is unclear, but the *swnw* Hery-shef-nakht (Chapter 6) was an overseer of the *hekay*. Two Old Kingdom *swnw* are known to have been funerary priests of Heka: Ipi (App. B, no. 4) and Ny-ankh-ra (App. B, no. 30). It is not clear how their role as funerary priests, even of Heka, could be relevant to their medical practice. Heka shared with Serqet (see below) the ability to seal up the mouths of snakes, and also to provide relief if a man was bitten.

Priests of Serqet

Priests of Serqet were also magicians and undoubtedly practised medicine, particularly in preventing and treating attacks by snakes and scorpions (von Känel, 1984). The Brooklyn papyrus on snake bites (pp. 40 and 183) provides a pragmatic approach to the management of snake bite but was 'under the hand of the *kherep* priests of Serqet' with no mention of the *swnw*. Five known *swnw* were also *kherep* priests of Serqet: Ir-en-akhty (App. B, no. 7), Khuy (App. B, no. 49), Nemty-em-hat (App. B, no. 66), an anonymous *wer swnw* (App. B, no. 83) and Psamtek-soneb (App. B, no. 145). Amen-mose (p. 135) was a *kherep* priest of Serqet but not a *swnw*, and believed to have been a worker–doctor in the necropolis workmen's village of Deir el-Medina (Kitchen, 1986). Ny-ankh-ra (App. B, no. 30) held the title *imy-khet* of Serqet.

Serqet (also known as Selket, or Selkis in Greek) was a goddess of great antiquity known from the First Dynasty of the Old Kingdom. She was identified with the scorpion, and is usually represented with this creature on her head (fig. 5.2). In spite of this rather unappealing appendage, her appearance was generally attractive and her influence benign. The need to appease her gave her a major role in protection from scorpions and other venomous animals. She was one of the four protective goddesses of coffins and canopic jars (the others being Isis, Nephthys and Neith). Serqet's particular role was the protection of Qebhsenuef the son of Horus who was specifically concerned with the canopic jar containing the intestines (see Table 3.1).

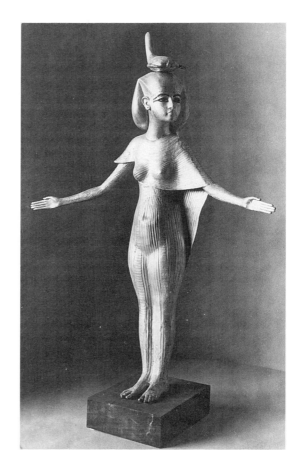

5.2 The scorpion goddess Serqet, whose priests had a special role in the treatment of bites by venomous animals. She is seen here as a guardian of the canopic chest of Tutankhamun, 18th Dynasty. (Cairo Museum, JdE 60686)

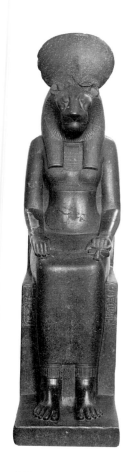

Serqet's name is the feminine active participle of the archaic causative verb *sereq*, meaning 'to cause to breathe'. This may well relate to the rapid and deep breathing which is a common effect of a scorpion sting. Alternatively, it might describe her role in curing victims of respiratory failure which is a rare complication of a sting.

The recto of the Chester Beatty papyrus VII, written in the reign of Ramses II, contains a number of magical spells for protection against scorpions. Most invoke various wives of Horus whom Gardiner (1935) suggested might be merely appellations of Serqet, who is actually named in the eighth spell:

'Someone approaches me.'
'It is not I who approach you, it is Wepet-sepu, wife of Horus, who approaches you.'
'You poisons, come forth to me. I am Serqet.'

Sekhmet and her priests

Sekhmet was the lion-headed goddess (fig. 5.3) who, with her husband Ptah and son Nefertem, completed the Memphite Triad. Her name is derived directly from the word for power, *sekhem*, with the addition of the feminine termination '*t*'. She symbolised power and might, spreading terror before her, and had the capacity to bring pestilence. In the *Tale of Sinuhe*, Amunenshi, an Asiatic ruler, compared fear of the pharaoh Senusret I (Twelfth Dynasty) with that of 'Sekhmet in the year of pestilence'. As in the case of Serqet, the need to appease Sekhmet resulted in her acquiring an important role in healing. This was so strong that her priests were considered parallel, though possibly somewhat inferior, to the *swnw* in the practice of medicine (von Känel, 1984). The Ebers papyrus (854a; p. 113), the Edwin Smith papyrus (Case 1, gloss A) and the Hatnub graffito (p. 129) all testify to the medical role of her priests. It is also possible that priests of Sekhmet functioned as veterinary surgeons (p. 119).

Deities concerned with childbirth

There is no direct evidence of the involvement of the *swnw* in childbirth, and it seems very likely that magic was a popular means of seeking a favourable outcome. The grotesque dwarf god Bes (fig. 5.4) was believed to exert a particularly favourable influ-

5.3 (above) The lion-headed goddess Sekhmet, whose priests had a special role in healing. This statue is from the temple of Mut in Karnak, reign of Amenhotep III, 18th Dynasty. (British Museum, EA 63)

5.4 (right) A relief showing four representations of the protective god Bes from the Late Period (c. 600 BC). (British Museum, EA 1178)

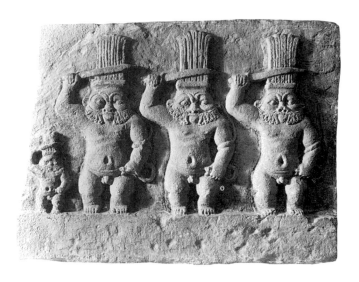

ence in pregnancy and childbirth, and he was frequently represented in the *mammisi* or birth houses attached to temples (see below). However, his protective and curative powers were more far-ranging, and his image was a favourite amulet both carried by the living and buried with the dead. Furthermore, his head usually appears above 'Horus the Saviour' on cippi (see below).

Taweret (the great one) was a goddess with the head of a hippopotamus, the legs and arms of a lion, the tail of a crocodile and a body embellished with pendulous human breasts (fig. 5.5). In spite of these improbable attributes, Taweret had a special role in helping women in childbirth. Like Bes, she was a favourite subject for amulets.

Meskhenet, whose symbol of two loops on top of a vertical stroke represents the two-horned uterus of a heifer, was the goddess of childbirth, the same Egyptian word, without the goddess determinative, meaning birthing stool. The magical childbirth featured in the Westcar papyrus (Chapter 9) describes her role alongside Heqet, Isis and Nephthys. Heqet was the frog goddess, and the title 'servant of Heqet' might possibly indicate 'midwife' (Hart, 1986), although there is no definite Egyptian word for midwife and no account of their work. The very important goddess Isis, the sister–wife of Osiris and mother of Horus, replaced Hathor (see below) in the role of divine mother, and is depicted suckling Horus-the-Child in innumerable small statuettes, representing the king (the living Horus) receiving divine milk. In addition, she was the tutelary goddess for the canopic jar containing the liver of the deceased. Nephthys shared with her sister Isis the role of protecting the king and was also the tutelary goddess for the canopic jar which contained the lungs.

The birth house or *mammisi*. Many temples from the Ptolemaic period, such as those at Edfu, Dendera and Philae, feature a *mammisi*, freestanding buildings decorated with birth scenes of deities and kings. The temple of Hathor at Dendera, for example, shows the birth of Ihy, the child of Horus and Hathor. Although there is no evidence that the *mammisi* were used for obstetric purposes, it is nevertheless conceivable that they were visited by those advanced in pregnancy in the hope of securing divine assistance in the birth of their child. However, the cult of the divine child was an affair of state rather than part of daily life.

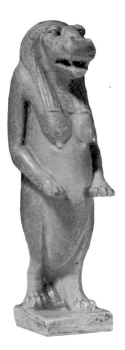

5.5 An amulet of the protective goddess Taweret, from the Third Intermediate Period, c. 1000 BC. (British Museum, EA 64592)

Other deities

Thoth (Greek form of the Egyptian name Djehuty) was of central significance to Egyptian medicine and magic because of his role as the god of the scribes. He came to embody all literary achievements and the 'house of life' (*per ankh*) was under his protection (p. 131). No less important to healing was his special ability to write and also to recite what was written. For this reason he was frequently invoked in healing incantations (see below). Thoth is commonly represented either as a baboon (*Papio cynocephalus*) or as an ibis (*Ibis religiosa*). He appears with the head of the ibis, or occasionally a baboon, mounted on a human body in the scene showing the weighing of the heart from the *Book of the Dead* (fig. 5.6).

The benign cow goddess Hathor had a special role as symbolic mother of the kings dating back to the Old Kingdom, where she appeared to be the successor to unnamed cow goddesses of predynastic times. There is a statue of Hathor suckling Amenhotep II, but Hathor's role as divine mother of the kings was later shared by Isis.

The ithyphallic god Min, attested already in the Predynastic Period, was the symbol of reproduction, both animal and vegetable. Amun-Kamutef was an ithyphallic manifestation of Amun, who had a very similar appearance to Min. The lettuce (*Lactuca sativa*) was closely associated with Min, and also featured in the aftermath of the homosexual assault of Seth on Horus. Thus the lettuce acquired the reputation of being aphrodisiac.

In the Late Period, two deified mortals acquired a reputation as healers, although neither is known to have been a *swnw* during his lifetime. Imhotep and Amenhotep-son-of-Hapu, officials under Djoser and Amenhotep III respectively, were deified long after their deaths, and their shrines became healing cult centres (see Chapter 6).

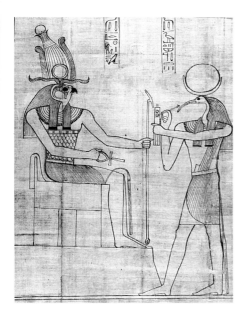

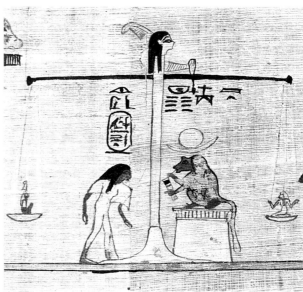

5.6 The god of writing, Thoth, had a special role in medicine. He is shown above (left) drawn on papyrus as an ibis-headed scribe, in the hieratic funerary papyrus of Nes-ta-nebet-asheru, 21st Dynasty, c. 950 BC (British Museum, EA 10554, sheet 63) and (right), less commonly, as a baboon-form scribe, in the *Book of the Dead* of Nodjmet, 21st Dynasty, c. 1065 BC. (British Museum, EA 10541)

Demons as causes of disease

The medical papyri make specific mention of malign influences which enter the body from the outside. The Ebers papyrus (854f) is quite specific as to the side of the body:

> The breath of life enters into the right ear and the breath of death enters into the left ear.*

*The significance of the left side is considered in Chapter 3.

Case 8 in the Edwin Smith papyrus describes an extensive skull fracture with intact scalp. Gloss D clearly describes the entry of an entirely extraneous malign influence from outside the body:

> As for something entering from outside, it means the breath of an outside god or death. It is not an entering of that which is created by his flesh.

A clue to the nature of such an influence is found in a misplaced gloss (Ebers 855y):

> As to *neba* entering from the outside, it means his heart is *neba* because of [something] entering from outside.

The meaning of *neba* is unknown. The phrase 'entering from outside' is identical in format to Case 8 of the Edwin Smith papyrus but, in its second appearance in this text, is embellished by a god-like determinative and Westendorf (1992) refers to these entities as 'sickness-demons'. Other examples include the untranslatable *nesiet*-disease caused by a demon which enters the body through the eye. Ebers 209 refers directly to the belly being attacked by the *nesiet* demon. Ebers 854e is another misplaced gloss which ascribes deafness to breathing air from the 'beheading demon' (*heseq*).

Reference has already been made to the introduction of poison/semen (*metut*) by an incubus, sometimes in the form of a donkey (*aa*), but based upon the homosexual assault of Seth on Horus. In a related category is *aaa*, and in Chapter 3 it was explained why such a meaning is preferred to the alternative proposal of 'haematuria due to schistosomiasis'. We may note here that the medical papyri contain eight remedies to drive out the *aaa* of a god, a goddess, a dead man or a dead woman. Berlin 189 provided a spell for this purpose.

Incantations

Magical papyri and those medical papyri with a substantial magical component sometimes establish their authenticity by a statement that they were found under the feet of a statue of a god. Thus, for example, one section of the Ebers papyrus (856a) states that the book was found under the feet of [the statue of] Anubis in Letopolis and was then brought to a king of the First Dynasty. This would imply an archaic, if not divine, origin and greatly increase the authority of the contents.

The significance of names

Many incantations and spells specifically identified a being who could benefit the supplicant. It was believed that knowing someone's name, and particularly their secret name, gave one power over them, a concept which is not entirely unfamiliar today. This can be seen in those parts of the *Book of the Dead* concerned with overcoming the various obstacles which were placed in the path of the deceased in the underworld. The following example is taken from Chapter 125 of the papyrus of Ani (Faulkner, 1972):

> 'We will not let you enter by us,' say the door-posts of this door, 'unless you tell
> our name.'
> '"Plummet of truth" is your name.'
> 'I will not let you enter by me,' says the right-hand leaf of this door, 'unless you
> tell my name.'
> '"Scale-pan which weighs truth" is your name.' [and so on]

In one myth, included in a magico-medical text, Isis went to great lengths to determine Ra's secret name and so gain power over him (Chester Beatty XI). Using the god's own spittle, she fashioned a snake which bit Ra, causing him great pain, and she then offered to alleviate his suffering with magic in exchange for divulging his own secret name. He was eventually obliged to comply with this request, and so Isis became 'the mistress of the gods who knew Ra by his own name'.

Special protection was obtained by identifying each part of the body with a named god, as in the following excerpt from Spell 42 of the *Book of the Dead*, which follows identification of the deceased with Ra:

> My hair is Nun; my face is Ra; my eyes are Hathor; my ears are Wepwawet; . . .
> my lips are Anubis; my molars are Serqet; my incisors are Isis [and so on]

A similar practice is followed in the incantation for protection of a cat stung by a scorpion in the Metternich stela (see below).

Incantations as therapy

There is great variation in the format of incantations used for healing, and the simplest is addressed directly to the disease or the disease-demon itself, without involvement of deities or drugs. Ebers 131 is such a spell against *wekhedu*, an important pathological entity, with supernatural overtones, considered in Chapter 3:

> An incantation [against] *wekhedu*: . . . I trample Busiris; I throw down Mendes; I ascend to the sky to see what is done therein. Nothing will be done in Abydos until the driving out of the [evil] influence of a god, a goddess, male *wekhedu*, female *wekhedut*, and so on, and the influence and all evil things that are in this my body, in this my flesh and in these my limbs. . . . I will not say: I will not repeat: Perish as you came into being! Words to be said four times and spat out over the site of the disease. Really effective: a million times.

Usually, however, a deity is invoked at the same time, as in this example from the Metternich stela for use against the venom of snake bite (Spruch IIa):

> Flow out, poison. Come forth. Go forth on to the ground. Horus will exorcise you. He will punish you. He will spit you out. . . .

Most incantations were intended to be used together with a conventional remedy and three such spells have pride of place at the beginning of the Ebers' papyrus. The following is an extract from Ebers 1:

> I have come from Heliopolis with the great ones of the great house, the lords of protection and the rulers of eternity. I have also come from Sais with the mother of the gods. They have given me their protection. I have utterances that the lord of the universe has composed to eliminate the doings of a god, a goddess, a dead man, a dead woman, etc. that are in this my head, in these my vertebrae, in these my shoulders, in this my flesh, in these my limbs . . .
> To be recited during the application of a remedy on any member of a sick man. Really excellent: a million times.

It is followed by Ebers 2, which is an incantation for loosening bandages. Ebers 3 makes very clear the power of the combination of magic and medicine:

> Incantation for drinking a remedy: The remedy comes, and there comes that which drives [evil] things from this my heart and these my limbs. Strong is magic in combination with a medicine and vice versa. Do you remember then that Horus and Seth were taken to the great palace of Heliopolis when Seth's testicles were discussed with Horus? He was healthy (*wadj*) as [when] he was on earth. He did everything which he wished, like the gods which were there.
> Words to be spoken when the medicine is drunk. Really excellent: a million times.

Although the details and significance of the incantation are obscure, there is a very clear intention of reinforcing the effect of a remedy with magic, and this could only benefit a patient. In many situations, the power of suggestion would have far outweighed any therapeutic benefit from the drugs which were used.

More commonly, incantations relate to a particular disease and the use of specifically prescribed drugs. Typical of this genre is Ebers 61, which is contained within a list of seventeen remedies to eliminate the *hefat*-worm from the belly (see Chapter 3). The other sixteen remedies are not accompanied by incantations:

> Another [remedy]: Sedge (*isw*), 5 ro; *shames*-plant 1/4; cook in honey and eat.

Their incantation: May the burden [of illness] be loosened; may weariness be turned aside, which 'one who is on his belly' (i.e. worm or snake) has placed in my belly, that the god has created, that an enemy has created. What is harmful to it (the worm), may the god loosen, namely what he has made in this my belly.

Ebers 385 contains a great spell 'to eliminate a collection of water in the eyes'. This invoked the eyes of Horus and Atum and claimed to be effective against many conditions, including *wekhedu* and *wekhedut* of the eye. It was to be recited over green eye-paint which, with honey and cyperus grass (*giw*), was to be applied to the eye. It was designated 'really efficient'.

The practice of reciting incantations while taking medicines was widespread in the ancient world and continued over thousands of years. The elder Pliny (xxviii, 3) in the first century AD asked the question:

Have words and formulated incantations any effect? ... All our wisest men reject belief in them, although as a body the public at all times believe in them unconsciously.

The recto of the Edwin Smith surgical papyrus deals mainly with trauma where the cause of the injury would generally be all too obvious and there would seem to be no necessity to ascribe the condition to occult powers. It is therefore hardly surprising that there is only one incantation in the treatment of the forty-eight injuries described. This is included in the treatment of Case 9, a wound of the forehead in which the shell of the skull has been smashed. After describing the local application of the egg of an ostrich (a sympathetic remedy) triturated with grease, the papyrus continues:

That which is to be said as a charm over this remedy: Repelled is the enemy that is in the wound! Cast out is the [evil] that is in the blood, the adversary of Horus, [on every] side of the mouth of Isis. This temple does not fall down; there is no enemy of the vessel therein. I am under the protection of Isis; my rescue is the son of Osiris.

The verso of the Edwin Smith papyrus contains eight incantations unrelated to the surgical papyrus on the recto. The first is intended to counteract the 'wind of the pestilence of the year', which may relate to an annual epidemic on the epagomenal days, the dangerous low point of the year. It is directed to the benign deities Osiris, Horus, Nekhbet, Isis and Nephthys, whose protection is sought against a range of malign deities, including the son of Sekhmet (son of the 'disease-god' with divine determinative) and also of Hathor (who floods the rivers). The second incantation on the verso is another to ward off the 'wind of sickness', the disease-gods and the messengers of Sekhmet, and in it Horus is invoked. The third is again for protection against the pestilence of the year, but there is no mention of wind. Meskhenet is invoked:

I am the abomination that came forth out of Buto. O Meskhenet, who came forth out of Heliopolis. O men, O gods, O spirits, O dead, be you far from me. I am the abomination.

The seventh and eighth incantations define the conditions under which the incantation is to be pronounced. The seventh, for 'cleansing everything from pestilence' requires the incantation to be pronounced before a *nefret*-flower, bound to a piece of *des*-wood and tied with a strip of linen. The eighth incantation, for an unspecified purpose, specifies that the incantation be pronounced while holding a *shames*-flower in his hand.

Protection against dangerous animals

The *Book of the Dead* contains numerous incantations for the deceased to ward off dangerous creatures in the hereafter, including crocodiles (Spells 31 and 32) and snakes (Spells 33 to 39). The recto of the Chester Beatty papyrus VII contains incantations invoking the protection of Serqet against scorpions. Some of these incantations were available in the form of the cippus which is described in the following section.

In view of the dread with which the ancient Egyptians regarded snakes, it is remarkable that this creature should have had a well defined healing role in the civilisation of ancient Greece. Asklepios, the Greek god of medicine, carried a staff round which was entwined a snake, identified as the harmless *Elaphe longissima* (Jackson, 1988). The snake has retained its symbolism in healing to the present day, in spite of its malign influence on Eve in Genesis 3. The powers of healing attributed to the snake may have arisen from its air of mystery or because of the renewal of its skin, which symbolised rebirth. Snakes featured prominently in the healing dreams which occurred in the process of incubation or temple sleep (see below in relation to sanatoria).

Cippi and the Metternich stela

Many shrines in both temples and homes in the Late Period of ancient Egypt contained stelae known as cippi which were believed to confer protection from attack by certain animals, particularly snakes, scorpions and crocodiles. A typical cippus (fig. 5.7) shows Horus-the-Child, with side lock, standing on the backs of crocodiles, holding a variety of dangerous animals and thus symbolising his victory over malign

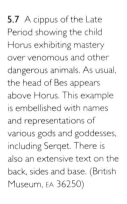

5.7 A cippus of the Late Period showing the child Horus exhibiting mastery over venomous and other dangerous animals. As usual, the head of Bes appears above Horus. This example is embellished with names and representations of various gods and goddesses, including Serqet. There is also an extensive text on the back, sides and base. (British Museum, EA 36250)

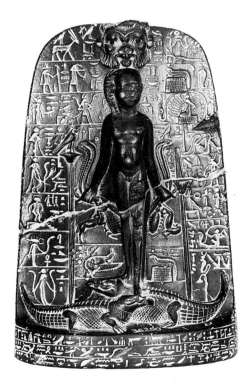

forces. In this guise he was known as Horus-the-Saviour (*shed*). The head of Bes is often included above the relief of Horus to confer additional protection (see above). In his role as protector from harmful creatures, Horus succeeded the saviour god Shed who fulfilled a similar role in the New Kingdom.

Cippi provided a range of texts and incantations which could be recited both for prevention of attack and for relief in the event of a sting or bite. The effect of the incantation could be reinforced by the application of water which had been poured over the stela, thereby absorbing its magical texts and scenes. The incantations inscribed on a cippus were necessarily abbreviated and drawn from a body of texts which have features in common with the Pyramid Texts of the Old Kingdom. Thus, for example, Pyramid Text Utterance 378 says:

> I am Horus, the young child with his finger to his mouth; the sandal of Horus is what tramples the *nekhi* snake.

An essential feature of the incantations was that the patient must be identified with a god and particularly with Horus, and so cause the malign forces to reconsider the gravity of what they had done.

The most complete and least corrupt version of the texts is found on the unique and extremely elaborate Metternich stela in the Metropolitan Museum of Art in New York (fig. 5.8) (Scott, 1951; Sander-Hansen, 1956). It was commissioned by the priest Nes-Atum in the reign of Nectanebo II, the last pharaoh of the Thirtieth Dynasty, immediately before the second Persian conquest in 343 BC. Nes-Atum was an ancient Egyptian antiquarian and went to very considerable trouble to collect the best available texts from cippi and from the burial place of the Mnevis bulls in Heliopolis. His selection of texts was then engraved with meticulous care on a fine block of dark green greywacke, standing almost one metre high and covered on all sides with text. Following the usual pattern of a cippus, the upper part of the front has a panel carved in high relief showing the child Horus standing on the backs of crocodiles, grasping various noxious animals, while attendant deities are shown standing on snakes, all demonstrating their triumph over the powers of evil.

The first incantation is against snakes and is followed by an extraordinary spell for a cat stung by a scorpion, here identified with the cat goddess Bastet:

> O Ra, come to your daughter, whom the scorpion has stung on a lonely road.
> Her cries reach heaven; harken on your way . . .

The spell continues at considerable length and places each part of the cat's body under the protection of a different god: Ra himself is invoked to protect the head. This reflects the placing of the different parts of a deceased person under the protection of individual deities as described in Chapter 42 of the *Book of the Dead* (see above). A later spell on the stela, addressed to Bastet, seeks help for a sick cat. These texts add to the great body of evidence illustrating the special position of the cat in late Egyptian society (Malek, 1993).

The back of the Metternich stela (Spruch VI) contains the remarkable story of Isis, Horus and the scorpion, which provides the basis for most incantations against scorpion stings. It describes how Isis set out one evening accompanied by seven scorpions whose names were known to her and who had been assigned for her protection. Isis and her entourage were refused entry at the first house they encountered. The indignant scorpions conferred and then transferred all their venom to their leader, Tefen, who then stung the son of the mistress of the house. Isis hastened to massage the throat of the child and called upon the poison of Tefen to come forth from the child.

5.8 The Metternich stela, on which is engraved a wealth of magical texts for protection from bites of venomous animals (end of 30th Dynasty). The front includes a representation of the child Horus as in the cippus shown in fig. 5.7. (Metropolitan Museum of Art, New York, MMA 50.85, Fletcher Fund, 1950)

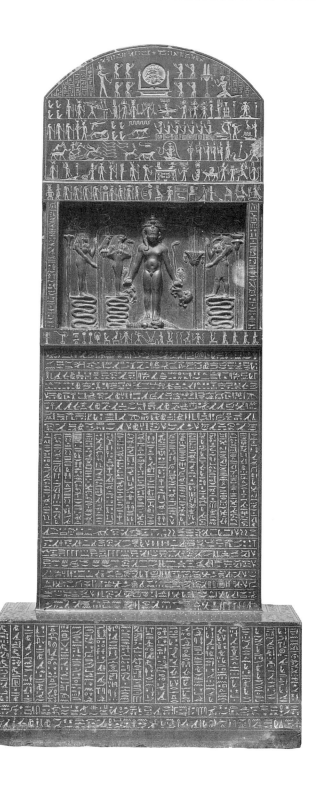

The story is then interrupted in order that those who might need to use the incantation can be instructed how to relate a stricken child to Isis' son Horus and so to proclaim:

May the child live and the poison die. As Horus will be cured for his mother
Isis, those who suffer will be cured likewise.

In the next part of the story, Isis (Spruch XIV) found Horus himself unconscious after being stung by a scorpion. She sought advice from Serqet, as the authority on scorpions, and then appealed to the gods, and Ra in particular, with these words:

Horus has been stung. O Ra; your son Horus has been stung who is without sin.

She then brought the solar barque to a standstill and this disruption of the equilibrium of the cosmos was so grave that Thoth was despatched to help her. This he did by means of the following spell:

Awake Horus. ... I am Thoth sent to cure you for your mother Isis and to cure
the sufferer likewise. ... The poison dies, its fire is drawn away.

Amulets

All collections of Egyptian antiquities bear testimony to the enormous popularity of amulets, worn by the living or buried with the dead (Andrews, 1994). They served many magical purposes, including preservation and protection of the body in life and after death. Petrie (1914) classified amulets as homopoeic, phylactic, theophoric, dynatic and ktematic, the first three categories having considerable relevance to medicine.

Homopoeic amulets portrayed living creatures (or their parts) from which the wearer hoped to assimilate their desirable attributes on the principle of *similia similibus*. These amulets included those in the shape of parts of the human body and others of animals with desirable characteristics such as strength, speed and sharp eyesight. In the former category are eyes, ears, the phallus and especially the heart. Favoured animals included the lion, cow, monkey and hedgehog.

Phylactic amulets were protective and included those of Bes, Taweret and the *wedjat* eye of Horus to which reference has already been made. A subcategory comprised the apotropaic amulets in the form of animals one desired to avoid, such as hippopotamus, crocodile and scorpion.

Theophoric (more correctly theomorphic) amulets covered most of the Egyptian pantheon, but specially relevant to medicine were Isis, Horus, Imhotep and Serqet, considered above. The amulet representing the girdle of Isis (Gardiner sign-list v 39) was reputed to staunch the flow of blood at miscarriage.

Sanatoria and incubation

In the context of ancient Egypt, the word 'sanatorium' describes a precinct where patients could be totally or partially immersed in healing holy water or practice incubation (temple sleep) in the hope of having a dream in which a deity would indicate a cure. The stela of Qen-her-khepeshef (see fig. 2.3) may give a very early account of such practices: '... I have spent the night in this forecourt. I have drunk the water. ...

My body has spent the night in the shadow of your face ...' (Quirke, 1992). Furthermore, this is a member of a family known to have been in possession of the Chester Beatty dream book. Otherwise, however, these practices are not proven before the Late Period, and the only archaeologically attested example is within the temple enclosure immediately to the west of the courtyard of the great temple of Hathor at Dendera (fig. 5.9). The main building is Ptolemaic and Roman but occupies the site of a much earlier temple. To the north is the *mammisi* or birth house and to the south is the well, beyond which lies the sacred lake. There is no evidence to suggest that the mud-brick sanatorium was used as a hospital for the practice of conventional medicine.

5.9 Plan of the 'sanatorium' associated with the Ptolemaic temple of Hathor in Dendera. The cubicles may be for the purpose of incubation, and surround a sacred pool.

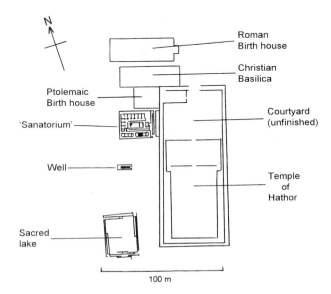

The structural remains show a number of cells around a sunken corridor. These are presumed to have been for incubation, and the corridor leads to a series of basins, which were filled with water from the sacred lake. The miraculous powers of the holy water could be made more efficacious by allowing it to flow over certain healing statues inscribed with appropriate texts. The basins could then be used for the immersion of parts of the body or even for total immersion. The dream book of the thirteenth century BC that features in the Chester Beatty papyrus III (British Museum 10683) lists a long series of dreams, noting which are good (*nefer*) and which are bad (*beyen*).

No healing statues have survived in Dendera, but a text on block is still in place in one cell. A complete example of a healing statue in black granite was found in Tell Atrib, belonging to a man called Djedhor (fig. 5.10). There is a small basin at the base where water would collect after being poured over the statue and its magical texts. The influence of the texts would be absorbed into the water and their effects obtained by drinking the water. The statue of Djedhor is holding a typical cippus (see above).

The sanatorium at Dendera appears to reflect much of the divine healing practised in ancient Greece, with which it would have been contemporary. The Greek god Asklepios, assisted by his daughter Hygieia, was the pre-eminent healing deity, and the major Asklepian sanctuaries were in Epidauros, Cos and Pergamum (Jackson, 1988). Ritual cleansing with water played a major part, and Greek experience of incubation is well documented (Edelstein and Edelstein, 1945). Suppliants would sleep in

5.10 The healing statue of Djedhor, from the Macedonian Period (Philip Arrhidaeus, c. 320 BC), found in Tell Atrib. In front of and below his feet is the basin for the collection of holy water. In front of his lower legs there is a typical cippus. (Cairo Museum, JdE 46341)

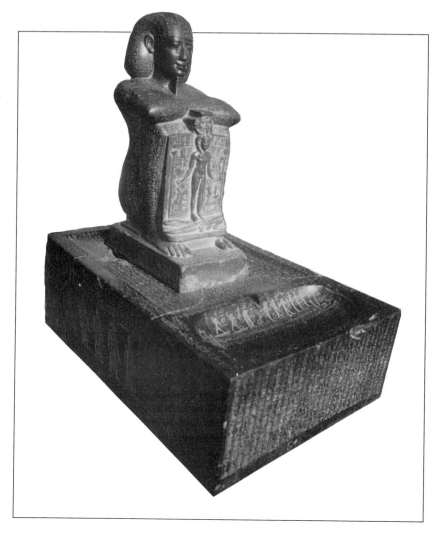

an *abaton* or sacred dormitory, which would seem to parallel the small rooms in Dendera, and priests were available to assist the patients in the interpretation of their dreams.

Conclusion

Magic and religion, inseparable in ancient Egypt, played a major role in treatment of the sick. Malign influences were thought to be the cause of many diseases, and it was common practice to invoke the help of a benign deity to counteract the malign influence. Sometimes a spell was recited in isolation and sometimes in conjunction with conventional medical therapy. Magicians and priests of various gods functioned as healers alongside the *swnw*, but protective gods were invoked directly by the use of amulets and by display of a cippus. With relatively few effective drugs and operations available, it would be wrong to underestimate the curative value of suggestion and expectation of cure which must have accompanied the use of magic.

CHAPTER SIX

The healers

Most people with pain, illness or injury will turn to another for help. In any human society, however simple its organisation, some will inevitably emerge as possessing, or appearing to possess, superior healing skills. These may be based on invoking the gods, on the exercise of magic, on the practice of what we recognise today as the art and science of conventional medicine, or on the use of so-called alternative forms of medicine such as osteopathy and homoeopathy.

There can be little doubt that doctors, priests and magicians were all involved in healing. The Ebers papyrus (854a) contains a misplaced gloss which makes this very clear (slightly different wording appears in the Edwin Smith papyrus, Case 1, Gloss A):

> There are vessels in him to all his limbs. As to these: If any doctor (*swnw*), any *wab* priest of Sekhmet or any magician (*sau*) places his two hands or his fingers on the head, on the back of the head, on the hands, on the place of the heart, on the two arms or on each of the two legs, he measures [or examines] the heart because of its vessels to all his limbs. It speaks from the vessels of all the limbs.

This passage contains convincing evidence that the relationship between the heart beat and the peripheral pulse was understood (see Chapter 3). However, the special relevance to our present discussion is the apparently parallel role of doctors, priests and magicians in what may be considered by us as conventional health care. Our forefathers would not have found this in the least surprising. Monks practised surgery until, in the twelfth century, it is said that the Pope forbade their shedding of blood. Thereafter they acted in an advisory capacity and, in Britain, some returned to active surgical practice after the Dissolution of the Monasteries in 1536. The Company of Barbers, incorporated in 1462, had a long tradition of surgery and indeed merged with the Guild of Surgeons in 1493. Their joint charter as the Company of Barber–Surgeons was granted by Henry VIII in 1540. Apothecaries were permitted to offer medical advice, and to this day a licentiate of the Society of Apothecaries is a registrable medical practitioner. In the Middle Ages there were journeying unqualified surgeons who specialised in such operations as cutting for stone in the bladder. Tight and monolithic control of medical practice is a recent development.

Who were the practitioners of conventional medicine?

It is difficult to define conventional medicine, and the process leads us into the pitfall of analysing the past in terms of modern concepts. It is perhaps better to start from the standpoint of ancient Egyptian medical practice, and then to see how we can relate to their ideas.

There is ample evidence in the Edwin Smith and parts of the Ebers papyri that ancient Egyptian healers had a three-phase approach to the management of their patients. First, they listened to their patients' symptoms and then examined them using their eyes and hands, as the following examples show:

> If you examine a man with obstruction of his stomach and it is irksome for him to eat bread. His belly is constricted and his heart is too feeble to go, like a man

suffering from heat/inflammation of the anus (sic). You should examine him lying down. You find his belly is hot and there is an obstruction in his stomach. (Ebers 188)

You should then place your hand on his stomach. You find his stomach dragging (sic). It goes and comes under your fingers. (Ebers 189)

You should then probe his wound although he shudders greatly. You then cause him to lift his face. ... He discharges blood from his two nostrils and from his two ears (Edwin Smith, Case 7)

Secondly, they reached their diagnosis and we find consistently in the Edwin Smith and occasionally in the Ebers papyri a formal pronouncement, often with a recapitulation of the important clinical findings. This section was introduced by the stock phrase 'You shall then say concerning him (or it)'. In the Edwin Smith papyrus, this section concluded with a declaration of whether the condition was to be treated, 'to be contended with', or not to be treated.

Sometimes it is difficult to follow the logic. The examination in Ebers 188 (cited above) is followed by the conclusion 'it is a case involving the liver'. On other occasions the logic is easy to follow and we can recognise jaw spasm, fractured base of skull and meningeal irritation in the following declaration which follows the examination in Edwin Smith Case 7 above:

One having a gaping wound in his head, penetrating to the bone. ...
The cord of his mandible [i.e. the temporalis muscle] is contracted; he discharges blood from his two nostrils and from his two ears; he suffers stiffness in his neck. An ailment with which I will contend.

It is clear that such passages were intended to guide the practitioner in reaching a diagnosis and deciding on a plan of action on the basis of a body of clinical experience, partly his own and partly from the oral and written experience of others. Transmission of the latter was the essential function of the medical papyri.

It was only after reaching a diagnosis and deciding on the overall approach that the healer proceeded to the third phase, which was treatment. This was mainly based on past experience of patients with similar conditions, and the Ebers papyrus often contains the phrase 'really excellent – a million times!' The whole three-phase approach could be repeated as the patient's condition changed, sometimes introduced with the phrase 'If you examine him after doing this' (Ebers 189).

This formal, structured and logical approach to the patient is very clearly recognisable as the basis of our current approach to a patient. It has been followed in unbroken succession through the Hippocratic school, Galen and on to the doctor of today. The differences over the passage of centuries have been in the understanding of the nature and causes of disease, the accuracy of diagnosis with more sophisticated technology, and the effectiveness of treatment with modern drugs and the expanded scope of surgery. The underlying philosophy is unchanged.

Having defined at some length what is meant by conventional medicine, we turn to the equally difficult question of who, in ancient Egypt, practised in this manner. There seems little doubt that the most important was the *swnw*, an Egyptian word usually translated as doctor or physician. However, it seems likely that he was not alone in the practice of conventional medicine, as suggested by the quotation at the beginning of this chapter. In particular, it now appears that certain priests did not restrict their ministrations to invoking the deities or practising magic but were involved in what we would regard as conventional medicine (see below). First, however, it is necessary to consider the *swnw* in further detail.

The doctor

There is ample evidence that the Egyptian word *swnw* (or <*sinw*>) should be translated as physician or doctor, meaning one who practised conventional medicine as defined above. Appendix B is a tabulation of known *swnw* of the pharaonic period drawn from the publications of Jonckheere (1958), van der Walle and de Meulenaere (1973), Ghaliounghui (1983), de Meulenaere (1986) and a personal communication from the last author (1994). Serial numbers in Appendix B cite references to these authors. After the Twenty-seventh Dynasty, the word *swnw* had come to mean embalmer as well as doctor and identification of profession is usually uncertain.

The phrase 'placing the hand' recurs so frequently in the medical papyri that it seems to be the hallmark of an ancient Egyptian doctor, as does the carrying of a stethoscope today. Westendorf (1992) raised the fundamental question of whether placing the hand was to establish the diagnosis or to cure by something analogous to the 'laying on of hands'. Perhaps it was both.

The Egyptian word for doctor

The hieroglyphic writing for *swnw* is shown in fig. 6.1. The word is conventionally pronounced in Britain as 'sewnew'. Jonckheere (1958) cited the full *scriptio plena* of the word with all the phonetic signs present (fig. 6.1a) and this also appears in the *Wörterbuch* of Erman and Grapow (1929), although not elsewhere to my knowledge. However, the related word *swnw*, meaning illness, is written out in the same form in the Berlin papyrus (161). This would seem to give strong support for the transliteration *swnw* as it appears in the *Grundriss*, VII 2 (Table 2.2). However, both Jonckheere (1958) and Westendorf (personal communication, 1990) prefer the transliteration 'sinw', which is closer to the Coptic word for doctor (*SAEIN*) and gives some indication of the likely pronunciation.

The fullest form of the word which is normally seen is in fig. 6.1b. In several unrelated words, the arrow (Gardiner sign-list T 11) is the triliteral phonetic for 'swn', while the pot or bowl (Gardiner sign-list W 24) is the very common biliteral phonetic 'nw'. The seated man is the male determinative (Gardiner sign-list A 1). For a female physician the male determinative is replaced with the feminine termination of the loaf (Gardiner sign-list X 1) which is the equivalent of the consonant 't'. Thus a lady doctor is a *swnwt* (fig. 6.1c). Whether this is a scribal error in the case of the lady Peseshet (Appendix B, no. 20) is considered below. The ancient Egyptians were somewhat relaxed about indicating plurality but, in the case of *swnw*, this may be shown either by three plural strokes or by three seated men determinatives.

It is possible that the arrow may also have the role of an ideogram, implying that the *swnw* was an 'arrow man', or one who was skilled at removing arrows from soldiers. This was a very difficult but important task (Mays, Parfitt and Hershman, 1994), which the *swnw* would have been expected to perform. It is often erroneously stated that the arrow is the doctor's lancet, and the pot his medicine jar. Many of the more elegant representations of the arrow leave no doubt that it is indeed an arrow, and two arrows are shown in a quiver (fig. 6.1d) on the coffins of the Middle Kingdom physicians Seni and Gua in the British Museum (see below).

Egyptian words are very commonly abbreviated, especially hieroglyphic inscriptions carved on stone, plaster or wood. The simplest designation of a doctor is simply an arrow, as in the wooden panel of Hesy-ra (see fig. 6.4). Often there is also the *nw* pot. It is less common to find the full writing as in fig. 6.1b.

The evidence for believing that *swnw* means 'doctor' is very strong indeed. Many ancient Egyptian words survive in Coptic, in which the word for 'physician' (*SAEIN*)

a)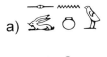

b)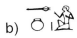

c)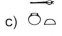

d)

6.1 Hieroglyphic writings of the word *swnw*, meaning physician or doctor. (a) The full writing, which was seldom used. (b) The fullest form which is normally seen. (c) Writing for *swnwt* (lady doctor) with the feminine termination 't', represented by the semicircular loaf (see fig. 6.5). (d) An unusual form in which the arrow is represented by a quiver with two arrows (see fig. 6.9).

is close to both *sinw* and *swnw*. Internal evidence from Egyptian papyri is also strong. In addition to the extract from the Ebers papyrus cited above, there are a number of passages which link the *swnw* to the care of the sick. The following are among the most convincing.

> [Thoth] ... imparts useful knowledge to the learned and to the *swnw* his followers, in order to free those whom his god wishes him to keep alive. (Ebers 1)

> ... You should then prepare a secret herb remedy which the *swnw* makes ... (Ebers 188)

> Manual of a collection of remedies of the *swnw*. (Chester Beatty VI, 8)

> And when you have fallen ill ... I will search for the chief *swnw* and he will prepare a remedy. (Papyrus Leyden I, 371)

The Berlin medical papyrus carries what appears at first sight to be the signature of a *swnw* (see p. 122):

> Sealed by the scribe of the god's words, chief of the skilful *swnw* Netjer-hetepu. (Berlin 163a)

The much damaged tomb inscription of Weshptah, vizier to Neferirkara (Fifth Dynasty) recounts how the pharaoh, while praising him, noticed that Weshptah did not hear him.

> [Weshptah was conveyed to] the residency, and his majesty caused the [royal] children, the companions, the lector priests and the chief *swnws* (plural) to go [there]. .... His majesty [had] brought to him a case of writings.

In spite of all, Weshptah died.

Further support for the meaning of *swnw* is provided by the inscription to Amenhotep-son-of-Hapu, the graffito from the Hatnub quarry concerning Hery-shef-nakht, and the statue inscription of the *swnw* Wedja-hor-resnet, all of which are reproduced below.

Titles of doctors

Probably the majority of doctors were designated simply as *swnw*. However, special titles were not uncommon, particularly among the very distinguished doctors who were granted burials with memorials which have survived. We can identify six special grades which, in other contexts, imply administrative authority (Table 6.1). It is very difficult to say what was the correct ranking order of these titles, if indeed there was a recognised hierarchical structure.

The most exalted title appears to be *kherep swnw*, which would mean controller or administrator of doctors. The only example is Medu-nefer (Appendix B, no. 28), a court ophthalmologist from the Old Kingdom. *Hery swnw* means one with authority over doctors, most examples being New Kingdom. The title *imy-r* is very common in other contexts and is usually translated as overseer. *Sehedj* is translated as inspector, and all fourteen examples of *sehedj swnw* are from the Old Kingdom. The most common special title is *wer swnw*, with fifty-two examples covering all periods. Egyptian adjectives normally follow nouns, and it is unlikely that *wer* is here the adjective 'great', but more likely the noun 'great one' or 'chief' with *swnw* following as an indirect genitive. Faulkner (1962) translates *wer swnw* as 'master physician'. *Wer* is commonly represented by its very common biliteral phonetic the swallow (Gardiner sign-list G 36) but, in seven of the *wer swnw* listed in Table 6.1, the sign is that of a

Table 6.1 Hierarchical titles of known doctors

	OLD KINGDOM AND FIRST INTERMEDIATE PERIOD	MIDDLE KINGDOM	SECOND INTERMEDIATE PERIOD AND NEW KINGDOM	THIRD INTERMEDIATE PERIOD AND LATE PERIOD
kherep swnw administrator of doctors	1	–	–	–
hery swnw one with authority over doctors	2	–	5	1
imy-r swnw overseer of doctors	2	1	1	–
sehedj swnw inspector of doctors	14	–	–	–
wer swnw chief of doctors	12	15	16	9
imy-r geswy depet per aa swnw overseer of the two sides of the boat of doctors of the palace	1	–	–	–
swnw doctor	30	5	25	6
foreign doctors	–	–	4	–
totals	62	21	51	16

stooping man leaning on a stick. Jonckheere (1958) interpreted this as Gardiner sign-list A 20, normally read as *semsu*, meaning eldest. He therefore proposed the title of 'doyen'. However, Ghaliounghui (1983) has pointed out that, in some cases, the stick is not forked and the sign thus appears to be Gardiner sign-list A 19, which can have the same meaning as the swallow. I have listed them all as *wer swnw*. Mereruka (Appendix B, no. 25) of the Sixth Dynasty had a unique title which is considered below.

Occasionally an administrative doctor's title was followed by the geographical limits of his authority, such as Upper or Lower Egypt or both. The physician Pu-ra (App. B, no. 95) of the New Kingdom was *wer swnw* in the Place of Truth, which means the necropolis.

Titles such as controller, inspector or overseer of doctors raise the interesting question of whether these persons were in fact doctors themselves. In the United Kingdom today it is quite usual for those in administrative charge of doctors to be lay persons, and this might very well have applied in ancient Egypt. This is of special interest in the case of the lady Peseshet (see below).

Doctors with royal connections

Not uncommon is the title of *swnw per aa*, which means doctor of the Great House or palace (Table 6.2). 'Court physician' is probably the best English translation. The hieroglyphs for great house normally precede *swnw* because of honorific transposition. By the New Kingdom, the phrase *per aa* had come to mean the king, and from *per aa* is derived the word 'pharaoh'. More specific is the title *swnw (n) nesu*, meaning doctor of the king, which has been found only in the Middle and New Kingdoms. *Swnw n neb tawy* means doctor to the lord of the two lands and must also refer to the

Table 6.2 Known doctors with royal connections

	OLD KINGDOM AND FIRST INTERMEDIATE PERIOD	MIDDLE KINGDOM	SECOND INTERMEDIATE PERIOD AND NEW KINGDOM	THIRD INTERMEDIATE PERIOD AND LATE PERIOD
sehedj swnw per aa inspector of palace doctors	3	–	–	–
wer swnw per aa chief of palace physicians	7	1	1	1
imy-r geswy depet per aa swnw overseer of the two sides of the boat of doctors of the palace	1	–	–	–
swnw per aa doctor of the palace	14	–	–	–
kherep swnw per aa administrator of doctors of the palace	1	–	–	–
sehedj swnw n nesu inspector of doctors to the king	1	–	–	–
wer swnw n nesu chief of doctors to the king	–	1	–	–
swnw n neb tawy doctor to the lord of the two lands	–	–	1	–
hery swnw n neb tawy one with authority over the doctors to the lord of the two lands	–	–	2	–
wer swnw n neb tawy chief of doctors to the lord of the two lands	–	–	1	1
swnw n nesu doctor to the king	–	–	1	–
wer swnw n per hemet nesu chief of doctors to the queen	–	–	1	–
swnw n per hemet nesu doctor to the queen	–	–	1	–

king himself. The title *swnw n per hemet nesut* means doctor to the house of the royal wife or queen. Two Old Kingdom *swnw* carry the title *rekh nesu* (known to the king).

Almost half of all known doctors and dentists in the Old Kingdom had a royal connection, and this probably reflects their privileged position, which resulted either in their being granted a tomb which has survived or that they should be mentioned in the tombs of important officials. After the Old Kingdom it became easier for common persons to achieve a substantial burial, and the proportion of known doctors with royal connections becomes much less.

Specialisation

About 430 BC Herodotus made his celebrated visit to Egypt and remarked on the

Table 6.3 Known specialists

	OLD KINGDOM AND FIRST INTERMEDIATE PERIOD	MIDDLE KINGDOM	SECOND INTERMEDIATE PERIOD AND NEW KINGDOM	THIRD INTERMEDIATE PERIOD AND LATE PERIOD
ophthalmologist	7*	–	–	2*
gastro-enterologist	2*	–	–	1*
proctologist	2*	–	–	–
dentist/doctor	3*	–	–	1
dentist only	2	–	–	–
swnw – supervisor of butchers	3	–	–	–
inspector of the liquids in the *netnetet*	2*	–	–	–
total involved in one or more specialties	16*	–	–	3*

*Indicates some practitioners involved in more than one specialty.

degree of specialisation he found. This is borne out by the qualifying words, usually parts of the body, which follow *swnw* on many stelae. Thus, for example, *swnw khet* means doctor of the abdomen, which we may interpret as gastro-enterologist, with three known examples. More common is the title *swnw irty* meaning doctor of the eyes or ophthalmologist, of whom nine are known.

Certain specialties are more difficult to interpret. The multi-specialist Ir-en-akhty (see below) carried the designation *neru pehuyt*, which can be translated literally as herdsman of the anus. It is perhaps significant that he was not *neru pehuyt per aa*. It would surely be inappropriate to imply that the royal palace required the services of a proctologist! Still more obscure was the title *aaa mu m-khenu netnetet*, usually translated as the interpreter of the liquids in the *netnetet* (which cannot at present be translated). Strangely, there are no known examples of specialists in the Middle and New Kingdoms. Most are in the Old Kingdom, but there are three in the Late Period when Herodotus made his visit (Table 6.3).

Dentists carried the separate title *ibeh*. Three of the five known dentists of the Old Kingdom also carried the title *swnw*, corresponding to the doubly qualified doctor/dentists of today. A small number of doctors recorded the fact that they were also scribes. This emphasises the dignity of the profession of scribe.

There is no clear indication in the papyri, or in funerary inscriptions, that surgery was a separate branch of medicine as it is today. The Ebers papyrus contains instructions for minor surgical interventions interspersed among prescriptions which would be used for typical medical conditions (see Chapter 8). Furthermore, there is no evidence for anything but the simplest repertoire of surgical procedures. However, Ebbell (1937) noted that the quotation from the predominantly medical Ebers papyrus (854a) at the beginning of this chapter lists the *swnw* before the *wab* priest of Sekhmet. He contrasted this with the corresponding passage in the Edwin Smith surgical papyrus, where the order was reversed. From this he hypothesised that the *swnw* was predominantly a physician and the *wab* priest of Sekhmet a surgeon.

The veterinary surgeon

Ghaliounghui (1983) suggested that the *wab* priest of Sekhmet might have a special role as a veterinary surgeon, for whom no Egyptian word has yet been identified, other than the epithet *rekh kau* (one who knows the bulls). He pointed out that it would be logical for priests to be concerned with the well-being of sacrificial or divine animals. There are three *swnw* from the Old Kingdom, who are portrayed supervising butchery. One of these is Wenen-nefer (Fifth Dynasty; App. B, no. 17) who was a *wab* priest of Sekhmet as well as a *sehedj swnw* (inspector of physicians) (Mariette, 1889). The other two have the hieroglyph for *wab* before *swnw*, but no mention of Sekhmet. However, the dominant hieroglyph of *wab* priest can also mean 'pure', perhaps designating something analogous to the modern concept of a public health doctor.

In the tomb of Petosiris at the beginning of the Ptolemaic period (Lefebvre, 1924) there is a reference to his 'herds being numerous in the stable thanks to the skill of the *wab* priest of Sekhmet' (58c, 26). However, the Kahun veterinary papyrus makes no mention of any role for *wab* priests of Sekhmet in the care of animals.

The graffito in the Hatnub quarry relating to Hery-shef-nakht (see below) also shows his colleague Aha-nakht, a *wab* priest of Sekhmet, without the title of *swnw*, but who appeared to share his medical duties. Aha-nakht carried the additional title of *rekh kau*.

Swnw with priestly titles

Many *swnw* carried priestly titles. There are four known *wab* (or *imy-r wab*) priests of Sekhmet (Table 6.4). Apart from Wenen-nefer (Appendix B, no. 17), involved in the butchery scene, there were Nedjemu (App. B, no. 73) and Hery-shef-nakht (App. B, no. 75) of the Middle Kingdom, and Amenhotep (App. B, no. 85) of the New Kingdom. Others carry such titles as *hem netjer* (servant of god) and *wab nesu* (royal priest). Other priestly titles are relevant to the practice of magic and are considered below and in Chapter 5.

Certain *swnw* in the New Kingdom were appointed to work in estates of gods. Amenhotep (App. B, no. 86) and Pahatyu (App. B, no. 93) were overseers of doctors in the estate of Amun; Innay (App. B, no. 87) was an overseer of doctors in the estate of Ptah; Pu-ra (App. B, no. 95) was a *wer swnw* in the Place of Truth (the necropolis).

Association of the *swnw* with magic

Chapter 5 discusses the role of magicians in the provision of health care. Here, we merely note instances of *swnw* who carried titles indicating their status as professional magicians (Table 6.4).

The word *sau* appeared in the quotation from the Ebers papyrus at the beginning of this chapter and is translated simply as 'magician'. This title was probably borne by two physicians: Akmu (App. B, no. 67) and another anonymous *swnw* (App. B, no. 82) of the Middle Kingdom (see Chapter 5).

Priesthoods of the god Heka and the goddess Serqet implied status as professional magicians (p. 99). *Heka* also means magicians and Hery-shef-nakht (App. B, no. 75) was overseer of *hekaw* (see below). The title *kherep* Serqet was borne by Ir-en-akhty (App. B, no. 7; see below), Khuy, another multi-specialist (App. B, no. 49), an anonymous *wer swnw* (App. B, no. 83), Nemty-em-hat (App. B, no. 66) and Psamtek-soneb (App. B, no. 145). Mereruka (App. B, no. 25) and Huy (App. B, no. 147) were lector priests (*khery-hebet*), a title closely associated with magic and, in particular, the recitation of spells and incantations (pp. 98–9).

Remuneration of the doctor and control of practice

We are not well informed on how doctors were remunerated for their services in the pharaonic period. Barter or money-barter (Janssen, 1975) was the normal practice before the introduction of money in the Late Period: Table 1.4 lists the calorific value

Table 6.4 Doctors holding priestly titles or connected with magic

	OLD KINGDOM AND FIRST INTERMEDIATE PERIOD	MIDDLE KINGDOM	SECOND INTERMEDIATE PERIOD AND NEW KINGDOM	THIRD INTERMEDIATE PERIOD AND LATE PERIOD
imy-r wab priest of Sekhmet	–	2	–	–
wab priest of Sekhmet	1	–	1	–
kherep of priest of Serqet	2	2	–	1
wab priest of the gods	–	–	–	1
imy-r wab priest of the court	1	–	–	–
wab priest of the king	4	–	–	–
wab priest	2	–	1	–
hem netjer priest	1	–	1	–
Magicians				
lector priest	1	–	–	1
imy-r magician (*hekaw*)	–	1	–	–
hem netjer priest of Hekaw	2	–	–	–
magician (*sau*)	–	2	–	–

of the rations for the doctor in the necropolis workers' village of Deir el-Medina in the Nineteenth Dynasty. Presumably these were in addition to his basic ration as a workman.

There is a little more information for the Ptolemaic Period. Writing in the first century BC, Diodorus Siculus (Book I, 82) said:

> On their military campaigns and their journeys in the country they all receive treatment without the payment of any private fee; for the physicians draw their support from public funds and administer their treatments in accordance with a written law which was composed in ancient times by many famous physicians. If they follow the rules of this law as they read them in the sacred book and yet are unable to save their patient, they are absolved from any charge and go unpunished; but if they go contrary to the law's prescriptions in any respect, they must submit to a trial with death as the penalty, the lawgiver holding that but few physicians would ever show themselves wiser than the mode of treatment which had been closely followed for a long period and had been originally prescribed by the ablest practitioners. (Loeb edition)

The general tenor accords well with the intense conservatism of the Egyptians, but it is unclear whether the state sponsored treatment was restricted to the military and civil servants. The tight control of standards of practice as outlined by Diodorus Siculus would have been extremely difficult to maintain, and it would be surprising if doctors did not receive some form of direct remuneration from treatment of the general public.

Legendary doctors

Djer

Djer (Athothis) was a pharaoh of the First Dynasty buried at Abydos approximately 3000 BC. Information on his role in medicine stems solely from the *History of Egypt* written by the Egyptian priest Manetho for the Greeks in the third century BC. The passage describing Djer as a physician and an anatomist is cited at the beginning of Chapter 3. It is hard to believe that a pharaoh would either have been a *swnw* or that he would have engaged in anatomical studies at that early date. There is no known Egyptian inscription which supports Manetho's claims for Athothis.

Imhotep

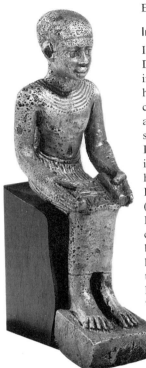

Imhotep was the royal chamberlain to King Netjerkhet (Djoser) of the Third Dynasty, and the architect of the step pyramid, the oldest surviving major stone building in the world. Africanus quoted Manetho, referring to Djoser, 'who because of his medical skill has the reputation of Asklepios among the Egyptians'. Eusebius' citation was similar. It is generally believed that this must have referred to Imhotep and not Djoser himself. Possibly by the Nineteenth, and certainly by the Twenty-seventh, Dynasty, Imhotep was deified as the 'son of Ptah'. During the Thirtieth Dynasty, in the inscription on a private statue belonging to Pasherentaihet, Imhotep is addressed as 'one who comes to the one who calls to him to cast off sickness and heal the body' (Wildung, 1977a, b). In the Ptolemaic Period, the Greeks identified Imhotep with Asklepios, their god of medicine. In the second century BC, Ptolemy VIII (Euergetes II) built a shrine to Imhotep at the great temple of Hatshepsut in Deir el-Bahri, which then became a place of pilgrimage by the sick. Figure 6.2 shows his typical representation in countless small statuettes. However, Imhotep's tomb has never been found and it is not known whether he held the title of *swnw*. Therefore, although he was clearly a polymath of great distinction, it is generally agreed by Egyptologists that he cannot, on currently available evidence, be considered as a *swnw*. Nevertheless, the great physician Sir William Osler pronounced in 1923 that Imhotep was 'the first figure of a physician to stand out clearly from the mists of antiquity'. It is sad that this cannot at present be confirmed, but his cult remains strong to this day (Estes, 1989).

6.2 Typical copper alloy statuette of Imhotep, deified long after his death, as a healer, seated with a papyrus roll on his knee (26th Dynasty). (British Museum, EA 11061)

Amenhotep-son-of-Hapu

The base of a statue was found at Karnak with the following remarkable inscription, placed by an otherwise unknown daughter of Psamtek I in the Twenty-sixth (Saite) Dynasty:

> O, Prince Amenhotep son of Hapu, justified [i.e. dead]. Come, O good doctor. Behold, I suffer in my eyes. Cause me to be well immediately because I made this [statue] for you ...

Amenhotep-son-of-Hapu was a royal scribe of great distinction under Amenhotep III (Eighteenth Dynasty) but there is no contemporary evidence that he held the title of *swnw*. The king established a regular funerary cult for Amenhotep-son-of-Hapu 'in recognition of his perfect character' (Wildung, 1977a, b) and it appears that he was deified by the time of the Twenty-sixth Dynasty.

Many healing shrines feature Imhotep and Amenhotep-son-of-Hapu side by side, and fig. 6.3 shows them in relief on the rear (east) wall of the Ptah temple at Karnak. Each had become recognisable with standard iconography.

6.3 (opposite) Imhotep (left) and Amenhotep-son-of-Hapu (right) were both deified long after their deaths and venerated as healers. This relief is on the outside of the rear (east) wall of the Ptah temple at Karnak (probably 26th Dynasty or later).

Netjer-hotep

Netjer-hotep is mentioned three times in Berlin 163 as a *swnw* who is the author of the papyrus (see Chapter 2). The name may merely symbolise one who appeases

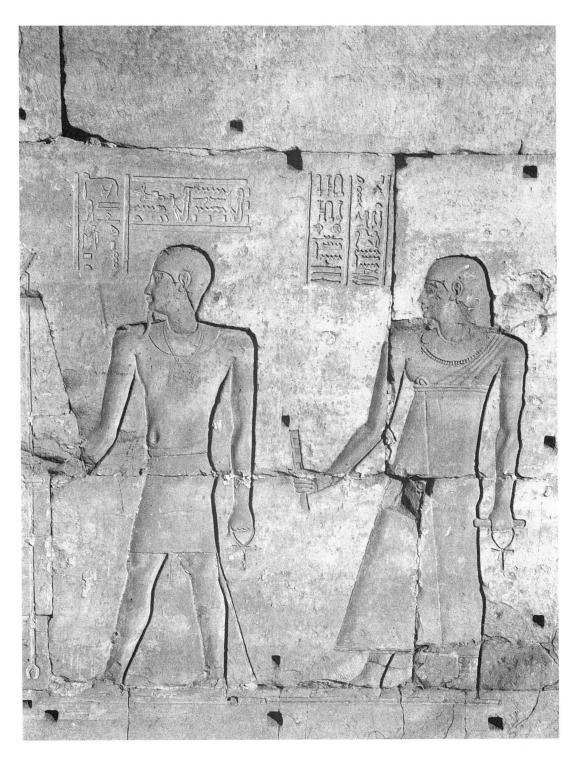

(*hetep*) malign gods (*netjer*) or disease-demons, and there is general agreement that his existence is unproven (Jonckheere, 1958).

None of these legendary doctors has been included in Appendix B.

Notes on ten selected pharaonic doctors

In this section I have selected ten doctors of special interest who will give some insight into the medical profession in pharaonic times. I have attempted to select examples from different social strata as well as from the various time periods of ancient Egypt. I have also tried to show some of the diverse circumstances by which they have become known to us.

Hesy-ra OLD KINGDOM, THIRD DYNASTY

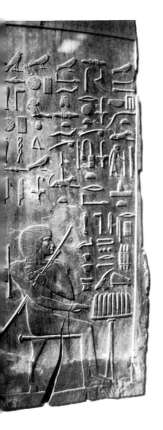

6.4 Wooden stela of Hesy-ra, 3rd Dynasty, showing (top right corner) his title as 'chief of dentists and doctors'. (Cairo Museum, JdE 28504)

Hesy-ra (Appendix B, no. 46) is unique in being the first authenticated doctor in the world (*c.* 2650 BC). A man of great distinction, he held many exalted titles under King Netjerkhet (Djoser) and would have been a contemporary of Imhotep. His tomb, north of the stepped pyramid of Djoser in Saqqara (s 2401; Porter and Moss, 1981), was described in detail by Quibell (1913). The tomb contained six magnificent wooden niche-stelae in a wonderful state of preservation and now in the Cairo Museum. The top right-hand corner of one of these (fig. 6.4) shows the swallow, tusk and arrow – *wer ibeh swnw* – 'chief of dentists and doctors' (see fig. 6.1).

It is difficult to see how Hesy-ra could have combined his many important posts with the practice of medicine and dentistry. Was *wer ibeh swnw* perhaps an honorary title? Was he a doctor who rose to higher things in later life, but remained sufficiently proud of his medical and dental qualifications to place them at the head of this stela? Was he perhaps a layman with an administrative role in the health services? The title *wer swnw* hardly suggests a purely administrative non-medical role, as might well be the case for *kherep* or *sehedj swnw* (see Table 6.1).

Peseshet OLD KINGDOM, FIFTH TO SIXTH DYNASTY

The lady Peseshet (Appendix B, no. 20) had her own stela in the tomb of Akhet-hotep, probably her son, in Giza (Hassan, 1932). In three places on the stela (fig. 6.5) we see the hieroglyphs *imy-r swnwt*, which present an interesting problem. The word for overseer is *imy-r*, *imy* being a *nisbe* adjective which should agree in gender and number with the noun which it qualifies. A female overseer should therefore be written *imt-r* or *imyt-r*, with '*t*' as the feminine termination. However, the Egyptians were none too meticulous in the use of the feminine termination in adjectives, and the same error occurs in Peseshet's title *imy-r hem-ka* 'overseer of the funerary priests'. Jonckheere (1958) believed the writing to be scribal errors for *imyt-r sinw(w)* 'directrice des médecins'. Majno (1975) preferred to read the title as it had been written and translated it as 'chief woman physician'. Ghaliounghui (1983) reconstructed to *imy(t)-r swnwt* and translated as 'lady director of lady physicians'.

With or without the terminal '*t*', *imy-r* must refer to Peseshet and mean '[female] overseer'. However, the Egyptians almost never used a feminine termination in error in a masculine word, and *swnwt* must surely mean female physician(s). Furthermore, it seems unlikely that a woman would have been the overseer of male doctors in the Old Kingdom. Therefore I believe that the title should read '[female] overseer of the female doctors'. It does not necessarily follow that Peseshet was herself a doctor, but I would like to believe that she was and so should have the distinction of being the first recorded lady doctor. No other Egyptian lady doctors are known until at least the Ptolemaic Period.

These distinctions are not purely academic. If Peseshet was *imyt-r swnwt* then we know that female doctors existed in the Old Kingdom, 4000 years before Elizabeth Garrett Anderson. If the reading is *imyt-r sinw*, as Jonckheere suggested, then Peseshet would seem to be the female overseer of the physicians and we could not be entirely certain that female doctors existed at that time.

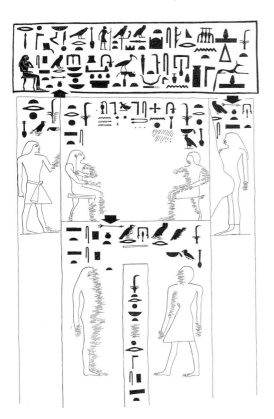

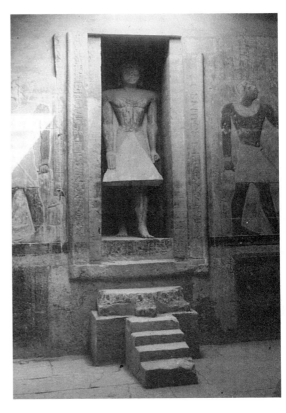

6.5 (above) Stela of the lady Peseshet, 5th to 6th Dynasty, showing her title of 'overseer of the female physicians' (indicated in three places by broad arrows). From the tomb of Akhet-hotep in Giza (Hassan, 1932).

6.6 (right) The ka of Mereruka shown striding from the false door of his 6th Dynasty tomb in Saqqara. His many titles included 'overseer of the two sides of the boat of the physicians of the great house' (i.e. the palace).

Mereruka OLD KINGDOM, SIXTH DYNASTY

Mereruka (Appendix B, no. 25) was vizier and son-in-law to King Teti. As might be expected, he was granted a splendid tomb immediately adjacent to the pyramid of Teti in Saqqara (fig. 6.6). The mastaba of Mereruka contains more strings of titles by far than any other tomb (Baer, 1960). Among these is the unique title *imy-r geswy depet swnw per aa*, which translates literally as 'overseer of the two sides of the boat of the doctors of the great house'. This would appear to be an adaptation of a nautical tradition which divided the crew of a ship into two teams of oarsmen, one for each side of the boat. Indeed, it is still customary in the British Royal Navy to divide a ship's crew into port and starboard watches. The words *imy-r geswy* are known in other administrative titles outside the field of medicine, and gangs of workers in the royal necropolis of the Valley of the Kings were so divided. However, the use of such a phrase in a medical context is unique, and curious to say the least.

Jonckheere (1958) and Ghaliounghui (1983) have reviewed the discussions of this title, the former including Mereruka in his listing of doctors and the latter excluding him. I have favoured his inclusion because I cannot see that his own personal standing as a *swnw* is any less certain than that of an *imy-r swnw*, a *kherep swnw* or a *sehedj swnw*. Nevertheless, it is hard to imagine the pharaoh's son-in-law practising medicine.

Ankh OLD KINGDOM, SIXTH DYNASTY

We have no knowledge of Ankh's tomb. He is, however, an example of the many doctors known to posterity only because of mention in a relief on the wall of someone else's tomb, in this case a tomb of exceptional interest from the medical point of view. Ankh (Appendix B, no. 12) is seen (fig. 6.7) bearing four ducks as offerings in the funerary procession of the tomb owner Ankh-ma-hor. In front of him is his title and name, *swnw per aa* Ankh. As court physician he might well have been a personal

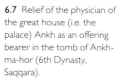

6.7 Relief of the physician of the great house (i.e. the palace) Ankh as an offering bearer in the tomb of Ankh-ma-hor (6th Dynasty, Saqqara).

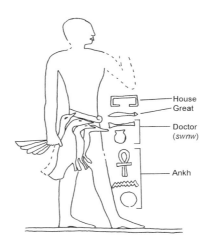

House
Great

Doctor
(*swnw*)

Ankh

friend of Ankh-ma-hor, or perhaps he was his doctor (or both). Those represented in reliefs were believed to be accessible to the tomb owner in the hereafter, and there might be distinct advantages in having your own doctor with you in the afterworld.

Ankh-ma-hor was, like Mereruka, vizier to Teti, and their mastaba tombs are close together immediately to the north of their master Teti's pyramid. Ankh-ma-hor possessed many important titles but none of direct relevance to medicine. Nevertheless, his tomb contains no fewer than seven items of medical interest to us today:

> Portrayal of the court physician Ankh (see above)
> Representation of a circumcision (see fig. 8.4)
> Scene of manipulation of toes and fingers (see fig. 6.14)
> Portrayal of a hydrocele (see fig. 4.15)
> Achondroplasiac dwarfs working as craftsmen (p. 78)
> Portrayal of obesity (see fig. 4.11)
> Portrayal of gynaecomastia (see fig. 4.11)

We are fortunate that Ankh-ma-hor should have chosen to display this remarkable concentration of items of medical interest. There is evidence that he went to great trouble in the planning, supervision and even the alterations to the reliefs in his tomb (see Badawy, 1978; Firth and Gunn, 1926).

Ir-en-akhty FIRST INTERMEDIATE PERIOD

Ir-en-akhty's false door (fig. 6.8) was found in Giza by Junker (1928). Interest lies particularly in the wide range of medical specialties which the deceased (Appendix B, no. 7) appeared to practise. Readings on the false door include the following:

> *swnw per aa* (appears five times): court physician
> *sehedj swnw per aa*: inspector of court physicians
> *swnw irty per aa*: court ophthalmologist
> *swnw khet per aa*: court gastro-enterologist
> *neru phuyt*: proctologist (lit. herdsman of the anus)
> *aaa mu m-khenu netetet*: interpreter of liquids in the *netetet*

6.8 False door of Ir-en-akhty (1st Intermediate Period), showing the modern equivalents for his remarkable range of medical specialties, mainly practised in the great house (i.e. the palace). The stela was found at Giza and described by Junker (1928).

Gua MIDDLE KINGDOM, ELEVENTH / TWELFTH DYNASTY

Seni (brother) MIDDLE KINGDOM, ELEVENTH / TWELFTH DYNASTY

Gua (Appendix B, no. 80) and Seni (App. B, no. 78) were both *wer swnw* and their beautiful wooden outer coffins, typical of the Middle Kingdom, lie beside one another in the British Museum (nos 30839 and 30840). In each case, the arrow of *swnw* is represented by a quiver containing two arrows (fig. 6.9). In one place on the coffin of Gua

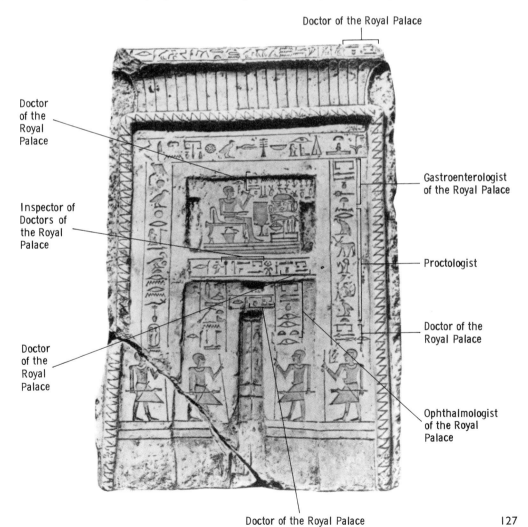

Doctor of the Royal Palace

Doctor of the Royal Palace

Doctor of the Royal Palace

Inspector of Doctors of the Royal Palace

Doctor of the Royal Palace

Gastroenterologist of the Royal Palace

Proctologist

Doctor of the Royal Palace

Ophthalmologist of the Royal Palace

Doctor of the Royal Palace

6.9 Inscription from the wooden coffin of the chief physician Gua, from el-Bersha, Middle Kingdom. The word for doctor is here abbreviated to the quiver shown under the swallow (see also fig. 6.1d). (British Museum, EA 30839)

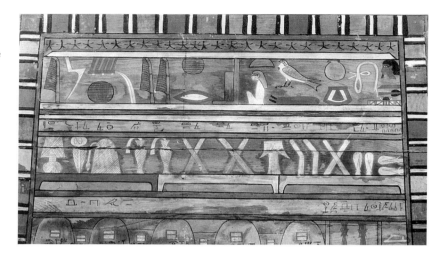

this looks like the semi-hieratic form of the roll of bread (Gardiner sign-list X 5), which is often used instead of the ear of an ox (Gardiner sign-list F 21), but elsewhere (and in the case of Seni) there can be no doubt that they are arrows (see Edwards, 1938).

Renef-seneb MIDDLE KINGDOM, TWELFTH DYNASTY

Renef-seneb (Appendix B, no. 74) held the title of *wer swnw* but, unlike some of the examples above, he appears to have been a plain working doctor in an uncongenial industrial environment. He is known solely because his name is included, along with more than a hundred other names, on a stela (no. 85) in a quarry in Sinai (Serabit el-Khadim), where he was presumably the doctor to the team (Gardiner, Peet and Cerny, 1952). It seems astonishing that he should share the same title as men such as Hesy-ra and Wedja-hor-resnet (below), who clearly moved in the highest circles in the land, yet still took pains to emphasise their title of *wer swnw*. Other stelae in the same location list two other *swnw*: Akmu (App. B, no. 67) and another, anonymous, man (App. B, no. 82), who probably carried the additional title of *sau* (magician).

Hery-shef-nakht MIDDLE KINGDOM, TWELFTH DYNASTY

Bearing an even more illustrious title than the previous example, Hery-shef-nakht (Appendix B, no. 75) was *wer swnw n nesu*, chief of the king's physicians. However, he is known to posterity only as a result of a hieratic graffito (fig. 6.10) in the Hatnub alabaster quarries, near Tell el-Amarna (Anthes, 1928). Hery-shef-nakht is unique in bearing the triple qualification as specified in the excerpt from the Ebers papyrus at the beginning of this chapter: he was *wer swnw*, *wab* priest of Sekhmet and also an overseer of magicians (*imy-r hekau*). The glimpse of his work is tantalisingly brief:

> Reading the papyrus rolls daily ... when he is sick, who places his hand on a man when he knows it [i.e. the illness], who is skilled in examining strongly.

The last word in this passage is *djerit*, which would appear to be derived from *djeri* meaning strong or strongly. Anthes translated this as 'by the hand' and the usual word for hand is *djeret*. Although the transliteration is similar, the hieroglyphs are quite different. Furthermore, there is no word corresponding to 'by'.

No less interesting is the fact that the graffito is shared by Hery-shef-nakht's apparent colleague Aha-nakht, shown smaller and therefore in a subordinate role. Aha-

6.10 Hieratic graffito from the alabaster quarries in Hatnub (12th Dynasty), showing the chief of the king's physicians Hery-shef-nakht and his colleague Aha-nakht (Anthes, 1928).

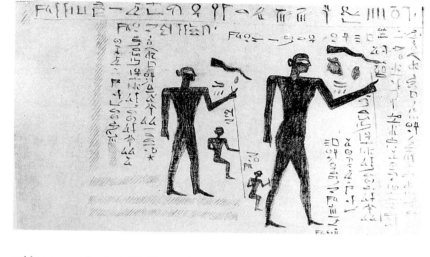

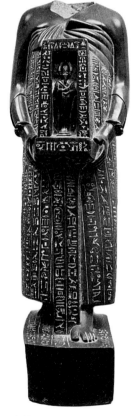

6.11 Statue of the chief physician Wedja-hor-resnet (27th Dynasty). His statue is engraved with an extensive curriculum vitae. The head was lost in antiquity, and inappropriate replacements have been added and removed from time to time. (Vatican Museum, 22690)

nakht was a *wab* priest of Sekhmet, though neither *swnw* nor magician. Nevertheless, he described his work in similar terms to Hery-shef-nakht as placing the hand and being skilled in so doing. There is, however, no mention of reading the papyrus roll daily (presumably reciting a spell) which perhaps accorded with Aha-nakht not being a magician. This scene provides exceptional and quite remarkable confirmation of the parallel role of the *swnw* and the *wab* priest of Sekhmet in providing conventional medical attention, as specified in the passage from the Ebers papyrus at the beginning of this chapter. Aha-nakht was also *rekh kau* (one who knows oxen) and therefore probably a vet (see above).

Wedja-hor-resnet LATE PERIOD, TWENTY-SEVENTH DYNASTY

Wedja-hor-resnet (Appendix B, no. 138) is depicted in a green basalt naophorus statue (inv. no. 22690) in the Vatican (fig. 6.11). The head, arms and shoulders depart from the Egyptian canon and were restored, probably in Roman times. There is an extensive inscription over the plinth, body and the naos, which gives a most important biographical account of the establishment of the Twenty-seventh (Persian) Dynasty by Cambyses (Cambyses II of Persia), who assigned to Wedja-hor-resnet the office of *wer swnw* (Lichtheim, 1980). He held many very important titles, including royal seal-bearer, sole companion to the king, administrator of the palace and commander of the royal navy. In spite of these very high offices he declared himself to be a *wer swnw* no fewer than ten times, and it is clear that he attached great importance to this title.

On the back plinth is an important statement concerning the command he received from Darius I (the second king of the Twenty-seventh Dynasty) to restore the *per ankh*, the 'House of Life', which had fallen into decay. The inscription continues: 'His majesty did this because he knew the virtue of this art to revive all that are sick …'. The extent to which this passage provides evidence that the *per ankh* functioned as a medical school is considered below.

Training of the doctor

Transmission of knowledge within the family

Countless stelae bear testimony to sons following the profession of their fathers. The Greek historian Diodorus Siculus, writing in the first century BC, said:

They are instructed from their childhood by their fathers or relatives, in the practices proper to each manner of life. ... they are the only people where all the craftsmen are forbidden to follow any other occupation ... than those ... handed down to them from their parents. (I, 74 & 81)

This finds some support in the following, rather obscure, extract from the Ebers papyrus (206):

You shall prepare for him medicines, secret to who is under the doctor, except for your own daughter.

The word for 'under' would here be in the sense of 'under the authority of' rather than 'under the treatment of'. With man and woman determinatives (not present here), the plural can mean 'relatives', and is so translated in the *Grundriss* (IV 1, 94). It is not clear why the passage should specify daughter rather than son but, whatever the true meaning of this difficult passage, it appears to support transmission of knowledge within the family.

Jonckheere and Ghaliounghui report no examples of sons following their father as a doctor in ancient Egypt, although Jonckheere (1958) reported two families, one of which contained two doctors and another with three, but without filiation between doctors. I am grateful to Professor Kitchen for drawing my attention to the Ashmolean stela (1883.14) of Iuny, which shows two known *wer swnw*: Huy (App. B, no. 110) and Khay (App. B, no. 113). What appeared to have escaped notice is that Khay was described, almost certainly in relation to Huy, as 'his son who causes his name to live' (fig. 6.12). Professor Kitchen also drew my attention to the Louvre stela

6.12 (below) Stela of Iuny showing, in the second register, the chief physician Huy and his son the chief physician Khay (19th Dynasty). See also fig. 6.13. (Ashmolean Museum, 1883.14)

6.13 (right) Another stela of Iuny showing, in the lower register, the chief physician Huy being offered incense by another of his sons, the physician Kha-em-waset (19th Dynasty). See also fig. 6.12. (Louvre, C 89)

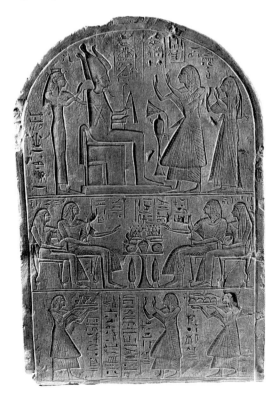

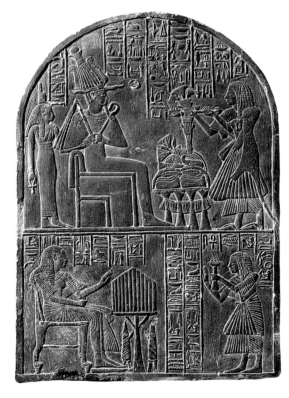

C 89 (fig. 6.13), which seemed to have escaped the notice of both Jonckheere and Ghaliounghui. This is a second stela belonging to Iuny and also features Huy, but here his name is caused to live by one who appears to be another of his sons, the *swnw* Kha-em-waset, first listed (App. B, no. 116) by de Meulenaere (1986).

The papyri as textbooks

There can be little doubt that the medical papyri (Chapter 2) fulfilled a role no less important than that of medical texts today. Many were in a format which simply listed remedies for named diseases, and these were clearly intended for reference because the drugs available to the ancient Egyptians were far too numerous to remember. They would therefore fill the role of textbooks of pharmacology or materia medica. On the other hand, in the Edwin Smith and parts of the Ebers papyri, the reader was taken systematically through the process of examining the patient, reaching a diagnosis and prescribing treatment, as described early in this chapter.

It is likely that master copies would be preserved in the *per ankh* (see below), and fortunate doctors would have their own copies. Surviving copies generally come from unknown tombs, which may well have belonged to doctors without progeny to whom they could have bequeathed their papyri. Reference to papyri would have required the *swnw* to be literate. It is difficult to know what proportion of the various social classes could read and write, but some *swnw* have recorded that they were also scribes. It cannot be said that the medical papyri were the exclusive property of the *swnw*. The Chester Beatty papyri (see Chapter 2) belonged to the archive of a non-medical family in Deir el-Medina.

Was the *per ankh* a medical school?

Strouhal (1992) and Reeves (1992) expressed the view that doctors received their training in the House of Life (*per ankh*), suggesting that it might have been something analogous to the modern medical school and those of Greece and Alexandria. The strongest evidence for this statement is found on the statue of Wedja-hor-resnet and is cited above. Gardiner (1938) described his cogent reasons for reconstructing a lacuna to read 'dealing with medicine' so that, according to his suggestion, the relevant part of the text on the back plinth should read:

> His Majesty King Darius commanded me to return to Egypt ... in order to restore the department[s] of the House[s] of Life [dealing with medicine] after [they had fallen] into decay. ... This his majesty did because he knew the virtue of this art to revive all that are sick ...

However, after an exhaustive review of the evidence, Gardiner concluded that the *per ankh* was neither a school nor a university, but was rather a scriptorium where books connected with religion and cognate matters were compiled. It seems unlikely that the *per ankh* was a medical school as the term is understood today.

The international reputation of Egyptian doctors

It is clear that Egyptian doctors were held in high regard by neighbouring countries. In response to a request, Ramses II despatched a doctor, known from Akkadian texts as Pariamakhu (App. B, no. 92), to the Hittite court 'to prepare herbs for Karunta, King of the land of Tarhuntas'. Other requests for medical help were less charitably received (Kitchen, 1982). The New Kingdom physician Neb-amen (App. B, no. 100) is portrayed receiving gifts for services rendered to a Syrian prince (Lefebvre, 1956).

Information arising outside Egypt is perhaps more convincing. In the *Odyssey*

(4, 229–32), Helen uses a drug which banishes pain and sorrow. This had been given to her by Polydamna, daughter of Thon, an Egyptian:

> For in that land the fruitful earth bears drugs in plenty, some good and some dangerous; and there every man is a physician and acquainted with such lore beyond all mankind.

Cyrus II, the Persian king who captured Babylon in 539 BC, was the father of Cambyses, who became the first king of the Twenty-seventh (Persian) Dynasty in 525 BC. Herodotus (III, 1) described how, before the Persian invasion, Cyrus had sent to the pharaoh Ahmose II (Amasis) for the services of the best ophthalmologist in Egypt. However, Egyptian doctors practising overseas were not always successful (see p. 206). In spite of their intense national pride, the Egyptians appeared to allow foreign doctors to practise and, in the New Kingdom, there are records of four unnamed Babylonian doctors (*asu*) (Jonckheere, 1958).

Paramedical staff

Pharmacists

On the assumption that the medical papyri were written for the *swnw*, it appears to be the general rule that they were expected to prepare their own medications. As a preface to the preparation of a medication, the typical phrase is 'then you shall prepare for him ...'. Occasionally, however, we find 'then you shall cause one to prepare for him ...'. The latter phrase implies the existence of those who were accustomed to prepare remedies. There is, however, no known Egyptian word for pharmacist.

There is an important ostracon from Deir el-Medina (BM 5634), which records absences from the work force in the fortieth year of the reign of Ramses II (Cerny and Gardiner, 1957). Line 21 of the recto lists the absences of Pa-hery-pedjet and appears to be continued on line 22 where he was absent 'with Khonsu' and 'with Horemwia' on certain days for the 'preparation of medicines'. The same ostracon records that both Khonsu and Horemwia were absent from their work because of sickness on five of the six days in question. Pa-hery-pedjet probably has the distinction of being the first known pharmacist.

Nurses

There are several Egyptian words for nurse, but most of these relate to wet-nursing or child care. The determinative hieroglyph is a woman suckling a child (Gardiner sign-list B 5), a woman seated on a chair with a child on her lap (Gardiner sign-list B 6) or the female breast (Gardiner sign-list D 27). However, the Egyptian word *khenmet* has the usual seated woman determinative, and is usually translated as 'dry-nurse'. I am unaware of any texts or reliefs which shed light on the work of such a nurse in relation to medicine.

Midwives

It is inconceivable that there were no women who were specially skilled and experienced at assisting with childbirth. In the book of Exodus (1: 15) the king of Egypt asked the Hebrew midwives Shiphrah and Puah to kill the male children whom they delivered. However, there is no known Egyptian word for midwife and no medical papyri deal with childbirth. In the only text describing childbirth (Westcar X, 8 et seq.), the mother is assisted by four goddesses and not by a midwife or doctor (pp. 192–4). However, this was a magical birth. Obstetrics is discussed further in Chapter 9.

Physiotherapists

It is again inconceivable that the Egyptians had not discovered the beneficial and pleasurable effects of manipulation and massage. In the Westcar papyrus (VII, 15), the magician Djedi had 'his servant at his head to smear him and another to rub his legs'. This sounds like a simple form of physiotherapy.

Figure 6.14 shows the remarkable scenes in the tombs of Ankh-ma-hor and Khentika, which appear to represent manipulation of fingers and toes. This could be manicure and pedicure, but the words of the patients and therapists shown in the figure suggest very strongly that a therapeutic effect is intended. Alternatively, it has been suggested that these scenes represent a form of reflexology, and current illustrations of this type of treatment certainly look remarkably like these tomb reliefs.

| Inspector of the treasury Heny | Make these pleasant, dear one | I shall act for your praise |

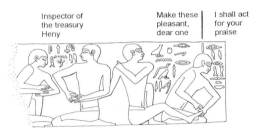

TOMB OF KHENTIKA

6.14 Scenes depicting physiotherapy or, alternatively, pedicure, manicure or grooming, in relation to initiation. The tombs of Khentika and Ankh-ma-hor are both 6th Dynasty and close to the pyramid of Teti at Saqqara.

[Making] pleasant dear one

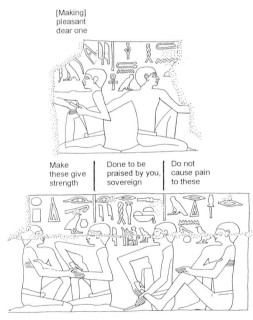

| Make these give strength | Done to be praised by you, sovereign | Do not cause pain to these |

TOMB OF ANKH-MA-HOR

Bandagers

The work of the embalmers has shown a remarkable degree of skill in the application of bandages. It is not entirely clear whether the word *wet* refers only to an embalmer or whether it can also be used to mean one who bandages the living. The essential reference is in the Edwin Smith papyrus (Gloss A in Case 9), which mentions the application of a 'bandage which is under the hand of the embalmer (*wet*)'. There is no difficulty over the word for bandage (*seshed*); the only question is whether the bandage was actually applied by a *wet* or if he merely supplied the bandage for use by the *swnw*. Breasted (1930) supported the latter view. Chapter 3 discusses the evidence for transfer of information from embalmers to *swnw*.

Swnw not previously listed

So thorough was the work of Jonckheere, Van de Walle, De Meulenaere and Ghaliounghui that it is difficult to find a *swnw* who had escaped their attention. The following, not previously listed to my knowledge, were kindly drawn to my attention by Richard Parkinson, Pierre Querinci and Rosalind Park.

Djuaw-khuf (Appendix B, no. 59) was a *sehedj* (inspector) of *swnw* and 'known to the king' (Hassan, 1960). He appears in a panel in the tomb of Wash-duaw who was inspector of the court physicians and also court ophthalmologist. It seems likely that Wash-duaw is the same as Wah-duaw (App. B, no. 15), listed under the latter name before the publication by Hassan. The tomb of Wash-duaw is in Giza and dated to the Fifth Dynasty of the Old Kindgom.

Sankhu-Ptah (App. B, no. 51) is briefly mentioned as an overseer of doctors in an illustration of a scene from his Sixth Dynasty tomb (Eggebrecht, 1984).

Tjau (App. B, no. 55) appears in a relief as a dependent of Hem-min, in the latter's tomb (M 43) at El-Hawawish, now dated to early Sixth Dynasty (Kanawati, 1985). The reading of the title of Tjau is uncertain but may be *iry-khet swnw* (overseer of doctors).

Anon. A hymn to Ra on the ostracon O.DM 1706 from Deir el-Medina mentions a *swnw* (App. B, no. 134) whose name is unfortunately lost in a lacuna (Mathieu, 1993):

> Praise to Ra when he goes to rest ... the divine barque from land to land for the deceased (the Osiris), the scribe and *swnw* ... who says: Adoration to you.
> O Ra ... adoration to you ... when you set in the sky ...

No *swnw* has been listed later than the Twenty-seventh Dynasty. The word certainly appears but, in the Ptolemaic Period, the meaning of *swnw* becomes unclear and can also mean embalmer.

The practice of conventional medicine by priests

There can be no doubt that certain priests practised medicine in a conventional manner as defined earlier in this chapter (von Känel, 1984).

Priests of Sekhmet

The quotation from the Ebers papyrus, repeated in the Edwin Smith papyrus and cited at the beginning of this chapter, makes no distinction between the work of the *swnw* and the *wab* priest of Sekhmet in placing the hand to feel the pulse. Independent evidence for their role in conventional medicine appears in the Hatnub graffito in the case of Aha-nakht. The juxtaposition of his figure to that of the *swnw* Hery-shef-nakht (fig. 6.10) implies that their roles were similar, and the text for Aha-nakht confirms this:

The scribe of the hall of judgement, Aha-nakht. I am a *wab* priest of Sekhmet, capable and skilled of his brotherhood, who places a hand on a man when he knows it [i.e. the illness], skilled in examining strongly and one who knows bulls.

This may be compared with the graffito of the *swnw* Hery-shef-nakht above. The phrase 'one who knows bulls' implies that Aha-nakht was also a veterinary surgeon. It seems very likely that the *wab* priests of Sekhmet practised conventional medicine and made use of the medical papyri in much the same way as the *swnw*.

Priests of Serqet

Serqet was the scorpion goddess and it was long believed that her priests had a special role in the treatment of bites and stings from venomous reptiles and insects. The stela of the foreman Baki (BM 265) from the necropolis workmen's village at Deir el-Medina shows Amenmose with the title *kherep* Serqet (Bierbrier, 1982). It is generally believed that he functioned as a 'village doctor' for Deir el-Medina, possibly under the supervision of a *swnw*, one having been identified from a record of payments on an ostracon (App. B, no. 132). There are numerous other inscriptions relating to 'Dr' Amenmose (Kitchen, 1986, 1987), showing his full titles to include 'servant of the place of truth (the necropolis) and *kherep* Serqet of the lord of the two lands (the king) in the place of eternity (the necropolis)'.

The most convincing evidence of the conventional medical role of *kherep* priests of Serqet comes from the papyrus on snake bites of the Brooklyn Museum (47,218.48 and 47,218.85), considered further in Chapters 2 and 8. The beginning of the first section is lost but the opening paragraph of the second section (no. 39) states:

> Beginning of the collection of remedies to drive out the poison of all snakes, all scorpions, all tarantulas and all serpents, which is in the hand of the *kherep* priests of Serqet, and to drive away all snakes and to seal their mouths.

What follows contains a number of spells, but these are far outnumbered by conventional remedies in a format typical of the medical papyri. Many of the remedies are grouped according to the species of snake which bit the patient, or to the signs and symptoms which the victim developed. This provides very convincing evidence that the healing role of the priests of Serqet was by no means restricted to invoking magic and the deities but also involved a pragmatic approach to the clinical problem in a manner essentially similar to that which we believe was followed by the *swnw*.

Conclusion

There can be no doubt that there was a professional class of doctors throughout the pharaonic period. They ranged from the highest social levels down to plain working doctors. The title of *swnw* was held in high esteem by men of exalted position who were unlikely to have worked as doctors.

The practice of medicine was not confined to the *swnw*; *wab* priests of Sekhmet and *kherep* priests of Serqet, together with various categories of magicians, were concerned in primary health care, although perhaps in an inferior capacity. The position of ancillary staff is less clear.

CHAPTER **SEVEN**

Drug therapy

The ancient Egyptian pharmacopoeia was weak by modern standards. The basis of treatment was mainly empirical rather than rational and, in most cases, aimed at the relief of symptoms rather than the eradication of the cause of the disease. To a large extent this was inevitable because the discovery of the nature of most internal complaints lay far in the future. It would, however, be useful here to consider the therapeutic options available in the second and third millennia BC.

Therapeutic options

The exercise of 'tender loving care' (TLC) has a measurable curative value for many conditions, particularly chronic pain and psychosomatic disorders. This effect is so powerful that formal investigation into the efficacy of a new therapeutic modality must be tested against a control group which is matched for equality of TLC. The negative confessions in Chapter 125 of the *Book of the Dead* indicate that the ancient Egyptians were not lacking in sympathy for the afflicted, and TLC would not have been in short supply from the doctor and probably the other healers as well.

The ancient Egyptians made great use of magic and invocation of the deities in the cure of disease. The range of techniques is outlined in Chapter 5, and there were many spells to be used with or without conventional remedies. Such practices have continued from the dawn of recorded history until the present time, and there are many conditions, particularly those mentioned in the previous paragraph, which would probably have been alleviated to some extent by spells, incantations, incubation and attempts to secure the intervention of benign gods.

Attention to diet would have been important to health and wellbeing. It is difficult to detect, in human remains or in the medical papyri, evidence of dietary disorders other than gross obesity and wasting. Nevertheless, it is reasonable to assume that the *swnw* would have given instructions on the improvement of diet where this was indicated. Many prescriptions in the medical papyri comprise or include normal dietary items, but the inference is that this was for a supposed therapeutic or adjuvant effect rather than correction of a deficient diet.

Surgery was an obvious therapeutic option and the scope is discussed in the following chapter. The Edwin Smith papyrus provides excellent evidence for the surgical treatment of injuries, including suturing of wounds, setting of fractures and reducing dislocated joints. However, prior to the Graeco-Roman Period there is no clear evidence of anything more than the simplest forms of elective surgical procedures, such as the incision of abscesses and probably the removal of small superficial tumours (see Chapter 8).

Some forms of massage and physical medicine were probably practised. Chapter 6 mentions evidence from the Westcar papyrus and it is possible that certain reliefs in tombs (see fig. 6.14) represent physiotherapy. The words of the participants support this interpretation, but it has also been suggested that the scenes show manicure and pedicure or even a type of reflexology representing the application of pressure to certain areas. There is certainly no evidence that any form of physical therapy was the prerogative of the *swnw*, and nothing in the medical texts links the *swnw* with any form of physiotherapy.

By far the commonest form of treatment recommended in the medical papyri was the use of drugs, drawn from a very wide range of animal, mineral and vegetable substances and administered in a variety of ways. The ancient Egyptians were renowned for their skill in this respect (pp. 131–2).

General principles

The ancient Egyptian approach to the use of drugs would have seemed entirely reasonable in the eighteenth and even the nineteenth century AD. Their practice seems so strange now because we are living in the midst of a therapeutic revolution, with the pace of change continuing to increase (Dollery, 1994; Sykes, 1994). It is useful to consider the major changes that we may better understand the past.

The first and most important change is that treatment is now directed, wherever possible, towards eradicating the cause of a disease rather than merely relieving symptoms. Secondly, there is less reliance on natural products as drugs, although almost 25 per cent of the active compounds in currently prescribed medicines were first identified in higher plants (Balandrin *et al.*, 1985). The active principles were identified, often synthesised, and then it became usual to design the molecule of a new drug for a specific purpose. It is no coincidence that, at the same time, a knowledge of botany ceased to be a requirement for medical students. The third aspect of the drug revolution has been improved methods for the assessment of efficacy and toxicity.

All of this is very far removed from the practice of ancient Egypt and, for that matter, Europe until about a hundred years ago. In pharaonic times, little was known of the aetiology of internal diseases and so it was seldom possible to direct treatment towards the cause of the disease. Furthermore, the only available drugs were natural products and a few simple chemical substances, with a very limited range of pharmacological effects. Even today, less than 10 per cent of the estimated 250,000 flowering plant species in the world have been examined scientifically for their potential in medicine (Editorial, 1994). If a plant has an active principle, it may be confined to one part, and be critically dependent on extraction procedures (see below). Finally, we should note that the ancient Egyptians' love of polypharmacy would have made it much more difficult to establish a genuine therapeutic effect for any particular drug.

Determining therapeutic efficacy is now known to be a far more difficult matter than was realised in the past. Expectation of cure may exert a very powerful effect, particularly in the relief of pain (Table 7.1). This factor, the 'placebo effect', must be

Table 7.1 An early demonstration of the placebo effect in providing pain relief after surgery (Beecher *et al.*, 1953)

SUBSTANCE ADMINISTERED	PATIENTS REPORTING PAIN RELIEF
aspirin (300 mg)	50%
placebo	40%
morphine (10 mg)	41%
placebo	32%
codeine (60 mg)	39%
placebo	34%

The differences in the percentages of patients reporting pain relief with active drug and placebo were statistically not significantly different.

eliminated in the assessment of a new drug. The basic principles of assessment include a comparison of the drug with an inactive 'placebo' given randomly, both patient and doctor being ignorant of ('blinded to') the true identity of the preparation which is administered. A drug must be tested in such a 'double-blind, placebo-controlled, cross-over, randomised' study before it can be said to be efficacious. Even side effects may occur in the placebo group. Thus, it would have been extremely difficult for the *swnw* to have arrived at a true assessment of the efficacy of most of his drugs, and his difficulties would have been greatly enhanced by the simultaneous use of a multiplicity of drugs, often concurrently with magical practice. Ebers 663 contains thirty-seven items and it is not clear which was thought to be the most important.

There is, however, a favourable aspect to the problem. Innumerable patients must have benefited purely from the placebo effect, even if the preparations were ineffective and the *swnw* was unaware of the concept. There is nothing wrong with this approach in the context of ancient Egypt. Furthermore, there is no reason why the placebo effect should be confined to medicines, and the attentions of a priest of Sekhmet or the spells of a magician might have increased expectation of cure, with or without the simultaneous administration of drugs by the *swnw*.

Magical considerations sometimes influenced the selection of a remedy. In ancient Egypt, as in most other parts of the ancient world, remedies were sometimes selected because they were derived from a substance, animal or plant that possessed characteristics which were deemed to be desirable in the state of the patient (*similia similibus*). In this connection Westendorf (1992) cited the prescription containing ostrich egg for a fractured skull in which the skull was equated to the shell of the egg (Edwin Smith, Case 9). This is clearly closer to magic than to rational medicine.

Collection, preparation and dosage of drugs

Collection

We are told little about how the healer obtained the raw materials for the preparation of his drugs. Certain animal products were taken from farm or domestic animals and this would have presented few problems. Others were from wild animals, including the lion, and would have required arrangements with hunters. The excrement of crocodile (used as a contraceptive: Kahun 21) might have been hazardous to collect. Virgin's urine (Ebers 729; Berlin 60, 64, 109) had considerable use, and one wonders whether there was a market for such a commodity. Certain drugs must have presented a real challenge to the collector as, for example, bile of tortoise (Ebers 347) and 'the excrement of flies which is on the wall' (Ebers 782).

Most of the mineral products in the pharmacopoeia were found in Egypt and must have been easily available. However, real lapis lazuli (*khesbedj maa*), used for certain eye conditions, was imported from Afghanistan and would have been expensive.

Drugs were prepared from a very wide range of plants. Many of these were food products (see Tables 1.1, 1.2 and 1.3) which would normally have ensured their availability. We do not know whether herb gardens were maintained for plants which were used exclusively for the extraction of drugs. Alternatively, collection would have required searching for the plants in the wild. We do not know whether this was undertaken by the healers themselves or by professional herb-gatherers, but Ebers 294 (parallel to Hearst 35) gives a brief glimpse of the gathering of an unknown herb *senutet*:

> Beginning of remedies to cause mucus (*setet*) to go down from the pelvis (*nephu*). A herb – *senutet* is its name – growing on its belly like the *kadet*-plant.

It produces a flower like the lotus. If one finds its leaves [looking] like white wood, then one should fetch it and rub it on the pelvis. Then it (the mucus) will go down immediately. Its fruit is given on bread to [those with] *wekhedu* to cause (it) to go down from the pelvis.*

*The difficult words *setet* and *wekhedu* are discussed in Chapter 3.

Preparation

The first remedy to be listed for a condition was usually introduced by the stock phrase 'You shall then prepare (*ir*) for him', implying that the healer was expected to undertake his own preparation of drugs. A variety of phrases were then used, including grind (*nedj*) and cook (*pes*). *Atekh* means literally to 'press through' and has the

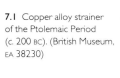

7.1 Copper alloy strainer of the Ptolemaic Period (*c.* 200 BC). (British Museum, EA 38230)

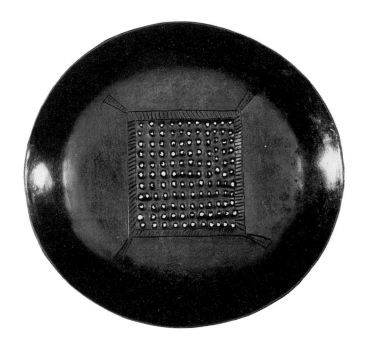

meanings of both 'mash' and 'strain'. Straining was achieved through perforated copper plates (fig. 7.1). Sometimes there are very specific instructions to prepare a homogenous mixture of the components of a preparation – 'as one thing' (*m khet wat*).

Active principles can be extracted from herbal preparations in water, alcohol or oil, depending on their relative solubilities in the three media. In many cases, the active drug in a herbal preparation is an alkaloid, a chemical grouping which includes atropine, nicotine, quinine and morphine. Most alkaloids are best extracted with alcohol, and wine or beer would have provided the strongest concentration of alcohol available in ancient Egypt. The word *sedjer* normally means a person 'spending the night' and the determinative shows a person lying in bed. Rather graphically, the same word is used to describe liquid extraction, as in the following:

You shall then prepare for him to drink: figs, 1/8; milk, 1/16; notched sycomore figs, 1/8; which have 'spent the night' in sweet beer, 1/10. Strain (*atekh*) and drink much so that he gets well immediately. (Ebers 202)

Oil was also used in preparation, frequently in combination with honey, as in this prescription for a man suffering from his stomach:

> You shall then make for him a remedy against it: haematite (ground up), *desh* (unknown) and carob, cook in oil and honey; to be eaten by a man at four dawns. (Ebers 197)

There is an extraordinary remedy of 'an old book boiled in oil' (Ebers 262). This was to cause a child to evacuate an accumulation of urine in its belly, but it is not clear whether this was intended to be serious therapeutics or a magical attempt to extract the wisdom from the old book.

The vehicles

The commonest vehicle for medicines was water, often specified as dew. A typical instruction is that a number of items should 'spend the night in dew' before being drunk (e.g. Ebers 19 and 21). The other main vehicles were honey, milk, oil, wine and beer, often with two of more of these used together. However, all five could well have been considered active drugs in their own right, particularly honey (see below). Oil or fat (*merhet*) was a precious commodity used extensively for lighting, apart from its culinary and medical uses. When used as a vehicle, the type of oil was seldom specified. Olive oil was unknown until introduced by the Greeks, and the main sources were the moringa tree (*baq*) and the fruit of *Balanites aegyptiaca* (*ished*). *Sefet* is an oil, possibly extracted from the fir tree (*ash*), with considerable medical use; it is one of the few of the seven sacred oils to have been identified. Castor oil is mentioned in several remedies as an active ingredient (see below). The earliest recorded use of linseed oil (from flax, *Linum usitatissimum*) is from the Ptolemaic Period (Manniche, 1989).

Wine (*irep*) was made from grapes, and it should have been possible to attain an alcohol concentration of 10–20 per cent, sufficient for the extraction of alkaloids. Ebers 287, a remedy to cause the heart (sic) to receive bread, requires that wine and wheat groats 'spend the night' before being drunk. However, there are no obvious instances of the use of wine to extract alkaloids of known potency from plants such as the water lily (see below). Apart from its use for extracting alkaloids, wine would have been a pleasant ingredient to offset other disagreeable components. Furthermore, mild intoxication would have eased the burden of many complaints.

There are many instances of beer (*henqet*) being prescribed to 'spend the night' with other components (e.g. Ebers 58, 63, 209, 210) which might have resulted in the extraction of alkaloids. Various qualities of beer were often specified. These might be 'beer which had perished' (*henqet net aq*, i.e. stale), 'sweet beer' (*henqet nedjmet*) or 'beer of special offering' (*henqet net hau-khet*), presumably of high quality. Sometimes the dregs or lees (*tahet*) were specified, and these might contain yeast.

Dosage

Weights were very seldom used in the preparation of remedies. Therefore, the balance shown amongst the instruments at Kom Ombo (see fig. 8.2) is highly unlikely to have any connection with pharaonic medicine. Volume was used almost exclusively and fig. 7.2 shows volume measures from the Petrie Museum (UC 26315). Table 7.2 lists the more common volume measurements, but considerable uncertainty exists. The *heqat* originally had a volume of approximately 4.5 litres, but was supplemented by the double and quadruple *heqat*, the latter first appearing in the Rhind Mathematical Papyrus (Second Intermediate Period). Unfortunately, it is not always clear whether, during and after the New Kingdom, *heqat* refers to the single, double or

Table 7.2 Volume measurements

EGYPTIAN NAME	MULTIPLE OR FRACTION OF SINGLE *HEQAT*	APPROXIMATE METRIC EQUIVALENT	
quadruple *heqat*	4	18	litres
double *heqat*	2	9	litres
single *heqat*	1	4.5	litres
henu	1/10	450	millilitres
ro	1/320	14	millilitres

The *heqat* was primarily a corn measure; *henu* also means 'jar'.

7.2 Small volume measures, each approximately double the capacity of the next smaller vessel (range 0.1–6.0 ml). They are from the 18th Dynasty and were found by Petrie in the South town of Nubt. (Petrie Museum, University College London, UC 26315)

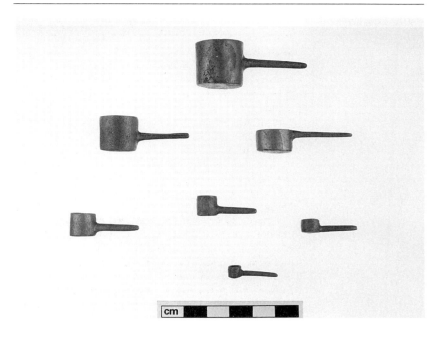

quadruple *heqat*. The *heqat* was clearly too large to have relevance to medicine and does not appear in the papyri as a measure. The *henu*, one-tenth of a *heqat* and approximately 450 ml (assuming the *heqat* to be single), is a more convenient measure for medical purposes, and appears not infrequently as the quantity of a raw material to be used for the preparation of a drug (Ebers 37), to specify the quantity of a component of a mixture (Ebers 323) or as the total dose of a mixture to be taken (Ebers 166).

Prescribing in *henu* measures leaves little doubt of the meaning:

> Another [remedy for cough (*seryt*)]: honey, 1 *henu*; ox-fat, 1 *henu*; water of
> *sa-r-em* (unknown), 2 *henu*; parched seed-corn of emmer, 1 *henu* ... (Ebers 323)

The smallest volume measure was the *ro*, 1/320 of a *heqat*, or about 14 ml, which is a convenient mouthful. It might be expected that prescriptions would often be written in multiples of *ro*s, designated as numerals <u>above</u> the *ro* sign, which is that of the mouth (Gardiner, 1957) (fig. 7.3). However, this system is not used in the extant medical papyri. Neither is the *dja*, which was rather more than 20 *ro*, and about 320 ml (Manniche, 1989).

Much the commonest method of formulating a compound prescription was by specifying fractional proportions for each component. The ancient Egyptians, in common with others in the ancient world, had strange conventions in their use of fractions. They could not conceive of a fraction in which the numerator was anything other than unity, and the denominator in the medical papyri is usually a power of two. Preferred fractions were therefore 1/2, 1/4, 1/8, 1/16, 1/32 and 1/64. Exceptions

The wedjat eye of Horus

7.3 Horus eye and hieroglyphic fractional notations as used in the prescription of drugs. Ro measures are shown with their equivalent as a fraction of a single heqat (4.5 litres).

to this rule were 1/3 and 2/3, and very occasionally 3/4. The usual method of writing fractions was to place the denominator <u>under</u> the mouth sign (fig. 7.3), which unfortunately was also used for *ro*, as in the previous paragraph. This raises the difficult question of whether they really meant *ro*, but the *Grundriss* and others have adhered to the strict interpretation as a fraction. Normally, 1/2 was written by the hieroglyph for 'side' (*ges*), and 1/4 was sometimes indicated by a cross with diagonal limbs. Many prescriptions were written in this format:

> You should then prepare for him strong remedies for drinking: fresh (type of) bread, cooked in oil and honey; wormwood/absinthe, 1/32; resin of the umbrella pine of Byblos (*peret-sheny*), 1/16; ? valerian (*shasha*) 1/8; add it together, cook together as one thing (*m khet wat*). To be drunk on four days. (Ebers 190)

Note that there is no indication of total quantities, only their relative proportions. Although this would ensure a uniform composition of the mixture, whatever the reference volume to which the fractions relate, there is no indication whatsoever of the total dose which the patient was to receive. This is, of course, totally contrary to modern practice, and it is difficult to understand how such a system could be used safely in the case of potentially toxic drugs. It may be that the reference volume was standardised, and so well known that there was no necessity to commit it to writing in the papyri.

Fractions could also be expressed in terms of the components of the Horus eye (fig. 7.3). The smallest of these is 1/64 and, as a fraction of a *heqat*, is 5 *ro* or 70 ml. The symbol for 1/64 could therefore be used to represent 5 *ro* (Ebers 318), 1/32 was similarly used to indicate 10 *ro* and 1/16 for 20 *ro* (Ebers 5, 6, 7, 219, etc.).

Routes of administration of drugs

There were five main routes of administration of drugs – oral, rectal, vaginal, external application and fumigation. The commonest was the oral route and typical instructions were as follows:

> To be eaten (*wenem*) by a man at four dawns. (Ebers 199)
> To be drunk (*sweri*) by a man. (Ebers 191)

Drugs might also be given as a suppository or enema (clyster) into the rectum. Herodotus (II, 76) commented on this practice in relation to their belief that all diseases came from their food. The instructions may relate to liquid or solid preparations thus:

> Poured (*wedeh*) into the anus (*pehwy*). (Ebers 143)
> Placed (*redi*) in the anus for four days. (Ebers 144)

Both *wedeh* and *redi* are very well attested words, widely used outside the medical papyri. In other cases there is a specific instruction to prepare the drug as a suppository:

> Made as a suppository (*met*) [and] placed (*redi*) in the anus. (Ebers 140)

The gynaecological papyri contain a number of remedies and contraceptives to be placed in the vagina:

> You should then prepare for it: new oil, 1 jar (*henu*), poured (*iweh*) into her vagina (*kat*). (Kahun 4)

Medicaments were applied directly to the skin for many reasons and not solely for local complaints such as injuries, snake bites and ulcers. Application of raw meat and then oil and honey to wounds was common practice (Chapter 8). Sometimes gynaecological patients were instructed to sit on the medication while naked (Ebers 797). Not infrequently there were specific instructions to bandage the medication in place:

> Grind and cook with the dregs of sweet beer. Bandage it on for four days so that he will recover immediately. (Ebers 200)

Local application was used extensively for diseases of the skin, hair, eyes, ears and anus. Examples are cited in the sections covering disease in these locations.

Fumigation was used for a range of problems, including snake bite and gynaecological complaints. The word for fumigate (*kap*) is well attested and, outside the medical papyri, is used to mean burning incense. The instructions were usually simple but sometimes we are left in no doubt as to the procedure which was to be undertaken:

> Dry human excrement (*shau*) added to terebinth-resin (*senetjer*). The woman is fumigated (*kap*) with it, causing the fumes (*hety*) to enter inside her vagina (*iuf*). (Ebers 793)

The word *iuf* normally means 'flesh' but was often used to mean the vagina (see Chapter 3).

The ancient Egyptian pharmacopoeia

The ancient Egyptian pharmacopoeia included hundreds of items, many of which cannot be translated. They were recommended for a great variety of diseases of which the meaning is also obscure in many cases. Egyptian prescriptions typically start with a terse statement of the diagnosis followed by: 'You shall then prepare for him:'. A major concern is that many are followed by paragraphs headed simply 'Another remedy' or just 'Another'. One assumes that these remedies were intended for treatment of the last disease to be specified in the previous paragraphs. This relies upon generations of scribes copying the paragraphs in the correct sequence. Unfortunately, there is no firm basis for total confidence in their work.

Products of the Ricinus (castor oil) plant (*degem*) have the unique distinction of something approaching systematic discussion in an isolated section of the Ebers papyrus (251). The approach is quite different from the listing of other remedies in the medical papyri, and it is tempting to believe that this section is a remnant of a lost general pharmacopoeia, perhaps related to one of the books listed by Clement (Chapter 2). This unique section is therefore cited in full:

> Knowledge of what is made from (or done with) the Ricinus plant, as that which was found in ancient writings and as that which is useful to mankind.
>
> a) One crushes its roots in water, to place on a head which is sick; he will then become well immediately, like one who is not ill.
> b) A little of its fruit (beans) is chewed with beer by a man with *wehi*-condition in his faeces. This is an elimination of disease from the belly of a man.
> c) The hair of a woman is also caused to grow by its fruit (beans); it is ground and made into one thing and added to oil; then the woman should anoint her head with it.
> d) Its oil (*merhet*) is also prepared from its fruit (beans), to anoint [a man] with the *wehau*-skin disease, affected with *itjetjet* and *hewau*, which is painful.
> The *riumu* come to a standstill like one to whom nothing has happened. But he is treated with ointment likewise for ten days, being anointed very early so that they are eliminated.
> Really excellent, a million times.

The significance of this passage is sadly diminished by the various pathological states which cannot at present be translated, and there is surprisingly no mention of its use for constipation, although this application is made clear in Ebers 25 (see below). Somewhat similar, though much less comprehensive, is consideration of the onion in the Brooklyn papyrus on snake bites (see Chapters 2 and 8).

> Para. 41: Very good remedies to be made for those suffering from all snake bites: Onion, ground finely in beer. Eat and spit out for one day. (then follows an incantation)
> Para. 42: As for the onion, it should be in the hand of the priest of Serqet, wherever he is. It is that which kills the venom of every snake, male or female. If one grinds it in water and one smears a man with it, the snake will not bite him. If one grinds it in beer and sprinkles it all over the house one day in the new year, no serpent male or female will penetrate therein.

Then follow many remedies for specific snake bites, in the usual format, with many containing onions.

Thanks to the determinatives at the end of the Egyptian words for drugs, they can usually be classified into mineral, animal or vegetable, the scheme which will be followed below. *Wörterbuch der Ägyptischen Drogennamen, Grundriss*, vol. VI (von Deines and Grapow, 1959) cites the key sections of the various medical papyri where specific remedies are employed.

It is far from simple to relate the items in the Egyptian pharmacopoeia to the diseases they were intended to cure. The major difficulty is in translating the name of many of the diseases and some 80 per cent of the botanical species. One suspects that some of the more outlandish animal preparations might well be popular names for a plant as, for example, snapdragon is today. The problems are further confounded by polypharmacy, with as many as thirty-seven items in a single remedy. It is often unclear whether a constituent is an active principle, a vehicle or merely added for its taste. Honey, for example, might be effective in all three categories. Many drugs, *djaret* for example, were used so extensively that it is impossible to define what pharmacological effect was intended. Furthermore, many substances were used for their supposed magical properties and we look in vain for any intended pharmacological basis. Nevertheless, the overall materia medica was not too dissimilar in character from that carried by the Egyptian folk healer of the present (Estes, 1989).

Unintentional medication

Quite apart from the best intentions of the healers, there must be many instances of powerful drugs which were administered unintentionally. Armelagos and Mills (1993) describe how Debra Martin detected the antibiotic tetracycline by serendipity, while examining a thin section of bone from the Roman Period. It seems likely that tetracycline was formed in the brewing process, as a result of contamination with an airborne streptomycete, and then ingested with the beer. A constant intake of this antibiotic might have influenced the pattern of bacterial infection.

Drugs of mineral origin

A wide range of minerals were employed and, in this section of the pharmacopoeia, there are the least difficulties in identifying the drug (Table 7.3).

Natron (*hesmen*)

Natron was deposited as a mixture of evaporites in areas which had previously been flooded, and subsequently evaporated to dryness as a result of climatic changes. The material was freely available and used extensively in mummification. The composition of natron varies greatly from one location to another (Garner, 1979) but the major constituents are sodium chloride ($NaCl$), sodium sulphate (Na_2SO_4), sodium carbonate (Na_2CO_3) and sodium bicarbonate ($NaHCO_3$). Its use in the solid state or as a paste would have a powerful osmotic effect, drawing out fluid and reducing swelling. This would have a role similar to that of Glauber's salts which is pure sodium sulphate. Natron was generally alkaline, depending on the proportion of sodium carbonate.

Its most extensive use was as an external application, often under a bandage. Perhaps the clearest and most logical use is in Hearst 140 (= Ebers 557):

> Another remedy to draw (literally: to bring) pus (*ryt*): *ipshenen* (unknown), 1; natron, 1; clay (or ? gypsum) from the potter's kiln, 1; carob, 1; terebinth resin, 1; bring flour of date (*nyt net benri*); make as one thing and bandage with it.

Ignoring the other components, natron would be appropriate for superficial sepsis.

Table 7.3 Remedies of mineral origin

COMMON NAME	EGYPTIAN NAME	COMPOSITION
alabaster	*shes*	calcium carbonate
alum	*ibnu*	potassium/aluminium sulphate/hydroxide
black eye-paint (galena)	*mesdemet*	lead sulphide
brick	*djebet*	various
calamine (?)	*hetem*	zinc oxide (suggested only by Ebbell, 1937)
chalcedony (?)	*seheret*	silicon dioxide
chalcopyrite (?)	*gesfen*[1]	copper/iron sulphide
clay	*im, deben* *besen*[2]	aluminium silicate
copper	*hemet*	copper – usually as hammering flakes
dew	*iadet*	water
glass flux (?)	*tjehenet*	
granite	*mat*	complex mixture
green eye-paint (malachite)	*wadju*	cupric carbonate/hydroxide
gypsum	*besen*[2]	hydrated calcium sulphate
haematite (blood stone)	*dedi*	iron oxide (Fe_2O_3)
lapis lazuli[3]	*khesbedj*	sodium/aluminium silicate and sodium sulphate
naphtha ?	*merhet khast*	desert oil, ? bitumen
natron	*hesmen*	sodium chloride, sulphate, carbonate, bicarbonate
Nile mud	*qah*	various
ochre	*sety*	hydrated iron oxide and clay
orpiment (?)	*sia*	arsenic sulphide
red lead	*peresh*	red oxide of lead
red mineral (?)	*tjeru*	? red ink
red natron	*hesmen djeser*	sodium chloride, sulphate, carbonate, bicarbonate
red ochre	*menshet*	hydrated iron oxide and clay
salt of Lower Egypt	*hemat*	sodium chloride
stone	*inr*	various
unknown mineral	*kesenti*	–
unknown mineral	*imru*	–

1 Aufrère (1984) suggested that *gesfen* might be decomposing chalcopyrite. Others have suggested it is asafoetida (see Table 7.5), although it never carries a plant determinative.
2 Faulkner (1962), but not the *Grundriss* or Lesko (1982–90), gives gypsum (?) for *besen*.
3 Probably not found in Egypt.

Ebers 595 also prescribes natron for drawing out pus. It was sometimes prescribed with common salt.

Natron was seldom recommended to be taken by mouth. However, an exception is Ebers 856d, which describes the two *metu* (probably blood vessels) to the thigh (see Table 3.2). It continues thus:

If he is ill as to his thigh and his two legs tremble, then you shall say concerning it: It is this *shetbau* vessel of his thigh, which has received an illness. That which is done for it: vegetable mucilage, *saam*-plant, natron, cooked as one thing, to be drunk by a man for four days.

No quantities are specified and it is difficult to imagine a condition of the legs which might be relieved by taking natron internally.

Common salt (*hemat*)

Salt (sodium chloride) was often specified as salt of Lower Egypt, where perhaps it was obtained by evaporation from sea water. Its main effect at high concentrations would be osmotic as for natron but, in a solution of approximately 1 per cent, its osmotic pressure is close to that of body fluids. Warm salt solutions are mildly emetic. It was often included in prescriptions with many components and perhaps was added mainly for its taste. Salt had a very wide use, being taken by mouth, by enema, as an anal suppository, and as a local application to the eyes, ears and especially to the skin, where it was often held in place by a bandage.

Malachite (*wadju*)

The usual Egyptian word for malachite is *shesmet* but this does not appear in the medical papyri. There are, however, many remedies containing green eye-paint (*wadju*), which depended on finely powdered malachite for its green colour. It was used extensively for eye diseases (Chapter 9). Majno (1975) produced convincing evidence that powdered malachite would inhibit the growth of the important pathogenic bacterium *Staphylococcus aureus*, no doubt due to traces of copper passing into solution. Estes (1989) produced further convincing evidence of the efficacy of cupric carbonate/hydroxide (the principal compound in malachite, see Table 7.3) in preventing growth of *Staphylococcus aureus* and *Pseudomonas aeruginosa*. Ebers 491 prescribes *wadju* as a dressing for a burn which has become foul, and Edwin Smith 46 to draw out inflammation (*seref*) from the mouth of a wound in the breast. It would, however, be hard to say whether the Egyptians recognised the anti-bacterial effect or were merely influenced by the decorative appearance of malachite.

Lapis lazuli (*khesbedj*)

Unlike all other minerals in Table 7.3, lapis lazuli was not found in Egypt and was imported chiefly from Badakshan in Afghanistan. It was a precious commodity which would raise the expectation of cure. Its medical use was confined to the eyes. Being virtually insoluble in body fluids, there is no obvious basis for any therapeutic effect.

Imru and gypsum

Imru is an unidentified mineral which is only known from eight cases in the Edwin Smith papyrus, seven of which are bony fractures and dislocations. It was recommended that the patient should be bandaged with *imru* and it is very tempting to believe that *imru* was something akin to 'gesso' (whiting and glue), used extensively in the preparation of mummy cartonnage, which would have been excellent as a splint. Gypsum or plaster of Paris (*besen* ?) was employed for plastering in building operations from the Early Dynastic Period (Lucas and Harris, 1989), but its mention in the medical papyri does not extend to the stabilisation of fractures or dislocations.

Other insoluble minerals

Many of the minerals in Table 7.3 are virtually insoluble in body fluids, including, for example, chalcedony, granite and haematite. It seems inconceivable that these substances can have exerted any pharmacological effect. By virtue of their mechanical properties they would be highly irritant when introduced into the eye, as for example in Ebers 382 which prescribes finely ground granite sprinkled over both eyes to eliminate white spots. It seems likely that such minerals were used in the hope of assimilating desirable qualities such as strength, durability and beauty.

Drugs of animal origin

The ancient Egyptian pharmacopoeia contained a wide range of animal products. Sometimes there was a sound pharmacological basis for the benefit which was expected. In other cases the substance simply provided a convenient vehicle for other constituents. In certain cases the remedy was based on characteristics of the donor animal, which were deemed desirable.

Honey (bit)

Few medicaments had wider use in ancient Egypt than honey. It was used both externally and internally in hundreds of the remedies in the medical papyri. This was partly as a vehicle (see above) and partly for its own intrinsic properties when applied externally or taken internally. It is largely composed of sugars (mainly glucose and fructose), and was of particular value in a society where the sugar beet and cane sugar were unknown. Its sweetness was clearly intended as a linctus to relieve cough in Ebers 323 (cited above, under 'Dosage'). Honey has powerful anti-bacterial and anti-fungal properties which are mainly due to the osmotic effect of high concentrations of sugar (Estes, 1989; Zumla and Lulat, 1989).

Much interest has centred on its use on open wounds (see Chapter 8). The osmotic effect would reduce swelling but, more importantly, bacteria do not grow in honey (Majno, 1975). Honey has been demonstrated to accelerate wound healing (Bergman et al., 1983) and similar benefits follow its use on burns and ulcers. Internal use on children with gastro-enteritis shortened the duration of diarrhoea (Haffejee and Moosa, 1985). Its use on open wounds appears to have been fully justified, and Zumla and Lulat concluded that the therapeutic potential of honey is grossly under-utilized. However, the Egyptians' use of honey in dental care could hardly have been justified (Chapter 9).

Milk (irtet)

Milk also had extensive use, often as a convenient vehicle, a role which is indicated by failure to specify the proportion in a mixture. The following is a remedy for an obstruction of the stomach (Ebers 193):

> tiam (unknown plant), 1/16; grains from umbrella pine of Byblos (peret-sheny), 1/16; ? valerian (shasha), 1/8; cyperus grass of the island (gyw n iw), 1/16; cyperus grass of the garden (gyw n hesep), 1/16; wine and milk; to be eaten and swallowed with sweet beer, to make him well immediately.

It seems likely that the unspecified amounts of wine and milk are included merely to act as a vehicle to make the other ingredients easier to take. The origin of the milk is unspecified but on other occasions it is indicated as the cow (Kahun 3), ass (Ebers 98) or 'human' (remetj). If the milk is of human origin, it is often specified as 'milk of one who has born a male [child]' (e.g. Ebers 109). This implies that some varieties of milk were thought to have healing properties of their own, which is difficult to substantiate.

Remedies containing milk were most commonly taken by mouth but also as an enema (Ebers 157), to be poured into the vagina (Ebers 819), or applied to the eyes (Ebers 368), the ears (as curds: Ebers 765) or the skin (Ebers 109).

Excrement (hes)

Excrement was prescribed from a range of species, including cat, ass, birds, lizard, crocodile, fly and man (see Ebers 793, above). Happily, such remedies were usually applied externally, but ingestion was recommended for excrement of *idu*-bird (Ebers 326) and fly (Ebers 782). External application included application of excrement from lizard, crocodile, pelican and human infant to the eyes (Ebers 344–70). It is difficult to discern any pharmacological basis for this practice.

Blood (senef)

Blood of a wide range of species was recommended, mainly as a component of external applications. Ebers 425, a remedy to prevent an eyelash growing into the eye after it has been pulled out, included blood of ox, ass, pig, dog and goat. Other remedies included the blood of lizard and bat (Ebers 424) and flies (Ebers 857). In all, the *Grundriss* lists blood from twenty-one species used as a medication.

Urine (mwyt)

Urine was used as a vehicle for medicines, although generally only for an enema or external application:

> Another [remedy] to drive out the *ashyt* disease (unknown): carob (*djaret*), salt of Lower Egypt (*hemat*), boiled in urine: applied to it. (Hearst 39)

Ramesseum papyrus III (A, 19–20) prescribed human urine to be placed in the eyes.

Placenta (mut-remetj)

The Egyptian word for placenta means literally 'mother of mankind'. Placenta of cat was one ingredient of a mixture recommended to prevent hair turning grey (Ebers 453).

Bile (weded, benef)

Cow was the preferred species, but goat bile (Ebers 433) was recommended for the treatment of a human bite (see Chapter 8). Bile of the unidentified *abedju*-fish was also used for strengthening the eyesight (Ebers 405), and pig bile (probably) for any evil thing in the eye (Ebers 392). Bile of unspecified origin (*benef*) was one component of a mixture prescribed for an infected wound of the breast (Edwin Smith 41) and ox bile for an abscess of the breast (Edwin Smith 46). Bile was seldom taken internally but that of the *gu*-bull was used for treatment of the unidentified *pened*-worm (Ebers 75).

Animal fat (adj, merhet)

The word *adj* was used exclusively to mean animal fat, whereas *merhet* could mean both animal fat and oils of vegetable origin (see above). There is reference above to the very common preparation of a mixture of drugs 'boiled with oil (*merhet*) and honey', which almost certainly relates to a vegetable oil. We can, however, be certain that an animal fat was intended when the species is indicated.

Animal fats had an extensive use in the prescriptions, partly because of their suitability to make a greasy ointment and partly in the hope of transferring some desirable characteristic of the animal. Perhaps the most remarkable example is Ebers 465:

> Another [remedy] to cause hair to grow on a bald person: fat of lion, 1; fat of hippopotamus, 1; fat of crocodile, 1; fat of cat, 1; fat of snake, 1; fat of ibex, 1; make as one thing, smear (or anoint) the head of the bald person with it.

It is interesting to contemplate the cost of this remedy and the powerful element of suggestion which would accompany its use. However, in this case there is no comment on efficacy, which sometimes took such forms as 'really effective – a million times!'.

Other species included antelope, ass, fish, goose, ostrich, ox, mouse and sheep. Preparations including animal fat could be taken internally or as an enema but were most frequently used for external application.

Meat (iuf)

Fresh meat was widely prescribed for application to a wound on the first day (see Chapter 8). This recalls the folk remedy of applying a steak to a black eye. Meat can provide blood clotting factors, and pioneer neurosurgeons used fresh pigeon breast meat to control oozing (Majno, 1975).

The prescription of meat to be taken by mouth may be an example of dietary treatment. An obscure section of the Ebers papyrus (284–93) comprises remedies to cause the heart to receive bread. It is likely that 'bread' refers to food in general, and the distinction between heart (ib) and stomach – literally 'mouth of the heart' (r-ib) – is often uncertain. This group of prescriptions abounds with nutritious items and three include 'fat meat'.

Liver (miset)

Of all the animal products, the most useful might be liver, which contains 90 per cent of the body store of vitamin B_{12} essential for the prevention of megaloblastic (pernicious or Addisonian) anaemia. The liver store is very large, being more than one thousand times the daily requirement. Raw liver by mouth and later injection of liver extract were the basis of therapy for megaloblastic (pernicious) anaemia before the discovery of vitamin B_{12}. However, there is nothing in the medical texts which can be identified with megaloblastic anaemia for which liver is recommended.

The second major therapeutic implication is deficiency of vitamin A causing night blindness, which can be treated by ingestion of liver, a rich source of vitamin A. There is one instance of raw liver being recommended for taking by mouth, for 'a woman who cannot see' (Kahun 1) and one of local application of cooked liver for a case of sharu-blindness (Ebers 351). Both texts are considered further in Chapter 9, but in neither case is there any firm basis for believing that the use of liver was a logical attempt to treat night blindness.

In Ebers 267 is a recommendation for oral administration of ox liver (not specified to be raw) for 'accumulations' (henau) in the urine.

Other internal organs

Testicles of a fallow ass, ground and added to wine, are recommended for the unexplained nesyt eye disease (Ebers 756). The heart (haty) of the mesha-bird appears once as 'another remedy' to kill the pened-worm (Ebers 81). The brain (amem) of various species appears as an external remedy.

The mouse (penu)

Hearst 149 recommends a mouse cooked in oil as 'another remedy' for local application to prevent hair turning grey. For reasons which are far from clear, the mouse had a long history in the preparation of medicines, particularly for the relief of cough (Dawson, 1924). In 1747, John Wesley, in his Primitive Physic, recommended for 'chin-cough or hooping cough (sic)':

Catch a mouse, kill it, put it in the oven and roast it till it's burnt to a cinder, take it out and pound it to a powder in a basin of milk and give it to a child to drink.

Drugs of vegetable origin

The ancient Egyptian healers made extensive use of herbs and other plants. They were well placed to exploit an environment which supported a wide range of indigenous plants (pp.131–2), but they also imported certain species from countries such as Lebanon.

Identification

A great number of plant species appear by their Egyptian name in the medical papyri. When the plant or tree determinatives (Gardiner sign-list M 2 and M 1) appear at the end of the word, we can be reasonably certain that we are dealing with a botanical species. However, some plant names carry the pellet determinative (Gardiner sign-list N 33) which more commonly indicates a mineral but, in the case of a plant, may indicate a seed, fruit or root. Fortunately, parallel readings often show the plant determinative.

In many cases there is general agreement on identification, and examples are shown in Tables 1.1, 1.2, 1.3 and 7.4. Positive identifications usually result from sources outside the medical papyri such as the non-medical papyri, labelled illustrations in tombs or sometimes, very rarely, a labelled jar with residual contents. There remain, however, a large number of plant remedies for which there is no general agreement on identification of the species: some may have become extinct or at least disappeared from the Nile Valley since the pharaonic period. Germer (1993) estimated that it was possible to identify only 20 per cent of some 160 plant products mentioned in the medical texts.

There are three major difficulties in recognising a species and assessing its role in therapy. First, the disease for which they were prescribed is often known only by an Egyptian word which itself cannot be translated. In such cases we cannot use the disease to assist in interpreting the plant name. The second problem is knowing which part of the plant was used and when it was gathered. This was sometimes specified but usually it was not. Many active principles are confined to one part of a plant and the concentration may show a diurnal or annual variation.

The third problem is that, even when we can be certain of the identification of a plant, we may still know little of the pharmacological effects of the compounds it contains (see Appendix C). Certain plants have been very thoroughly investigated, particularly when they contain potent drugs, many in the class of alkaloids. Familiar examples are morphine in the opium poppy (*Papaver somniferum*), atropine in deadly nightshade (*Atropa belladonna*), strychnine in *Strychnos nux-vomica*, cocaine in the leaves of the coca plant (*Erythroxylum coca*), curare in the vine *Chondrodendron tomentosum* and digoxin in the leaves of the foxglove *Digitalis purpurea*. Other plants contain antibiotics and anti-fungals. These few examples are sufficient to illustrate the range of potent drugs and poisons to be found in common plants. However, at the time of writing, the therapeutic potential of more than 90 per cent of botanical species remains to be studied systematically (Editorial, 1994).

Sources

In the last century, Loret made many identifications of botanical species, summarized in *La Flore pharaonique* (1892). Much later, Warren Dawson attempted to translate twenty-four Egyptian words of medical interest, including twelve plant names in a

Table 7.4 Herbal remedies with considerable agreement for the meaning of the Egyptian word

COMMON NAME	EGYPTIAN NAME	LINNEAN NAME	MEANING SUPPORTED BY
Common remedies			
acacia	*shendet*	*Acacia nilotica*	C,D,F,G,Gh,L,M
barley	*it*	*Hordeum vulgare*	D,F,G,Gh,M
bean	*iwryt*	*Vigna sinensis*	C,D,F,G,Gh,L,M
bryony	*khasyt*	*Bryonia dioica*	C,D,F,Gh,M
castor oil	*degem*	*Ricinus communis*	C,D,F,G,Gh,L,M
Christ thorn	*nebes*	*Zizyphus spina-Christi*	C,D,F,G,Gh,L,M
cinnamon	*ti-shepses*	*Cinnamonium zeylanicum* or *Laurus cinnamonium*	C,D,Gh,L,M
coriander	*shaw*	*Coriandrum sativum*	C,D,F,Gh,M
cyperus grass	*giw*	*Cyperus esculentus*	C,D,Gh,L,M
date	*bener(et)*	*Phoenix dactylifera*	C,D,F,G,Gh,L,M
emmer	*bedet*	*Triticum dicoccum*	C,D,F,G,Gh,M
fig	*dab*	*Ficus carica*	C,D,F,G,Gh,L,M
grape	*iareret*	*Vitis vinifera*	C,D,F,G,Gh,L,M
hemp	*shemshem(et)*	*Cannabis sativa*	C,D,F,Gh,M
juniper	*wan*	*Juniperus phoenicea / drupacea*	C,D,F,G,Gh,M
leek	*iaqet*	*Allium kurrat / porrum*	C,D,F,G,Gh,M
linseed/flax	*mehy*	*Linum usitatissimum*	C,D,F,G,Gh,L,M
lotus	*seshen*	*Nymphaea lotus*	C,D,F,G,Gh,L,M
moringa	*baq*	*Moringa pterygosperma*	C,D,F,G,L,M
onion	*hedju*	*Allium cepa*	C,D,F,G,Gh,L,M
pea	*tehu* or *peret-tehu*	*Pisum sativum*	C,D,F,Gh,M
pomegranate	*inhemen*	*Punica granatum*	C,D,F,G,Gh,M
raisin	*wenshi*	*Vitis vinifera*	D,G,Gh,M
seed corn of ?emmer (q.v.)	*mymy*	*Triticum dicoccum*	C,D,F
sycomore fig	*nehet*	*Ficus sycomorus*	C,D,F,G,Gh,L,M
(when notched)	*neqaut*		C,D,F,Gh,M
tamarisk	*iser*	*Tamarix nilotica / articulata*	C,D,F,G,Gh,L,M
watermelon	*bededu-ka*	*Citrullus lanatus*	C,D,F,L,M
willow	*tjeret*	*Salix safsaf*	C,D,F,G,Gh,M
wormwood (absinthe)	*sam*	*Artemisia absinthium*	A,C,M
Plants of limited use for medicines in the pharaonic period			
carob	*nedjem*	*Ceratonia siliqua*	C,F,G,L,M
dill	*imset*	*Anethum graveolens*	C,D,G,Gh,M
papyrus	*mehyt*	*Cyperus papyrus*	C,D,F,G,M
persea	*shawabu*	*Mimusops laurifolis*	C,D,G,M

A Aufrère (1983–9)
C Charpentier (1981)
D *Drogennamen* of the *Grundriss* (Table 2.2)
F Faulkner (1962)
G Germer (1979)
Gh Ghaliounghui (1987)
L Loret (1892)
M Manniche (1989)

series of papers in the *Journal of Egyptian Archaeology* (1932–5). Some new inter-pretations of Egyptian plant names were used in translations of medical texts by Ebbell (1937) and Lefebvre (1956). The next landmark, in 1959, was the *Wörterbuch der Ägyptischen Drogennamen* of the *Grundriss* series (Table 2.2), which gives most of the citations of the plants in the medical texts. Since then there has been the general Middle Egyptian/English dictionary of Faulkner (1962), *Food: the Gift of Osiris* (vol. II) by Darby, Ghaliounghui and Grivetti (1977), the appropriately cautious doctoral thesis of Germer (1979), and Charpentier's immense compilation of sources relating to all known botanical species in ancient Egypt (1981). Between 1983 and 1989, Aufrère published a series of twenty-seven studies of the lexicology of different natural substances in the *Bulletin de l'Institut Français d'Archéologie Orientale*, concentrating on those about which there had been disagreement and doubt. He placed emphasis on tracing Egyptian words through demotic to Coptic, and then seeking reconciliation with Graeco-Roman work, Pliny and Dioscorides in particu-lar. Finally, there is *An Ancient Egyptian Herbal* by Manniche (1989) and a review by Germer (1993). However, much uncertainty still remains.

Table 7.4 lists herbal remedies with a reasonable consensus for the meaning of the ancient Egyptian name. Tables 1.1, 1.2 and 1.3 list plants used as food but which may also have medical applications, noted in the last columns of each. Table 7.5 contains words which are less certain or for which alternative meanings have been attributed. Finally Table 7.6 lists words which cannot yet be translated with any confidence.

Although the number of positive identifications increases slowly, we are left with many Egyptian words we cannot translate and, conversely, certain species likely to have been used for medical purposes for which the Egyptian word is unknown. The Egyptian word for colocynth was believed to be *djaret*, but this is now thought by Charpentier (1981), Aufrère (1983) and Manniche (1989) to mean carob. Fennel was also native to Egypt and very likely to have had a medical use, although its Egyptian name remains unknown and the Coptic name has not provided a clue. Most authors from Dawson to Charpentier have proposed for *afet* / *afay* the meaning of clover (*Melilotus officinalis*). However, Aufrère (1986) argued cogently in favour of the wild or prickly lettuce (*Lactuca virosa*), noting that the usual word for the cos lettuce (*abu*) does not appear in the medical papyri. It would be surprising if the Egyptian doctors had not made use of lettuce, which was closely associated with the ithyphallic god Min and so might be expected to increase virility. Senna was used in Coptic medicine, but no word for it is known in ancient Egyptian. Only Ebbell (1937) has suggested that *gengenet* means senna, which must surely have been popular with the ancient Egyptians. It is surprising that the likely Egyptian word for garlic (*kheten*) does not appear in pharaonic remedies.

Narcotics, sedatives and pain relief

We have no clear evidence that the ancient Egyptians made use of the narcotics which were available to them. Opium, cannabis and mandrake were probably known by the New Kingdom, but the papyri are silent on the obvious uses to which one would expect them to be put.

Opium. One of the most difficult identifications has been that of opium, of which morphine is the most important component. It has been proposed that *shepen* is the Egyptian word for the opium poppy (*Papaver somniferum*), but the solitary reference to its internal administration is Ebers 782:

Remedy for driving out 'much crying' (*ashaut*): *shepnen* of *shepen*, flies'

Table 7.5 Herbal remedies of less certain interpretation, or for which alternative meanings have been attributed to the Egyptian word

EGYPTIAN WORD	MEANING WHICH NOW SEEMS MOST LIKELY	PROPOSED ALTERNATIVE MEANINGS
saam	*Ambrosia maritima* (A)	chaste tree (C,M)
inset	aniseed (*Pimpinella anisum*) (L,D?,M?)	
ished	*Balanites aegyptiaca* (C)	persea (M)
djaret	carob (*Ceratonia siliqua*) (A,C,M)	colocynth (D,Da)
matet	celery (*Apium graveolens*) (A,C,D,G,Gh)	mandrake (Da,F)
gesfen	asafoetida (*Ferula foetida*) (C,M)	? chalcopyrite (A)[1]
innek	conyza (*Erigeron aegypticus*) (A,C,L)	? thyme (F,G)
bebet	conyza, variety of (A)	fleabane (*Inula graveolens*) (C,D,F,M)
tepnen	cumin (*Cuminum cyminum*) (C,F,M,Gh)	caraway (D,G)
wah	earth almonds (tiger nuts), rhizome of cyperus grass (*Cyperus esculentus*) (C,G,M)	carob (F)
sheny-ta	earth almonds (tiger nuts), rhizome of cyperus grass (*Cyperus esculentus*) (C,M)	fenugreek (Da)
hemau	fenugreek (C) (*Trigonella foenum-graecum*)	
hemayet	fenugreek (M)	pod of fruit (D)
ash	fir tree (*Abies cilicica*) (C,G,M)	cedar (F), pine (D)
kad(et)	Hederacea, variety of, ? *Hedera helix* (A)	
iber	ladanum (resin of *Cistus creticus*) (C,E,D)	
afet / afay	lettuce (*Lactuca virosa*) (A,M)	clover (*Melilotus officinalis*) (C,D,F,G,Gh)
shespet[2]	melon (*Cucumis melo*) (C,G,M)	cucumber (D,F,Gh)
khet-des	myrtle (*Myrtus communis*) (A,E)	
shepen	opium poppy (*Papaver somniferum*) (C,Gh,L,?M)	
shames	pyrethrum (*Anacyclus pyrethrum*) (A)	
peret-sheny	grains from umbrella pine of Byblos (C)	*Pinus pinea* (E)
sut (1)	(grains of) wheat[3] (C,D,F)	
(2)	unknown symbolic plant of Northern Egypt, probably a rush or reed (C,D,F)	

1 See Table 7.3.

2 *Shespet* is also used with a direct or indirect genitive before other plants, and must also mean a part of these plants. The cucumber (*Cucumis melo* var. Chate or *Cucumis sativus*) is closely related to the melon. The Assyrians, Greeks and Romans called melons 'ripe cucumbers' (Manniche, 1989).

3 *Sut* (1) and *sut* (2) are homophones but are two entirely different words with different hieroglyphic writing.

A Aufrère (1983–9)
C Charpentier (1981)
D *Drogennamen* of the *Grundriss* (Table 2.2)
Da Dawson (1929, 1933 and 1934a)
E Ebbell (1937)
F Faulkner (1962)
G Germer (1979)
Gh Ghaliounghui (1987)
L Lefebvre (1956)
M Manniche (1989)

excrement which is on the wall, make into one thing, mash and eat for four days. It stops immediately.

As for much crying (*ashaut*) it means a child who is crying (*ashut*).

There is no question that opium is a highly effective remedy for stopping children crying, and was used extensively for this purpose in England during the nineteenth

Table 7.6 The commoner plant remedies which cannot, at present, be translated with any certainty from the Egyptian

EGYPTIAN WORD	POSSIBLE MEANING
aaamu	–
amau	–
besbes	–
deshru	unknown part of corn fruit (*sekhet*) (D)
gengenet	senna (E)
heden	–
iaw	–
ibu	–
ineb	–
kabet	–
kesbet	–
khet-awa	–
mendji	–
mikat	–
nehed	–
niaia or *niwiw*	–
pakh-serit or *pakh-setet*	–
sa-wer	–
sekhet	–
semyt	probably a generic term for vegetables
shasha	valerian (Gh)
shenef(et)	–
tentem	–
tiam	–
tjun	–
wam	–

D *Drogennamen* of the *Grundriss* (Table 2.2)
E Ebbell (1937)
Gh Ghaliounghui (1987)

century. Lefebvre (1956) translated *shepnen nu shepen* as 'graines de pavot', and this was followed by Charpentier (1981) who gave 'poppy, *Papaver somniferum album*' for *shepen* and 'poppy seeds' for *shepnen*. Ghaliounghui (1987) accepted this interpretation. However, the seeds of *Papaver somniferum* contain only a little morphine, which is normally prepared from the juice which exudes when the seed pod is incised. Furthermore, the opium poppy was not native to Egypt, and there is no firm collateral evidence that it was known in Egypt until after the time that the Ebers papyrus was written (Bisset *et al.*, 1994).

Merrillees (1962) proposed that base ring juglets (type BRI,I) were used to import opium from Cyprus in about 1500 BC. This view is based partly on the resemblance of such juglets, when inverted, to a poppy head (fig. 7.4) and partly upon the supposed identification of morphine in an Egyptian alabaster juglet of similar shape from the undisturbed tomb of Kha (Nineteenth Dynasty) (Muzio, 1925). However, Bisset and his colleagues, using modern analytical techniques, were unable to detect morphine in six of the juglets from Kha's tomb, which were clearly of Egyptian and not Cypriot origin.

7.4 Typical Cypriot base ring juglet (type BRI, IA,a,iv) of the type which may have been used to import opium into Egypt during the 18th Dynasty. An inverted seed pod of *Papaver somniferum* is shown alongside to demonstrate the resemblance which Merrillees (1962) suggested advertised the contents of the juglet. (From the author's collection)

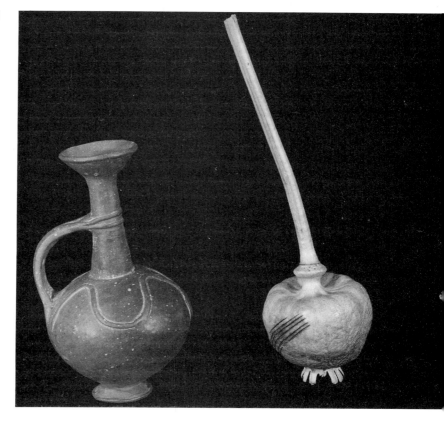

This supports the reluctance of Germer (1979) and the *Drogennamen* of the *Grundriss* to accept *shepen* as the opium poppy. If the ancient Egyptians were aware of the properties of opium, it seems inconceivable that they would have confined its use to that described in a single paragraph of the Ebers papyrus. *Shepnen* appears a few times in the medical papyri as a local application, but *shepen* never appears again, not even among the 200 drugs listed in the Vindob papyrus (D.6257) from Croco-dilopolis, written in the second century AD, by which time the properties of morphine were well known to the Greeks and Romans.

Cannabis (*Cannabis sativa*). There is general agreement with the view of Dawson (1934a) that *shemshemet* means cannabis, and the identification was strongly supported by the use of hemp in rope making. As a drug, it has remained in active use ever since pharaonic times. It does not appear very often in the medical papyri, but it was administered by mouth, rectum, vagina, bandaged to the skin, applied to the eyes and by fumigation. However, these applications provide no clear evidence of awareness of the effects of cannabis on the central nervous system.

Mandrake (*Mandragora officinalis*). The Egyptian word for mandrake originally proposed by Dawson (1933) was *matet*, now believed to mean celery (Table 7.5). *Rermet* is now accepted as mandrake by Charpentier (1981) and Manniche (1989). The London and Leiden papyrus of the third century AD (see Chapter 2) contains the

7.5 Stela of Ity, 12th Dynasty, showing two ladies characteristically 'sniffing the lotus' in the lower right hand corner. (British Museum, EA 586)

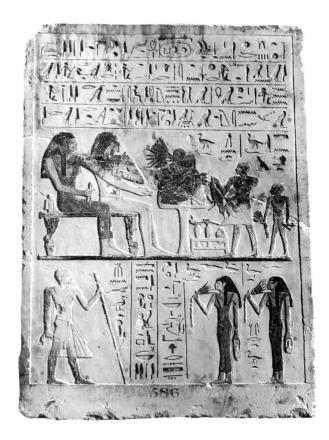

word *mantraguru* in demotic, clearly a form of Mandragora. The characteristic fruit is widely portrayed from the Amarna Period onwards in the New Kingdom, where its use was probably decorative.

The root contains the alkaloids *l*-hyoscyamine and *l*-hyoscine and traces of mandragorine. An alcoholic extract of the root has powerful sedative properties and can produce unconsciousness. However, there is no evidence that these properties were known in the pharaonic period and *rermet* does not appear in the medical papyri or the *Drogennamen* of the *Grundriss*.

The 'lotus' (*Nymphaea caerulea*, *Nymphaea lotos* and *Nelumbo nucifera*). There has been much confusion regarding the botanical species commonly referred to as 'lotus'. The two *Nymphaea* species are actually blue and white water lilies respectively, and native to Egypt (Harer, 1985). *Nelumbo nucifera* is the true (pink) lotus, but was probably not imported until the Persian Period. The Egyptian word *seshen* may cover all three species, although it could only mean the water lilies before the Persian Period.

Nymphaea contains four narcotic alkaloids which are concentrated in the flower and the rhizome but absent from seeds, stem and leaf. These alkaloids are soluble in alcohol but not in water. The effects can be experienced either by ingesting the roots or flowers, or by drinking wine in which they have been soaked. Harer has suggested that placing lotus blossoms in wine would produce a narcotic-laced wine or that a wine-extract of blossoms might be added to wine, as some depictions suggest. He also points out that an uninhibited young lady in the Turin erotic papyrus (no. 55001; Omlin, 1968) is always shown with a lotus above her head. However, it would not be possible to obtain any effect from sniffing the lotus blossom, as is so often depicted (fig. 7.5).

Internal medication in the medical papyri is always with the *khau* of the lotus, for which Faulkner gives the meaning 'flowers' and the *Grundriss* 'leaves'. The former would contain the alkaloids; the latter would not. Ebers 209 is a remedy for an obstruction in the right half of the belly, and the *khau* of the lotus which, together with fifteen other ingredients including beer, had to 'spend the night' before being strained and drunk. Ebers 479 is another remedy 'to treat the liver', possibly jaundice as it appears among remedies for skin diseases. This also includes *khau* of lotus, which here has 'spent the night' with wine and beer, conditions which might permit extraction of the alkaloids. Chester Beatty VI, 13 contains the use of *khau* of lotus (without beer or wine) as an enema.

Other analgesics. Without opiates or other narcotics, there would appear to have been limited opportunities for the symptomatic relief of severe pain. An unidentified part of the willow (*tjeret*) was recommended for internal use 'to cause the heart (sic) to receive bread' in Ebers 293. However, it is difficult to say whether this resulted in the effective administration of salicylates, derived from the glycoside salicin which is concentrated in the bark of the willow tree. Willow was otherwise used for surface application. The most effective analgesic would seem to have been alcohol, and Darby, Ghaliounghui and Grivetti (1977) have provided convincing evidence that intoxication was known and understood.

Incense and resins

Fumigation frequently involved the use of two varieties of incense: *senetjer* was probably terebinth resin in the pharaonic period but acquired a more general meaning in the Ptolemaic Period (Charpentier, 1981; Ghaliounghui, 1987); *antyu* was translated by Faulkner (1962) and others as myrrh. However, more recent work suggests a non-specific word meaning resin in general (Charpentier, 1981; Ghaliounghui, 1987). Both resins, particularly *senetjer*, were also prescribed to be taken by mouth.

Remedies for the gastro-intestinal system

About a quarter of all prescriptions in the Ebers papyrus were intended for the gastro-intestinal system. This is in line with the observations of Herodotus (II, 76):

> Every month for three successive days, they purge themselves for their health's sake, with emetics and clysters, in the belief that all diseases come from the food a man eats.

This accords with their concept of *wekhedu*, the toxin which could arise in the bowels and spread to the rest of the body through the *metu* (Chapter 3).

It is often difficult to distinguish between micturition and defecation with words such as *khaa*, *wesesh*, *pekha* and *wekha* which carry the general meaning of evacuate, but purgatives are clearly indicated in the following two passages:

> Another remedy for the belly: earth almonds (*sheny-ta*), 1/4; *gengenet*-plant, 1/4; wormwood (*sam*), 1/4; sweet beer, 15 *ro*; made into one thing, cook, strain and drink for one day. It is to cause a man to evacuate (*wesesh*) all which is in his belly. (Ebers 24)

Earth almonds or tiger nuts (the rhizome of *Cyperus esculentus*) were a staple item

Table 7.7 Some drugs which appear to have been used as aperients, with examples of their use

EGYPTIAN NAME	ENGLISH NAME	EXAMPLES
bener	date	Ebers 11,13,19,22,28
dab	fig	Ebers 6,17
degem	ricinus fruit	Ebers 25
djaret	? carob	Ebers 8,10,17
gengenet-plant	unknown[1]	Ebers 11,13,24,28,31
giw	cyperus grass	Ebers 19
hemat	salt of Lower Egypt	Ebers 13,23
ineb-plant	unknown	Ebers 16
ished-fruit	? balanites	Ebers 17
kesbet-tree	unknown	Ebers 16
khasyt	bryony	Ebers 19
neqawt	notched sycomore fig[2]	Ebers 7,18
peret-sheny	? grains from umbrella pine of Byblos	Ebers 23,29
sam	wormwood	Ebers 8,24
senetjer	incense (terebinth)	Ebers 23
shasha	? valerian	Ebers 26
shau	coriander	Ebers 19
shenfet-plant	unknown	Ebers 16
sheny-ta	? earth almond	Ebers 9,10,11,12,14,22,24,28
tepnem	cumin	Ebers 17
tiam-plant	unknown	Ebers 17,23
wadju	malachite	Ebers 15
wah	earth almond	Ebers 22
wam-plant	unknown	Ebers 16
wan	juniper	Ebers 23
The vehicles		
bit	honey	Ebers 7,8,9,10,11,12,14,16,22,23,28,29
henqet	beer	Ebers 9,14,15,19,24,29
iadet	dew	Ebers 19
irep	wine	Ebers 9,12
irtet	milk	Ebers 18
merhet	oil/fat	Ebers 11,17

1 Ebbell (1937) proposed senna for *gengenet*.
2 The sycomore fig was notched to allow the parasite *Crasipes longinus* to escape.

of diet, and wormwood has no particular laxative properties (Table 7.7). *Gengenet* appears many times in a similar context but Ebbell's reading as senna has not been confirmed. It also appears in Ebers 31 ('another [medicine] to drive out excrement (*hes*)').

Ebers 25 shows clearly that they were aware of the purgative properties of the castor-oil plant:

Another for the purging (*wekha*) of the belly and to drive out suffering from the belly of a man. Fruits/seeds (*peret*) of ricinus (*degem*), chewed (*wesha*) and swallowed with beer so that everything which is in his belly comes forth.

Table 7.8 Some remedies taken internally for disorders of the urinary system

EGYPTIAN NAME	ENGLISH NAME	EXAMPLES
For urine too plentiful or too often		
bi n sut	groats of wheat	Ebers 274,275,277,279
bit	honey	Ebers 277,278,280
giw	cyperus grass	Ebers 264
henqet	beer	Ebers 264,278
iaret	grapes	Ebers 278
ished	? balanites	Ebers 274,279
peret wan	juniper berries	Ebers 278
qemyt (& payt)*	gum	Ebers 275,277,279,280
sety	ochre	Ebers 274,277,279
To eliminate 'hurrying' of the urine		
giw	cyperus grass	Ebers 276 = 281
henqet	beer	Ebers 276 = 281
peret-sheny	? grains from umbrella pine of Byblos	Ebers 276 = 281
To put the urine in order		
bener wadj	fresh dates	Ebers 266,271,283
bit	honey	Ebers 263
giw	cyperus grass	Ebers 283
henqet	beer	Ebers 271
khasyt	bryony	Ebers 263,271,283
peret-sheny	? grains from umbrella pine of Byblos	Ebers 271,283
peret wan	juniper berries	Ebers 263,266
sety	ochre	Ebers 283
To eliminate heat in the bladder when he suffers from retention of urine		
baq	moringa oil	Ebers 265
bit	honey	Ebers 265
hemat	salt of Lower Egypt	Ebers 265
henqet nedjem	sweet beer	Ebers 265

*Qemyt is the word for gum in the Hearst papyri. Parallel passages in Ebers use the unfamiliar word payt in the same place, and it is assumed to have the same meaning as qemyt.
Ebers 277 = Hearst 63; Ebers 278 = Hearst 64; Ebers 279 = Hearst 66; Ebers 280 = Hearst 65

Section b of Ebers 251, cited in full above, says that if the fruit is chewed with beer by someone with the wehy-symptom in his faeces, there would be an elimination of suffering. The meaning of the wehy-symptom is unclear but Ebbell (1937) proposed diarrhoea and Lefebvre (1956) constipation, both feasible indications for a laxative.

Ebers (188–208) describes many cases of obstruction in the stomach (r-ib) and, whatever the precise interpretation of r-ib, it is clear that at least some of the sections describe constipation. Some of the drugs which appear to have been used as an aperient are listed in Table 7.7. Surprisingly, it is very difficult to identify drugs which were intended to prevent diarrhoea, but Ebers 44 gives a remedy to prevent 'evacuation' (weseshet).

It is much easier to distinguish the drugs which were prescribed to kill intestinal parasites, even though the Egyptian names cannot be related with certainty to specific

Table 7.9 Some drugs used for treatment of coughing (*seryt*)

Mineral products	
alum (*ibnu*)*	salt of Lower Egypt
ochre	*tcheru*-mineral
Animal products	
bone marrow	honey
cream/curd	milk
fat of goose	oil/fat (*merhet*)
fat of ox	tooth of pig
fat of pig	
Vegetable products	
acacia gum	flour
acacia leaves	gum
beer (various types)	lettuce (*afa*)
behen (Moringa) oil	peas
carob (*djaret*)	raisins
cumin	vegetable mucilage
date flour	water of yeast wheat
dates (pounded)	wine
earth almonds	wormwood*
emmer seeds (flour of)	yeast? (*sermet*)
figs	

fresh (kind of) bread, cooked in oil and honey
grains from umbrella pine of Byblos (*peret-sheny*)

aaamu-plant*	*meni*-resin*
amau-plant*	*meqeret* of the shore
aut-ib (? sandarac)*	*niaia*-plant
gengenet-plant	*senetjer*-resin
ished (*Balanites aegyptica*)	*shasha* (? valerian)
kerek	*shenef(et)*
khet-des-tree	*tiam*-plant*
mehut	

All were to be taken by mouth except, in some cases, for the drugs marked with an asterisk, which were to be heated and the fumes 'swallowed' through a reed.

Most remedies for cough are in: Ebers 190, 305–25; Berlin 29, 31–4, 36–47; Hearst 61

worms (see Table 4.1). Extracts of wormwood and pomegranate are known to be effective against some worms but there were many other items of unknown efficacy.

Remedies for the urinary system

There are substantial difficulties in defining disorders of the urinary system in the papyri (see Chapter 4). Furthermore, the proposed treatments do little to support the inferred diagnoses. Table 7.8 lists some of the components of the remedies under the headings of the disorders identified in Chapter 4.

Remedies for the relief of cough

Fortunately, the Egyptian word for cough (*seryt*) is well attested and we can note the remedies which are recommended (Table 7.9). Symptomatic relief of cough is either by a suppressant or by an expectorant. True cough suppressants are generally opiates, and there is no clear evidence of their use for this purpose. Some relief may be gained from sweet liquids, and honey, carob (*djaret*) and dates featured very prominently. *Djaret* was formerly read as colocynth which is a purgative, but has no particular properties in relation to cough. Expectorants increase bronchial mucus secretion and so make the cough more productive. They tend to be emetic in higher dosage (e.g. ipecacuanha). Wormwood/absinthe (*sam*) causes vomiting with habitual use of large dose, and appears three times for oral administration in Table 7.9.

Discussion of gynaecological and ophthalmic remedies is deferred to Chapter 9.

Conclusions

The extensive Egyptian pharmacopoeia contained items of mineral, animal and vegetable origin, dispensed by volume and not by weight. Most drugs in the first two categories can be identified from sources outside the medical papyri. However, many were sympathetic remedies, unlikely to have major therapeutic effects, although, in some cases, valuable therapeutic effects would have been obtained. About 160 plant products were used, but barely 20 per cent of these can be identified with certainty. Conversely, we do not know the Egyptian names for many herbal drugs which were probably used. Several identified vegetable drugs have proven therapeutic efficacy (Appendix C), and have remained in use until the present. Sadly we must remain ignorant of the effects of the many unidentified drugs.

CHAPTER EIGHT

Surgery, trauma and dangerous animals

Surgery

There is no convincing evidence that the specialty of surgery was separate from that of general medicine in ancient Egypt. Chapter 6 considered the rather flimsy evidence suggesting that perhaps the *wab* priests of Sekhmet undertook surgery, leaving the *swnw* to concentrate on internal medicine. This seems unlikely because of the very limited scope of surgery. There can be no doubt of their excellent management of injuries (considered below), but we know very little about surgery being used to relieve conditions which did not result from trauma. Apart from the celebrated circumcision scenes in the tomb of Ankh-ma-hor and in the precinct of Mut in Karnak, there are no depictions of surgery such as those which have revealed so much about surgical practice in the Middle Ages. There are no accounts of major surgery which can compare with those of Celsus for the Roman Period.

Surgical instruments

Graeco-Roman medicine has left us a wealth of surgical instruments, many of them superbly designed. In contrast, no one has found instruments which were unequivocally surgical from the pharaonic period. Some cosmetic instruments could have been used for surgery but there is no evidence of such use. Nevertheless, the device of presumed toiletry function from the tomb of Kha (fig. 8.1) clearly shows that they possessed the technical skills which would be needed to make very sophisticated surgical instruments.

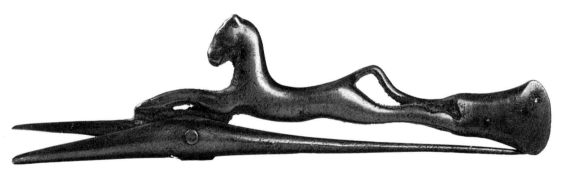

8.1 Presumed toilet instrument of unknown function from the undisturbed tomb of Kha, Deir el-Medina, 18th Dynasty. (Egyptian Museum, Turin)

There is a celebrated group of instruments carved in relief at the temple of Kom Ombo. The great temple itself is double, dedicated to both Horus-the-elder and Sobek, and dates from the Ptolemaic Period, Ptolemy VI (Philometor) being the earliest king to be represented in the decorations. However, there is an outer enclosure wall, dating from the second half of the second century AD, which forms a corridor around the temple. Near the north-western corner of the corridor, on the inner aspect of the outer wall, is the relief shown in fig. 8.2, which has been the source of endless discussion. Opinions have been divided on whether they are surgical or non-medical instruments, perhaps representing a foundation deposit. The surrounding reliefs are typically Egyptian, and there is no overt reference to the instruments, which are mounted on an offering table. Nevertheless, the relief closely resembles many well

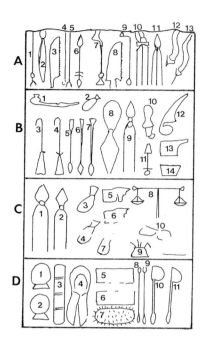

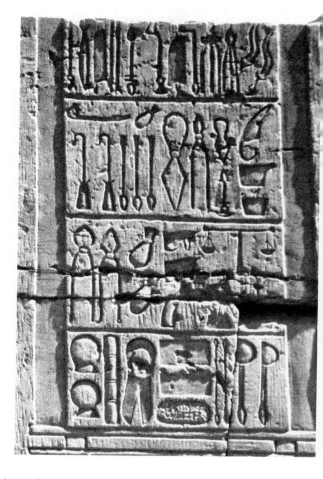

authenticated depictions of Roman surgical instruments (Tabanelli, 1958; Berger, 1970; Cassar, 1974). There is always a grey area of overlap between certain surgical instruments and others which are used for household purposes. However, many of the items shown in fig. 8.2 can be identified unequivocally as Roman surgical instruments which have been found in medical locations (Künzl, 1983; Jackson, 1986, 1990) or shown on the tomb of a surgeon (Tabanelli, 1958).

Positive identifications are listed in the legend to fig. 8.2. Perhaps the most convincing are D10 and 11, which clearly display the combination of a bellied iron blade and moulded handle with leaf-shaped dissector terminal, so characteristic of Roman scalpels. D3 is a typical Roman tubular copper-alloy box for surgical instruments or medicaments, as described by Jackson (1986). D7 is probably a sponge. The balance (C8) is a most powerful argument against the instruments being Egyptian, because their drugs were dispensed by volume and not by weight (see Chapter 7). Identification as Roman surgical instruments accords with the Antonine date of the wall.

The medical papyri make many references to 'knife treatment' (*djua*) and the ancient Egyptians had at least four words for knives which were used in surgical procedures – *des*, *khepet* and *shas* with knife determinatives, and *hemem* with a metal determinative (usually copper). However, the essential differences in the use of these

8.2 The instruments shown on the inner aspect of the northern part of the outer enclosure wall of the temple of Kom Ombo (Roman Period). Letters and numbers refer to the key diagram; numbers in parentheses refer to figure numbers in the publications listed below.

Identifications with a high level of probability: A1: Bifurcated sharp hook (2.4ᶜ). A8: Saw blade (5.7ᶜ). B2: Flask or clyster. B3&4: Hooks (2.1ᶜ, 57.15–18ᵃ). B5,6&7: Scoop-probe (cyathiscomele) (3.2ᵃ). B8: Cranioclast/craniotribe (29ᵈ). c1&2: Tooth forceps (5.2ᶜ) or bone forceps (5.4ᶜ). c3&4: Flask or clyster. c8: Balance. D1&2: Cupping vessels (1.3ᶜ, 55.7ᵃ, 70ᵉ). D3: Case for instruments (5.36ᵇ, 84ᵃ, 10.6ᶜ). D4: Shears (1.5ᶜ). D5&6: Bandages or bandage boxes (84ᵃ). D7: Sponge. D8&9: Double-ended probes (dipyrenes) (4.7&8ᶜ, 4.27ᵇ). D10&11: Scalpels (1.6ᶜ, 56.1–5ᵃ).

Less certain identifications: A2: Tooth forceps (5.2ᶜ), bone forceps (5.4ᶜ) or spring forceps (57.12ᵃ, 3.5ᶜ). A3: Saw blade (5.7ᶜ) or knife blade. A4: Probe (4.6ᶜ). A5: Bifurcated sharp hook (2.4ᶜ). A7&9: Cautery (7.4ᶜ, 58.14ᵃ). A10&11: Trivalve specula (81ᵃ, 8ᶜ). A12&13: Catheters for adult males (6.2ᶜ). B9: Tooth forceps (5.2ᶜ), bone forceps (5.4ᶜ) or uvula forceps. B12: knife. B13&14: bowl or mortar.

References: ᵃ Künzl (1983); ᵇ Jackson (1986); ᶜ Jackson (1990); ᵈ Habrich, Künzl and Zimmermann (1991); ᵉ Berger (1970).

instruments are not at all clear, except that the *khepet*-knife is mentioned only in relation to the ear (Ebers 767). It is quite likely that flint knives continued to be used well into the Bronze Age, and Egyptian flint knapping skills were equal to the best in the world. Miller (personal communication, 1994) has pointed out that a freshly flaked flint knife would be sterile and could be discarded after use. This would anticipate the disposable scalpel of today. Zipporah, the wife of Moses, circumcised her son with a sharp flint picked from the ground while on the journey from Midian to Egypt (Exodus 4: 25). In the *Tale of the Two Brothers*, Bata castrated himself with a *sefet*-knife: the word does not appear in the medical papyri but the related word *sef* (to cut) appears in Ebers 766. There is one reference to the use of a reed (*sut*) 'for making the knife-treatment' (Ebers 876; see below). Ebers 875 refers to the *henu*-instrument which appears to be a type of forceps although with a leather determinative (see below). The word *teshtesh* is used in the Brooklyn papyrus on snake bites (72a and 81), apparently here meaning 'incise': the *des*-knife was specified for this purpose in 72a.

The *pesesh-kef* knife was fish-tailed and not unlike the hieroglyph for the bicornuate uterus (fig. 3.5; Gardiner sign-list F 45). It appeared as a flint knife in the Predynastic Period, and later became part of the stylised set of instruments provided for the 'opening of the mouth' ceremony, allowing a mummy to partake of food offerings. A spell in the Pyramid texts states that the *pesesh-kef* is 'to make firm (*semem*) the lower jaw'. Roth (1992) and Harer (1994) have advanced the view that the *pesesh-kef* was used to cut the umbilical cord, and this could have magical significance in the re-birth of the dead. It closely resembles the headdress of Meskhenet, a goddess important in childbirth as a personification of the birth-brick (see Chapter 5).

Leca (1988) showed a collection of surgical instruments (his Plate XI), probably for ophthalmic use, but of a much later date than the pharaonic period.

Surgical procedures outside the field of trauma

There is no convincing evidence that the ancient Egyptians undertook anything beyond the very simplest surgical operations. There are no accounts in the medical papyri, nor is there evidence in mummies, to indicate the formidable operations of the first century AD, as described by the Roman author Celsus. Rowling (1989) estimated that 30,000 mummies had been examined without a single surgical scar being reported. The only illustrations of surgical procedures are the circumcision scene (see below), some aspects of industrial medicine in the tomb of Ipwy (see below) and a soldier of Ramses II portrayed at Abu Simbel having his leg treated.

The Edwin Smith papyrus is an instructional text for the management of trauma to the upper part of the body. Unfortunately, very little comparable material has survived in the field of surgery not connected with trauma. The nearest approach is the final section of the Ebers papyrus (863–77) and a few cases from the Edwin Smith papyrus. The surgical section of the Ebers papyrus dealing with swellings and tumours is summarised in Table 8.1, and begins with a condition, described in paragraph 863 as 'a swelling of flesh (*haw*) of any of the limbs (*at*) of a man', suggesting a solid tumour. The treatment (*sahemem*) cannot at present be translated.

The next paragraph, 864, merits extended citation:

Instructions for a swelling (*aat*) of the coverings of the 'brow' (*wepet*) of his abdomen. If you examine a swelling of the coverings of the 'brow' of his abdomen above his umbilicus. Then you should place your finger on it and you should palpate his abdomen ... That which comes into being comes forth when he coughs.

Table 8.1 Swellings and tumours listed in the Ebers papyrus (863–77)

PARAGRAPH	CONTENTS		RECOMMENDED TREATMENT
	EGYPTIAN	ENGLISH	
aat swellings			
863	*haw*	flesh	*sahemem* (meaning unknown)
864	*hebesu*	covering (?)	heat and *sahemem*
865	*mu*	water	pierce with a *hemem*-knife
866	*sefet* of *metu*	swelling of vessels	knife treatment (*djua*)
867	*adj*	fat	knife treatment (*djua*)
868	*sa*	meaning unknown	knife treatment (*djua*)
869	*ryt*	pus	knife treatment (*djua*)
870	*sheny*	hair	knife treatment (*djua*)
871	*wekhedu*	pus in this context	knife treatment (*djua*)
872	*metu*	vessels	treatment with heated knife
873	*metu*	vessels	not to be treated
873	of Khonsu	of Khonsu	spell
874	of Khonsu	of Khonsu	not to be treated
875	–	not specified	treatment with *des*-knife, *shas*-knife and *henu*-instrument
sefet swellings			
876	*metu*	haematoma ?	knife treatment with a reed burn if it bleeds
anut swelling of Khonsu			
877	of Khonsu	of Khonsu	no surgical treatment

This appears to be a classic description of an umbilical or an epigastric hernia (see Chapter 4), the former being illustrated in many paintings and reliefs of servants and workmen (fig. 8.3). The word *wepet* has many meanings other than brow, but the phrase 'above the umbilicus' seems to exclude the more common inguinal hernia (fig. 4.15). The text follows with the pronouncement and treatment:

> Then you shall say concerning it 'This is a swelling of the coverings of his abdomen, an illness which I will treat'. It is the heat of his bladder in front of his belly which creates it. Falling to the ground, [it] returns likewise. You should heat (*shemem*) it to imprison it in his belly. You treat it like the *sahemem* treatment.

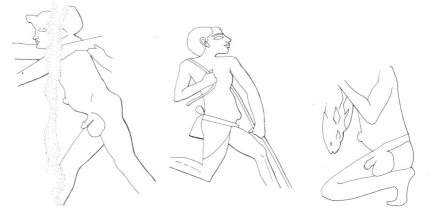

8.3 Three examples of umbilical hernia in tomb reliefs of the 6th Dynasty from Saqqara. Centre: from the tomb of Ptah-hotep. Left and right: from the tomb of Mehu.

Although the passage is unclear, it is possible that they had noticed that this type of hernia tends to disappear when the patient lies down. It is unclear whether it was intended that gentle heat should be used to relax the abdomen to facilitate reduction of the hernia, or whether the cautery should be used to create scarring in the hope of occluding the neck of the hernia.

Paragraph 865 refers to a swelling of the lower part of the abdomen with 'the water of his abdomen going up and down'. This would be an apt description of ascites (effusion of fluid into the peritoneal cavity). The recommended treatment is to pierce (*tjehen*) the swelling with a *hemem*-knife, similar treatment being advocated for ascites in the first century AD by Celsus (VII, 15, 1).

Paragraph 866 is the first concerned with swellings of the *metu*. This difficult word is discussed in detail in Chapter 3 and may refer to various parts of the body which are long and thin, such as blood vessels, ducts, tendons, muscles and possibly nerves. It is tempting to believe that this paragraph refers to a vascular tumour such as a haemangioma, but there is no confirmation in the description of the clinical findings. Following the usual declaration, it is recommended that the condition be treated with 'the knife treatment' (*djua*). This is a very common phrase in the medical papyri (Table 8.1) and was translated by Ebbell (1937) as the performance of an operation. Paragraph 872 also describes a swelling of the *metu*, but one which is 'rounded and hard under your fingers'. It is recommended that the knife be heated (*seshemem*, causative of *shemem*, see above) before using the knife treatment – then 'the bleeding is not great'. This supports the diagnosis of haemangioma. Paragraph 873 is again a swelling of the *metu*, and in this case it is said that 'they make many knots', which might be a cavernous haemangioma. Perhaps recognising the danger of serious haemorrhage, the instructions say 'do not put a hand on anything like this'.

Paragraph 867 refers to a swelling of fat (*adj*), which comes and goes under the fingers. This must presumably refer to a subcutaneous lipoma, usually quite mobile, which would be seen to be composed of fat after it had been removed. The knife treatment was recommended, followed by the customary treatment of a wound. There is no specific mention of suturing although this might be understood as included in the treatment of a wound. Surgical suturing is never mentioned in the Ebers papyrus, but is frequently recommended in the treatment of lacerations in the Edwin Smith papyrus (see below).

Paragraph 868 refers to a swelling of *sa* (with the goose biliteral), a word usually meaning son but here with a flesh determinative. It is said to be 'like the skin of his flesh, solid under the finger, large and painful'. It is unclear what is meant, but the knife treatment was recommended.

Paragraphs 869 and 871 describe swellings which are probably abscesses. They are cited in Chapter 4, where the differential diagnosis is considered. In both cases the knife treatment is recommended. They contrast with a breast abscess in Edwin Smith, Case 46, where the knife treatment is not recommended, probably because fluid is already exuding.

Paragraph 870 describes a swelling of hair (*sheny*) also to be treated with the knife treatment. This could perhaps be a dermoid cyst, lined with skin appendages including hair, or possibly a pilonidal sinus which sometimes contains hair and is located in the midline on the back at the bottom of the spine. The ancient Egyptians would certainly have been struck by the appearance of hair. Alternatively, *sheny* might be a genitive of location to describe something like a sebaceous cyst of the scalp.

The second part of paragraph 873 makes brief reference to a swelling (*aat*) of Khonsu, and treatment is restricted to a spell. The following paragraph (874) also deals with a swelling (*aat*) of Khonsu, which is 'terrible/rough (*neha*) and has made many swellings in it (or him)'. The treatment is succinct 'you should not do anything to it'. Paragraph 877 gives instructions for treating an '*anut* of the Khonsu-slaughtering'. *Anut* is a word which does not appear elsewhere but it is compared to any swelling (*shefet*). No surgical treatment is recommended. There are several possible interpretations of the 'Khonsu tumour', which might be a cancer, cutaneous leprosy, bubonic plague or even neurofibromatosis. The *swnw* would be well advised to leave these alone.

Some further detail on the application of the knife treatment is given in section c) of paragraph 875, cited in full in Chapter 4 in relation to possible removal of a guinea-worm. Parts of this paragraph are very difficult to interpret but it introduces two new instruments, the *shas*-knife and the *henu*-instrument. The word for grasp (*nedjer*) is well established and we can visualise the surgeon holding the part to be removed with a *henu*-instrument, held in one hand, while his other hand wields the *des*- or *shas*-knife, as is current practice with forceps and scalpel. Unfortunately, the nature of the *henu*- and *henuyt*-instruments remains obscure. It is tempting to believe that they were some type of forceps but the leather determinative for *henu* makes its construction problematical.

Paragraph 876 is concerned with *sefet* of the *metu*. *Sefet* is an unknown word which must be distinguished from *shefet* meaning 'swelling'. However, the examination records that it is red and rounded (or raised) like [the result of] a blow from a stick. If *metu* here refers to blood vessels, the description would accord with a haematoma (effusion of blood under the skin) and this was the interpretation of Ebbell (1937). The treatment is very clearly stated: 'You shall then use the knife treatment with a scirpus reed (*sut*), used for the knife treatment'. This evokes the drainage of the haematoma through multiple small skin punctures, a procedure which would carry danger of introducing infection.

Although most of the Edwin Smith papyrus is concerned with trauma (considered below), three cases refer to swellings, ulcers and infections of the breast (Cases 39, 45 and 46). Unfamiliar words are used and their meaning can seldom be verified from parallel use elsewhere. However, there is a clear picture of hard and soft swellings which are painful and which may contain fluid. Although the descriptions could apply to breast tumours or abscesses, their appearance within the Edwin Smith papyrus suggests that they are probably secondary infections of wounds. Either no treatment or else local applications are recommended, and in no case is there any suggestion that the knife treatment be used. In fact, the usual word for knife treatment (*djua*) does not appear at all in the Edwin Smith papyrus.

There is no mention of any form of anaesthesia for the procedures outlined above. This accords with the fearful accounts of surgery described by Celsus, and the concept of painless surgery lay millennia in the future. There is no evidence that the Egyptians used any drugs, other than alcohol, which could numb the senses to the required extent (see Chapter 7).

Trephining

Trephining (or trepanning) is undertaken today mainly to provide access to the brain. However, it is well documented to have been employed in antiquity, particularly in France, Jericho and Peru, with long-term survival of the patients as judged by the healing of the bone edges. Until quite recently, it has still been employed by folk doctors in Africa, without anaesthesia, for a wide variety of indications, and most patients have recovered (Hayes, 1962). Several procedures have been described. Four saw cuts can be made, followed by breaking out the contained square of bone. Alternatively, a circular area can be removed by twisting a sharp convex blade of metal or flint, leaving edges which are bevelled on the outside. Simple scraping can produce a hole which tends to be oval, again with bevelled edges. Finally a ring of holes can be drilled prior to breaking out the contained area of bone. In all cases the greatest care must be taken not to open the dura mater, because exposure of the brain would be fatal.

The surviving papyri make no mention of trephining but the evidence from mummies and skeletons is less clear. In most cases, holes in skulls from ancient Egypt are due to lethal trauma or natural thinning of the parietal bone, which lacks the characteristic edges of a trephine. However, Breasted (1930) in his Addendum 3, cited a personal communication of the discovery of a trepanned skull from one of the 'deep pits at Lisht' which 'belonged undoubtedly to one of the nobler families of the Twelfth Dynasty'. Ghaliounghui (1973) reported that the hole in the skull of Princess Horsiesnest Meritaten (kept in the Anatomy Department of the Cairo Faculty of Medicine) had well healed edges and an appearance consistent with the use of hammer and chisel, or a convex scraper with a wide radius as in the second method described above. Similar appearances were found in the frontal bone of a child. It would therefore appear that trephining was known to the ancient Egyptians, but there are very few surviving examples.

Tracheostomy ?

Ghaliounghui also drew attention to two slabs from the First Dynasty, discovered by Petrie and relating one to King Aha and one to King Djer. Each shows a kneeling figure with his arms behind his back, while another person points something looking like a dagger at the upper part of the front of his chest. Petrie interpreted this as ritual sacrifice but Vikentieff (1949–50) suggested it might be performance of a tracheostomy. This can only be surmise and seems very unlikely because the setting is that of a ritual and the point of the instrument is aimed too low for a tracheostomy. Human sacrifice is a plausible alternative explanation.

Circumcision

The procedure is very clearly shown in the famous relief (fig. 8.4) on the east thickness of the doorway to the tomb of Ankh-ma-hor, vizier and overseer of all the works of King Teti (Old Kingdom, Sixth Dynasty, c. 2345 BC). There are traces of a much damaged but similar scene in the precinct of Mut in Karnak. The seated figure in the centre of fig. 8.4 is apparently a *hem-ka* (funerary) priest, and the words in front of his head have usually been interpreted to mean that he is circumcising (*seb*), the word being close to the Coptic equivalent and not in doubt. Above are his words addressed to his assistant 'Hold him fast; do not let him fall!' The obsequious assistant replies 'I shall act for your praise.' The scene on the right is less easy to understand. The operator is saying: '[I] will make it comfortable (well, pleasant or sweet)', to which the patient responds: 'Rub it well in order that it may be effective'. These remarks can hardly describe a circumcision and it has been suggested that some form of analgesia is being provided before the actual circumcision is undertaken. It is less easy to suggest what form the analgesia might take. Cocaine is extracted from a New World plant not imported to Europe until some four thousand years later, and ice was probably not available in Egypt of the Old Kingdom. It has been suggested that the object in the hand of the operator was the stone of Memphis (limestone) which would evolve carbon dioxide under the influence of vinegar. It is true that the inhalation of carbon dioxide in concentrations greater than about 20 per cent can cause loss of consciousness, but it has no local anaesthetic effect and the vinegar would hardly 'make it comfortable'.

It has never been clear why Ankh-ma-hor should have chosen to include this scene in his tomb, although it has many scenes of medical interest (see p. 126). It has been suggested that it might represent Ankh-ma-hor's own circumcision or perhaps he simply wanted the facility of circumcision to be available for himself and his family in the hereafter. There is evidence that he took particular interest in his tomb decoration and many scenes were replastered and then recut. It is also unclear why a funerary priest should be undertaking the procedure.

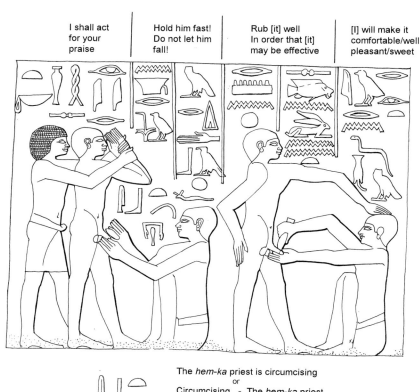

| I shall act for your praise | Hold him fast! Do not let him fall! | Rub [it] well In order that [it] may be effective | [I] will make it comfortable/well pleasant/sweet |

8.4 The circumcision in the tomb of Ankh-ma-hor, 6th Dynasty, Saqqara. Various interpretations of this scene are discussed in the text.

The *hem-ka* priest is circumcising
or
Circumcising - The *hem-ka* priest
or
Circumcising the *hem-ka priest*
or
One is circumcising the *hem-ka* priest

An entirely new proposal was advanced in 1991 by Ann Macy Roth. She pointed out that the words in front of the seated man are actually *sebet hem-ka*, whereas the verb to circumcise would be simply *seb* if the phrase meant 'the *hem-ka* priest is circumcising', with the subject following the verb as is normal. *Sebet* might be the infinitive followed by *hem-ka* as the object, i.e. 'circumcising the *hem-ka* priest'. Alternatively, *sebet* might perhaps be the common contraction for *seb.tw* meaning 'one circumcises', with *hem-ka* as the object, i.e. 'one is circumcising the *hem-ka* priest', which is the usual manner of indicating the passive mood – 'the *hem-ka* priest is being circumcised'. Either interpretation gives the *hem-ka* priest as the patient and not the operator. The proposal is then that the scene is an initiation ceremony for the *hem-ka* priest, perhaps one of Ankh-ma-hor's sons. This now makes sense of the scene on the right which is then interpreted as shaving the pubic hair for ritual purity. The words of the operator can be read as '[I] will make it pleasant (or sweet)', while the patient's words, 'rub it well, in order that it may be effective' would be entirely appropriate for the use of razors of that period. Further examination of photographs and the relief itself convinced Roth that the operator was using a razor rather than a knife. Shaving pubic hair is clearly shown in a relief in the tomb of Ni-ankh-khnum and Khnum-hotep, which includes the word for shave (*shaq*) in two places. It remains unclear who was performing the circumcision in the tomb of Ankh-ma-hor.

It seems very likely that circumcision was commonly undertaken for ritual initiation into manhood or phyles, rather than for medical reasons. Sponsoring circumcision was sometimes seen as a public benefaction, and a stela from Naga ed-Deir records a man called Wha who was circumcised with 120 others (Roth, 1991). Evidence from mummies indicates that it was by no means universal in the social classes who were mummified, and that it was undertaken in late puberty. One stela indicates that the owner 'achieved office before he was circumcised'. In contrast, Elliot Smith (1908) remarked in a footnote that, of the bodies in the prehistoric cemetery at Naga ed-Deir (Hearst Expedition), he found all the men were circumcised.

Surgery of the teeth and eyes is considered in Chapter 9.

Trauma

Ancient Egyptian concepts of traumatic lesions and their vocabulary were considered in Chapter 3. Here we consider their methods of treatment, for knowledge of which we depend mainly on the Edwin Smith papyrus (see Chapter 2). We are very fortunate that this papyrus has survived because almost no parallel passages have been found. The cause of trauma was usually obvious and therefore treatment was mainly pragmatic, with magic playing a minimal role. The papyrus is in the form of forty-eight illustrative cases of trauma, starting at the top of the head and proceeding downwards in an orderly fashion to finish in the middle of Case 48 which is a spinal injury (see fig. 2.2). However, this section of the book will be grouped by type of injury rather than by location.

Lacerations

The word for a wound is *webenu*, which might be superficial or deep. For a very deep and gaping wound the phrase is *webenu kefet*, the latter with a knife determinative. *Webenu* are present in twenty-four of the forty-eight cases in the Edwin Smith papyrus and, of these, eleven are graded as *kefet*.

The usual treatment for a wound was to bandage it with fresh meat on the first day. This is recommended in at least thirteen cases and probably two more where there are lacunae in the text. It was then recommended that the wound be bound with oil and honey, which might be expected to improve wound healing by two mechanisms. First, the osmotic effect of the sugars in the honey would draw fluid out of the damaged tissues and reduce swelling. Secondly, it is well recognised that bacteria do not grow in honey (see Chapter 7). Over all, honey would be expected to accelerate wound healing and this has indeed been demonstrated in controlled studies (Bergman *et al.*, 1983).

Stitching of wounds was recommended in the Edwin Smith papyrus in the following seven cases, where it seems entirely appropriate:

3 Gaping wound of the head (restored text)
10 Gaping wound above the eyebrows

14 Wound of the nostril
23 Flesh wound of the ear
26 Wound of the upper lip
28 Gaping wound of the throat
47 Gaping wound of the shoulder

The Egyptians were capable of superb needle-work from at least the Early Dynastic Period, the oldest surviving needles being predynastic (Petrie, 1917) (fig. 8.5). Gold needles in the Manchester Museum (4247 a and b) were dated to the First Dynasty by Petrie (1907). It is therefore remarkable that the word for sewing (*tep*) is extremely

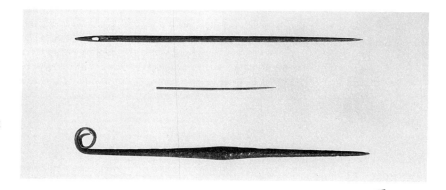

8.5 From the top downwards, a copper needle (UC 36154), a silver needle, broken at the eye (UC 36151), and a copper pin with loop head (UC 4301), all Predynastic and from Naqada. Below is an unprovenanced bird's bone needle case, containing fifteen copper alloy needles of the New Kingdom (UC 7721). All are shown actual size. (Petrie Museum, University College London)

uncommon, with a paucity of references in the *Wörterbuch* (Erman and Grapow, 1926–31). No word for 'sew' appears in the Egyptian–English dictionaries of Faulkner (1962) and Lesko (1982–90), nor in any of the medical papyri. The word in the Edwin Smith papyrus is *ider* and appears hardly anywhere else apart from the seven cases listed above. There has been no trace of surgical suturing in any mummy although there is a celebrated example of suturing having been used after death by embalmers in the Twenty-sixth Dynasty (see fig. 3.1). Their incisions were normally left open and covered by a flat metal plate.

Case 28 describes the use of stitching in challenging circumstances:

If you examine a man with a gaping wound of his throat, penetrating his pharynx, and if he drinks water, he chokes(?) [it] coming forth from the mouth of his wound. It is greatly inflamed and he develops fever because of it. You should then draw together that wound with stitching.

The suturing of a penetrating and infected wound of the pharynx would be a daunting prospect but might perhaps be the only chance of saving this man's life. It is declared to be an illness with which to contend, and the mention of a second examination indicates that the patient appeared to survive the suturing.

Sometimes the Edwin Smith recommends that the lips (*septy*) of a gash should be drawn together with bandaging. Case 11 uses the word *hayt* for bandage which it equates with the *seshed* linen bandage, obtainable from the embalmers. This is the very well known bandage used with such remarkable skill in the mummification procedure. In Chapter 3 it was explained that this was one of the few recorded points of contact between the *swnw* and the embalmers. Five other cases use the word *awy* which is explained in Gloss A of Case 10 and, probably with the same meaning, in the much damaged Gloss B of Case 2:

> As for two *awy* of linen, it means two *seshed*-bandages of linen which are applied to the two lips (*sepet*) of a gaping wound to cause one [lip] to be joined to the other.

Breasted (1930) advanced the very reasonable view that a bandage used in this manner might be adhesive, as is so widely used today for the treatment of minor lacerations. They would certainly have the technology to stick a *seshed* bandage to the skin, but no adhesive was used in the normal bandaging of a mummy. Bandaging was used to close lacerations in the following cases:

> 2 Gaping wound of the head
> 9 Gaping wound of the forehead
> 10 Gaping wound above the eyebrow
> 27 Gaping wound of the chin
> 47 Gaping wound of the shoulder

Infection of wounds must have been so common that it could have been regarded as a normal part of the healing process, as it was by Celsus in the first century AD. In the course of five examinations, Case 47 gives an excellent description of a wound of the shoulder which became infected but later recovered. Case 41 was also infected and the glosses give a clear description of the terms used.

> (A) As for 'an abnormality (*shemay*) of the wound (*webenu*) of his breast, which is inflamed (*nesry*)', it means that the wound which is in his breast is hesitating (*wedjef*), without closing up (lit. being veiled – *tjam*); high fever/inflammation (*shememet*) comes forth from it; its two lips are red and its mouth is open. . . . There is very great swelling. . . .

> (C) As for 'its two lips are ruddy', it means that its two lips are red like the colour of the *tjemset*-tree.

> (D) As for 'his flesh cannot receive a bandage', it means that his flesh will not receive the remedies because of the fever/inflammation (*shememet*) which is in his flesh.

No stitching had been used and there is a very clear picture of an ugly infected wound. Treatment was confined to local applications of various herbal remedies but including green pigment, with an unusual though phonetically plausible writing (*wadju*). Assuming this would have been a copper salt or perhaps powdered malachite, some anti-bacterial effect could be expected (see Chapter 7).

A section of the Ebers papyrus (510–41) contains a variety of remedies for wounds, including those resulting from a beating. No surgical treatment is recommended and the remedies consist of local applications, with oil and honey featuring in many of them. Paragraph 522 describes a sequential approach in which ox fat is applied on the first day, apparently to encourage the wound to become foul, but not too foul. This is reminiscent of the encouragement of 'laudable pus' in the days before antibiotics. Barley bread is recommended to dry the wound if it becomes too foul. The section of the Ebers papyrus dealing with the ears (764–81) contains a paragraph (766) which gives detailed instructions for a wound (*webenu*), comprising local applications and a supportive bandage.

Fractures

Injuries to bones are well described in the Edwin Smith papyrus, and the classification of fractures was considered in Chapter 3. We can identify simple closed fractures without a wound, and there are descriptions of comminuted, compound and impacted fractures. Perforation (*tehem*) of the skull is classically shown in the mummy of the unfortunate pharaoh Seqenenra, 'the hero' (Seventeenth Dynasty, *c.* 1600 BC) (fig. 8.6). Astonishingly, a recent X-ray analysis by Erhard Metzel has shown new growth of bone around the uppermost injury, indicating that he must have survived for at least a few months (Fleming and Fishman, 1980).

Diagnostic techniques. The Edwin Smith papyrus has relatively little to say on the diagnosis of a fracture. However, in six cases, there is reference to the elicitation of *nekhebkheb*, possibly an onomatopoeic word, thought by Breasted to mean crepitation, which is the sensation imparted when the fractured ends of a bone are moved against each other. This is unpleasant for the patient but is absolutely diagnostic of fracture, and was a valuable clinical sign before the introduction of radiography. It is mentioned in two patients with smashes (nose and cheek) and in three patients with the simpler *heseb*-fracture (mandible, humerus and ribs). Case 7 describes probing a scalp wound 'though he fears it greatly', searching for a fractured skull, a practice which continued well into this century before routine radiography became established.

A classic sign of fractured base of skull is bleeding from the ears and nostrils. This is reported in seven patients, and the observation was stressed in the formal declaration before pronouncing the prognosis which was always unfavourable. There can be little doubt that the dire significance of the sign was understood, as shown in the following seven cases:

4	Fractured skull	contend
5	Fractured skull	do not treat
7	Fractured skull	contend
8	Fractured skull	do not treat
17	Fractured maxilla	do not treat
21	Fractured temporal bone	contend
22	Fractured temporal bone	do not treat

In four patients it was remarked that they could not flex their neck to look at their breast. This is a well known sign of meningeal irritation (from blood or infection). This observation was also included in the formal declaration before the pronouncement of the prognosis, which was usually unfavourable:

3	Fractured skull	treat
4	Fractured skull	contend
5	Fractured skull	do not treat
7	Fractured skull	contend

Treatment of fractures. The Edwin Smith papyrus is unfortunately reticent on the reduction of fractures. A typical example is a fractured nose (Case 12), which is well described but lacks the essential information on how the shape of the nose was

8.6 Injuries to the forehead of the pharaoh Seqenenra, 17th Dynasty. (Cairo Museum, CG 61051; from Smith, 1912)

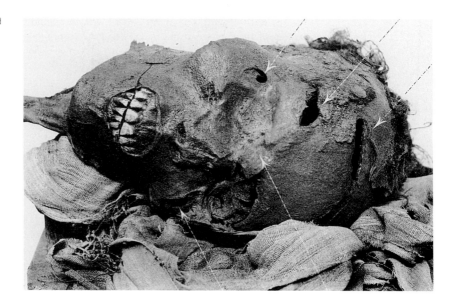

restored by reduction of the fracture. Nevertheless, the case contains much interesting detail which merits full citation:

TITLE
Instructions for a *heseb*-fracture in the chamber of his nose.

EXAMINATION
If you examine a man having a *heseb*-fracture in the chamber of his nose, and you find his face crooked and his face is flat; the swelling which is over it protrudes.

DIAGNOSIS
Then you shall say concerning him 'One suffering from a *heseb*-fracture in the chamber of his nose, an ailment which I will treat'.

TREATMENT
You should cause it to fall into its place. Clean out for him what is in his two nostrils with two swabs of linen, until every worm of blood, which coagulates in the interior of his nostrils, comes forth. Now afterwards, you put two swabs of linen, moistened with oil, placed in his two nostrils. You then place for him two stiff rolls of linen, bandaged on it. You should treat him afterwards with oil and honey and lint, every day until he is well.

Glosses define the 'chamber' of the nose as 'the middle of his nose [from] the bottom to the back, extending to between his eyebrows' – an explicit definition of the cavity of the nose. Another gloss explains that the 'worm of blood' is a simile, in which the blood clots are likened to the *anaret*-worm which 'exists in the waters'. Although it would have been interesting to know how they reduced the fracture, we note their use of linen moistened with oil which anticipates its modern equivalent of vaseline gauze. We also note the rolls of linen which are still used to maintain the restored shape of the nose under bandaging.

There is, however, one case in which the reduction of a fracture is explicitly described. Case 35 is concerned with a *heseb*-fracture of the clavicle:

8.7 Fractured radius and ulna with a splint, from a body in a tomb of the 5th Dynasty, Naga ed-Deir. Death had taken place before any healing of the bones had occurred. (From Smith, 1908)

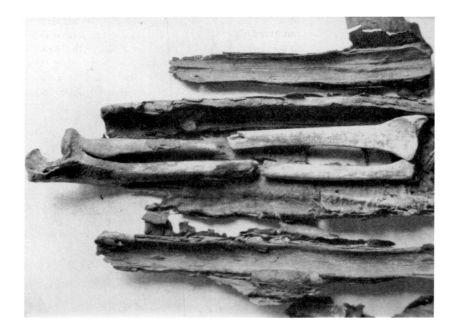

You should place him prostrate [on his back], [with] something folded which is in [between] his two shoulder blades. You should spread out his two shoulders in order to stretch apart (*dewen*) his two clavicles until that *heseb*-fracture falls into its place. You should then make for him two splints (*sesh*) of linen, and place them, one of them to the inside of his upper arm, and the other to the under side of his upper arm. You should bind it with *imru* and treat him afterwards with honey every day until he recovers.

The technique of reduction is thoroughly sound practice. Unfortunately, the account of the use of the splints makes little sense, probably because of a major scribal error (see below). *Imru* cannot be translated at present. However, it has a mineral determinative and might well be something equivalent to the modern plaster of Paris. Mummy cartonnage would certainly make an excellent splint. It is notoriously difficult to stabilise a fractured clavicle, but they usually unite without trouble.

Astonishingly, this treatment is repeated almost verbatim in Case 36 for a *heseb*-fracture of the humerus (*gab*, upper arm) for which the examination reads '... you find his upper arm is hanging down, crooked compared with its fellow...'. The only major difference in the treatment is that the word *gab* (humerus) is substituted for *bebwy* (clavicle), so the instructions read '... You should spread out his two shoulders in order to stretch apart his humerus until that break falls into its place...'. Traction is the standard procedure for fractured humerus, as there is often over-riding of the broken bones due to the pull of the triceps and biceps muscles. However, spreading out the shoulders is hardly the way to reduce a fractured humerus. Nevertheless, the application of the splints as described in Case 35 is appropriate for the fractured humerus (Case 36). My view is that this is a major scribal error, the first part of the treatment (the reduction) belonging to Case 35 and the second part (the splints) applying to Case 36.

Two sets of splints were found by the Hearst Expedition of the University of California to Naga ed-Deir, and were made available for study by Elliot Smith who published his findings in the *British Medical Journal* (1908). The splints were attached to bodies found in rock-cut tombs of the Fifth Dynasty (Old Kingdom, *c.* 2400 BC). The first was applied to a comminuted fracture of the middle of the femur of a girl aged about fourteen. The set comprised four wooden splints padded with linen bandages, the whole being bandaged in place and secured with a reef knot. Blood staining suggested the fracture was compound and there was no evidence of healing before the death of the patient. The splints extended from just above the fracture to well below the knee and Elliot Smith considered they would have been of little value. The second set (fig. 8.7) was applied to a compound fracture of radius and ulna (forearm), and comprised three pieces of bark (probably acacia) again wrapped in linen and bandaged to the arm. The wound appeared to have been plugged with vegetable fibre, presumably to staunch bleeding, but death had occurred before there was any sign of union between the bones. Elliot Smith considered that this splint would have been very effective for immobilising the bones.

Wood Jones published an account (1908) of the incidence of fractures found during the excavation of the area south of the first cataract, which was soon to be flooded by the first Aswan dam. There were 6000 bodies in burials ranging from 4000 BC to the first century AD. In comparison with modern times, there was a high incidence of fractures of forearm and clavicle which Elliot Smith attributed to blows from sticks (Table 8.2). Results of treatment were highly variable. Wood Jones (1908) published

Table 8.2 Incidence of fractures reported by Wood Jones (1908) from the excavation of the cemeteries at Aswan in 1907

SITE OF FRACTURE	INCIDENCE (%)
forearm (radius and ulna)	31.25
collar-bone (clavicle)	13.75
thigh (femur)	12.50
leg (tibia and fibula)	10.00
skull	7.50
upper arm (humerus)	6.20
face	4.38
ribs	4.38
pelvis	3.75
hand	3.12
foot	1.25
shoulder-blade (scapula)	1.25
breast-bone (sternum)	0.62
spine	nil
kneecap (patella)	nil

There were 6000 bodies, of which 200 had united fractures. Dates ranged from 4000 BC to AD 500.

illustrations of healed fractures of all six long bones of the limbs, in which it was barely possible to discern the fracture lines, so perfect was the alignment in every case (fig. 8.8). This is particularly impressive in the case of the oblique fracture of the femur, in which the pull of powerful muscles would have produced a tendency for the fragments to over-ride. It is not clear how the ancient Egyptians could have arranged sustained traction to prevent this. Most other results were far less satisfactory and there were many instances of gross shortening and misalignment.

8.8 Examples of healed fractures with excellent alignment, found in Nubia during rescue excavations before the raising of the first Aswan dam in 1908. (From Jones, 1908)

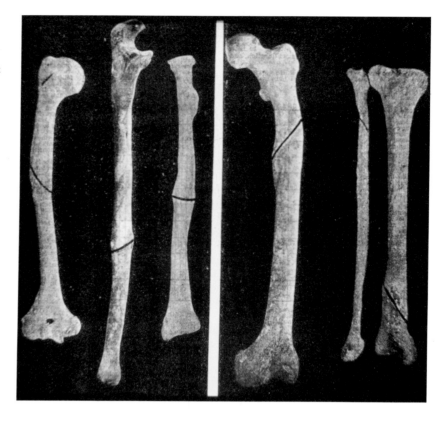

Injuries to joints

Chapter 3 considered the evidence for a very clear understanding of the concept of dislocation (*wenekh*) as things which were joined together and one becoming separated from the other. In contrast, a sprain (*nerut*) was defined as breaking open of members which nevertheless remain in their place.

Case 25 of the Edwin Smith papyrus is a classic account of dislocation of the jaw:

> If you examine a man having a dislocation (*wenekh*) in his mandible (*aret*, see fig. 3.4) and you find his mouth open and his mouth does not close for him, you then place your finger[s] on the back of the two rami of the mandible inside the mouth, your two claws (i.e. thumbs) under his chin and you cause them (i.e. the two mandibles) to fall so they lie in their [correct] place.

The fixed open mouth is diagnostic of a dislocated jaw, and the method of reduction is so close to the modern technique that the meaning of *wenekh* is not in doubt.

The tomb of Ipwy in Deir el-Medina contained a remarkable wall painting, now severely damaged, which showed a series of industrial accidents occurring (fig. 8.9, and see fig 3.6). At the top and on the right is a scene which looks very like the first stages of reduction of a dislocated shoulder, according to the classic method of Kocher. The arm is first externally rotated to stretch the pectoral muscles, the elbow is then brought forward in front of the chest and, finally, the hand is rapidly swept across to the opposite shoulder, when the shoulder should fall into place.

8.9 This manoeuvre from the tomb of Ipwy (see E/F in fig. 3.6) closely resembles the first stage of Kocher's method for reduction of a dislocated shoulder, demonstrated above by Mr Theo Welsh, FRCS.

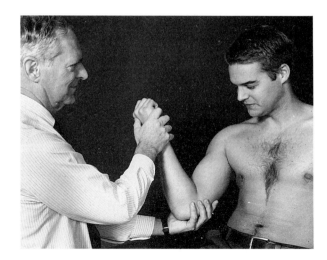

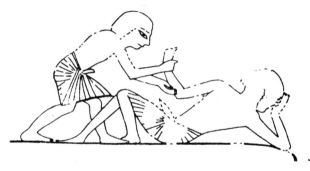

Neurological complications of trauma

The ancient Egyptians appeared to have no understanding of the function of the brain (Chapter 3) but, nevertheless, gave a graphic description of its exposure in a patient with a gaping wound of the head and a smash of the skull (see Chapter 3).

Edwin Smith, Case 8, describes a compound, comminuted fracture of the skull without a superficial wound. There is interesting detail of the sides of the body which are affected:

> You find there is a swelling rising on the outside of that smash which is in his skull. His eye is askew because of it, on his side with the injury which is in his skull. He walks limping with his sole on his side with that injury which is in his skull.

Walking is affected on the same side as the injury in spite of the fact that the tracts of the upper motor-neurons governing the muscles concerned cross to the opposite side in the brain stem. Therefore one would expect the disability to be on the opposite side to the injury. The usual explanation of the paradox in Case 8 is that the patient must have suffered the well known *contra-coup* injury, in which the brain is thrown against the opposite side of the skull and so injured on the side away from the superficial injury. Owing to the crossing of the upper motor-neurons, the muscular disability then appears on the same side as the injury. Alternatively, it may be no more than an error by a confused scribe!

In spite of the ancient Egyptians' apparent failure to appreciate the function of the brain, they did seem to understand the role of the spinal cord in transmitting information. Case 31 of the Edwin Smith papyrus describes a dislocation (*wenekh*) of the neck and the patient presents a clear picture of a high injury to the spinal column:

> You find him not knowing his two arms and his two legs because of it. His phallus is erect because of it and urine drips from his penis, without him knowing it. His flesh has received wind. An ejaculation befalls his penis.

All the main features of the condition are present, couched in classical Egyptian and using well established terminology. They are quite specific in saying that the neurological deficits are 'because of it' (i.e. the injury in the neck). There is no mention of a wound in this case, and therefore the most likely explanation of 'flesh receiving wind' is intestinal dilatation with gas (paralytic ileus), a well recognised complication of spinal injury. It is hardly surprising that this was a patient not to be treated. Case 33 (impacted fracture of the cervical vertebrae) has many features in common with Case 31 but the patient is speechless or unconscious (*degem*). Again he was a patient not to be treated.

Case 48 describes a sprain (*nerut*) of the vertebral column with pain when the legs are extended. Assuming this test was undertaken when the hips were flexed, it would be a diagnostic sign in favour of a prolapsed lumbar intervertebral disc with nerve involvement.

Firth (1915) reported a remarkable case of a copper alloy arrow-head found embedded in a middle or lower cervical vertebra. The specimen is from grave 762 in cemetery 98 of the Nubian Survey, and was dated to the New Kingdom. Recon-

8.10 A copper alloy arrow-head piercing a cervical vertebra, and which would have severed the spinal cord (see reconstruction drawing below). The specimen was found in a New Kingdom grave (98.762) in cemetery no. 98 at Dakka, 100 km south of Aswan, during the rescue excavations necessitated by the raising of the first Aswan dam (Firth, 1915). X-ray fluorescence by John Evans showed the body, but not the haft, of the arrow to be unalloyed copper. (Hunterian Museum of the Royal College of Surgeons of England)

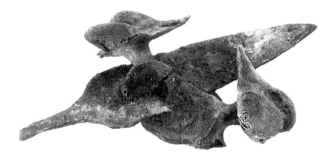

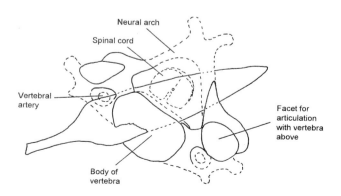

Neural arch

Spinal cord

Vertebral artery

Facet for articulation with vertebra above

Body of vertebra

struction shows that the arrow-head must have severed most of the spinal cord (fig. 8.10), resulting in instant paralysis of the body below the neck. Although this patient was beyond treatment, there must have been countless occasions when the *swnw* would have been expected to extract arrows from soldiers who had survived, for example, the injuries which befell the soldiers of Mentuhotep in the Eleventh Dynasty (Winlock, 1945). The Indian wars obliged military doctors in the United States to re-examine an age-old problem; Mays, Parfitt and Hershman (1994) have reviewed the contemporary literature from that period. Sadly, the medical papyri are silent on the treatment of arrow wounds.

Tetanus. There is a celebrated account of what appears to be the development of tetanus in Case 7, which also illustrates many of the points considered above. There is no finer case on which to conclude the section on trauma:

TITLE
Instructions for a gaping wound in his head, extending to the bone, penetrating the *tepau* of his skull.*
*See p. 50 for possible meanings of *tepau*.

FIRST EXAMINATION
... You should then probe his wound though he shudders greatly. You should then cause him to lift his face. It is painful for him to open his mouth. His heart beats too slowly (or weakly) for speech. You observe his saliva falling from his lips but not falling completely. He discharges blood from his two nostrils and from his two ears. He suffers stiffness in his neck. He does not find he can look at his two shoulders and his breast.

FIRST DIAGNOSIS AND PROGNOSIS
You shall say concerning him 'one having a gaping wound in his head extending to the bone and penetrating the *tepau* of his skull. The cord of his mandible is contracted; he discharges blood from his two nostrils and from his two ears; and he suffers stiffness in his neck – an ailment with which I will contend'.

FIRST TREATMENT
As soon as you find that man, the cord of his mandibles and his jaws are contracted, you should cause one to make for him something hot until he is comfortable and his mouth opens. You should then bind it with oil and honey until you know he has reached 'something' (*r rekh.k seper.f r khet*).

Already it seems likely that there is a fractured base of skull with meningeal irritation. Gloss B explains that the 'cord of the mandible' is probably the temporalis muscle (p. 51), one of the muscles which closes the mouth (see fig. 3.4), and there must be concern that the patient is developing tetanus (lock-jaw). The last phrase is puzzling, and Breasted translated it as 'until thou knowest that he has reached a decisive point'.

SECOND EXAMINATION
If you find [in] that man that his flesh has developed heat under the wound which is in the *tepau* of his skull. That man, he has developed toothache (sic) under that wound. You put your hand on him and you find his brow is wet with sweat. The muscles (*metu*) of his neck are taut, his face is flushed, his teeth and his back [? scribal omission here]. The odour of the chest (sic) of his head is like the excrement of small cattle. His mouth is bound, his two eyebrows drawn, his face is as if he was weeping.

SECOND DIAGNOSIS AND PROGNOSIS

You shall then say concerning him 'one having a gaping wound in his head extending to the bone and penetrating the *tepau* of his skull.

He has developed toothache; his mouth is bound; he suffers stiffness of his neck – an ailment not to be treated'.

Gloss I now explains that the final sentence of the second examination means that he cannot open his mouth, and his eyebrows and face are distorted in a manner which can be recognised as characteristic of the so-called risus sardonicus (the grimly jocular smile of tetanus). To his other troubles infection has been added, and the hopeless prognosis seems reasonable. The case lacks a time scale, but Westendorf (1992) has pointed out that the malodorous wound of the skull indicates that some considerable time has elapsed since the original injury, which would, of course, be necessary to allow for the incubation period of tetanus.

THIRD EXAMINATION

If, however, you now find that man, he has become pale and already shown exhaustion.

There is no third diagnosis and prognosis.

THIRD TREATMENT

You should then cause to be made for him a chisel of wood, padded with linen and placed in his mouth. You should then have made for him a drink of earth almonds (*wah*). His treatment is sitting down, placed between two supports which are of brick until you know he has arrived at something.

The chisel of wood seems to be the same as the boxwood wedge which is still occasionally used to open the mouth in spasm of the jaw. It is impressive that attempts should continue to be made to make the patient comfortable in spite of a prognosis which is (correctly) declared to be hopeless.

Burns

Fires were used for cooking and for a variety of industrial processes. Burns and scalds must have been common. The Ebers papyrus contains an important section (482–509) which is headed 'Beginning of the remedies for a burn', the word for a burn being *webdet* with a flame determinative. It begins immediately with a series of remedies to be applied consecutively as follows (Ebers 482):

day 1 black mud
day 2 excrement of small cattle (sheep, etc.), *sermet khepret*
day 3 resin of acacia, barley dough, carob (*djaret*), oil
day 4 wax, oil, cooked unwritten papyrus, *wah*-legume
day 5 carob, red ochre, *khes* part of *ima* tree, copper flakes

It is hard to see any logic in this progression. Black mud might perhaps cool the burn for a short time and so relieve the pain, but excrement of cattle on the second day would carry risk of serious infection. Oil would be soothing but does not appear until the third and fourth days. Cooling the burn would seem to be the obvious immediate treatment but is mentioned only in paragraph 484. A complex remedy (containing the ingredients of the fourth day above) is to be applied 'after it is cooled' but it is not clear whether it is the burn or the remedy which is to be cooled.

There follow a great number of remedies, without specification of the day on which they are to be applied. Honey appears in several and would reduce swelling and exert an anti-bacterial effect. Paragraph 491 includes copper flakes and malachite, which have a bactericidal effect (see Chapter 7). Oil appears in many. There remain many plant drugs for which no beneficial effect has been demonstrated, and the frequent appearance of excrement of various animals is disconcerting. However, perhaps we should not be too sceptical. The final paragraph (509) reads:

> Another [remedy]: barley bread, oil/fat and salt, mixed into one. Bandage with it often to make him well immediately. A true thing. I have seen it happen often for me.

Reliance on remedies was not total and this section of the Ebers papyrus contains two spells.

Snake bite

The snake has the distinction of being the first animal to interact with mankind in the Bible (Genesis 3: 1), and its evil reputation has continued ever since. Egyptian mythology abounds with stories of snakes. Every night the great serpent Aapep (Apophis) tried to obstruct the passage of the sun god through the underworld in the night barque. Similarly, all the deceased expected to be obstructed by snakes in their journey through the netherworld: there are several spells in the *Book of the Dead* to ward them off, and snakes being speared or cut with a knife feature in many vignettes. The ancient Egyptians lived in dread of snake bite as well as the sting of the scorpion. The frequent appearance of both snakes and scorpions in Egyptian mythology accords with the prominent role of magical incantations in the cure and prevention of snake bite, and this aspect of therapy has been considered in Chapter 5.

Until recently, little was known of the rational care of those who suffered from snake bites in ancient Egypt. The Edwin Smith papyrus has nothing to say on the subject and the Ebers papyrus confines its advice to methods for preventing a snake leaving its hole (Ebers 842–4). It is unlikely that the stomach complaint attributed to the '*betju*-snake' (Ebers 205) is in any way related to a true snake. Confusion arises because the snake determinative (Gardiner sign-list I 14) is also used for worms.

Publication of the Brooklyn Museum papyri 47,218.48 and 47,218.85 in 1989 came as a considerable surprise, as it presented an essentially pragmatic approach to snake bite although still not entirely free from magic. In a book published thirteen years after his death, Sauneron (1989) has provided a detailed exposition of the papyri, with a translation (into French). Although the existing copy of the papyri has been dated to about 300 BC, paragraph 42c claims, probably spuriously, that the original was discovered in the reign of Neferkara (Pepy II, Old Kingdom, Sixth Dynasty, c. 2200 BC). The two numbers refer to two parts of the same papyrus which was cut in half across the roll (see Chapter 2).

The Brooklyn papyri were undoubtedly a manual to guide those who were called upon to treat patients who had been bitten, and the logical approach to the problem is equalled only by the Edwin Smith papyrus. There is, however, no mention of the *swnw*, and the opening paragraph of the second section (p. 135) makes clear that it is intended for the use of the *kherep* priests of Serqet, whose role as healers has been discussed in Chapters 5 and 6.

Identification of the snake

The beginning of the first section of the Brooklyn papyri is unfortunately missing but the remaining paragraphs (14–38) name a total of twenty-one snakes and the

Table 8.3 Snakes listed in part I of the Brooklyn papyrus (47,218.48 and 47,218.85)

PARA.	EGYPTIAN NAME	DISTINCTIVE FEATURES	SEVERITY OF BITE	ASSOCIATED GOD	SPECIFIC TREATMENT (PARA.)
14	(lost)	(lost)	can be saved	none	–
15	Great serpent Aapep	entirely red, belly white, 4 teeth	dies quickly	none	–
16	*gany*	entirely black	dies quickly	Sobek	–
17	*ikher*	dark, comes to a man	dies quickly[1]	Kherybakef	–
18	*ka-en-am*	quail-coloured, big head, tail like mouse	can be saved	Sobek/Neith	–
19	*kedjuu*	small as a lizard	dies quickly	none	–
20	*sedbu*	red, yellow eyes	can be saved	none	48, 52
21	*nebed*[2]	green, belly white	non-lethal	Hathor	–
22	*fy tiam*	colour of *rer* snake	non-lethal	Geb	51
23	white *henep*[2]	entirely white, 4 teeth	may die	Serqet	78
24	red *henepu*[2]	white, red back, 3 teeth	can be saved	Seth	80
25	*neki*	2.4 m long	non-lethal	Ra	45, 47
26	*fy*	image of lotus on forehead	non-lethal	Horus	–
27	*fy* (blowing)	blue/green on neck unique crawling motion	can be saved	Horus	73
28	*fy* (horned)	quail-coloured	non-lethal	Horus	75
29	*fy* (small)	quail-coloured, no horns	can be saved	Horus	–
30	*fy*	no description	can be saved	Horus	–
31	*fy* (male)	like red *henepu* 24 above	can be saved	Seth/Geb	–
32	*hefaw arar*	sand coloured	non-lethal	Seth	–
33	*hefaw nefet*	quail coloured, makes loud blowing noise	can be saved	Horus	–
34	(lost)	entirely white	can be saved	Seth	–
35	*r-bedjadja*	black, 3 teeth	(lost)	Khonsu	53
36	*sedbu*	gold belly & neck, found in the fields	harmless	(lost)	52
37	(lost)	black, belly white	non-lethal	Hathor	–
38	*kar*	green, changes colour according to background	can be saved	Anubis	–

1 Can be saved if the snake is weak.
2 Female pronoun used throughout description.
Numbers of teeth refer to the bite wound.
The word *fy* may mean viper, or a snake resembling a viper.

chameleon (Table 8.3). Some of the missing names can be inferred from the second section of the papyri. Section one provides a brief description of the snake, the appearance of its bite and sometimes its habits. This is presumably intended to enable the healer to identify the snake from the description given by the patient, and then to give the appropriate prognosis and treatment.

The Egyptian word *hefaw* refers to snakes in general, while the word *fy* has been thought to refer to the family Viperidae, the vipers. However, several species of Colubridae look very like vipers (*Telescopus* species, for example) and the Egyptians had, of course, no concept of the current classification into Families. The Egyptian name *sebdu* appears to cover two different species but, in the case of paragraph 36, *sedbu* is qualified by the phrase 'one treads on it in the fields' and the descriptions have nothing in common. The associated deity is indicated by the phrase 'It stands for N', where N is the name of the god or goddess as listed in Table 8.3. The benign goddess Hathor is associated with at least one relatively harmless snake (*nebed*) whereas Sobek, the crocodile god, is associated with two very dangerous snakes (*gany* and *ka-en-am*). In the case of the red *henepu*, there is a departure from the usual form of words and the snake 'comes forth from the penis of Seth', a truly appalling provenance.

There are twenty-five paragraphs remaining out of the original thirty-eight in Section I of the papyrus, and Sauneron made several firm identifications. I am particularly indebted to David Warrell, Professor of Tropical Medicine and Infectious Diseases at Oxford, who has a special interest in venomous snakes and their bites: in a personal communication (1994), he has reconsidered those paragraphs where there is a possibility of identification from the tantalisingly brief descriptions in Section I (summarised in Table 8.3). It seems likely that, in some cases, females, immature forms and variants of a species have different Egyptian names.

Para. 14: If this snake, whose name is lost, differs from those in paras 27 and 28, the nature of the bite suggests the spitting cobra (*Naja pallida*).

Para. 15: Aapep is the great serpent which features so prominently in the *Book of the Dead* as a major hazard of the afterworld. A positive identification would be valuable, but no Egyptian snake fits the description. The largest and most rapidly fatal snake is the Egyptian cobra (*Naja haje*). However, if one ignores its venomous reputation, Aapep might be the 'racer' (*Coluber rhodorhachis*) or the hooded malpolon (*Malpolon moilensis*). Sauneron considered *Oligodon melanocephalus*, *Tarbophis obtusus* and *Zamenis diadema*, all with a generally red colour.

Para. 16: Warrell and Sauneron concurred that this might be the black desert cobra (*Walterinnesia aegyptia*). Warrell believed it could also be the burrowing asp (*Atractaspis microlepidota*).

Para. 18: This is most likely to be the Persian horned viper (*Pseudocerastes persicus*) as suggested by Sauneron, or possibly the hornless variant of the desert horned viper (*Cerastes cerastes*; see para. 28).

Para. 20: Sauneron suggested the viper *Echis coloratus* but this snake is usually lethal and does not have a yellow eye. Warrell suggested a python, the sand boa (*Eryx jaculus*), which fits the description and is non-venomous.

Para. 21: Possibly a harmless colubrid such as *Psammophis* or *Philothamnus*.

Para. 22: Sauneron proposed *Pseudocerastes persicus* (see para. 18), but Warrell did not consider there to be sufficient evidence.

Para. 23: Sauneron thought possibly *Telescopus obtusus*. Warrell thought it might be a pale variant of *Cerastes*.

Para. 25: Sauneron suggested *Naja pallida* (= *nigricollis*) but this rarely exceeds 2 m.

Para. 26: Warrell agreed with Sauneron that this is probably the viper *Echis pyramidum* (= *carinatus*), from the pattern on the forehead. However, *Echis* bites have a high fatality rate.

Para. 27: The Egyptian word for blowing (*tjau*) is clear, but *Echis carinatus*, suggested by Sauneron, makes a noise by rasping its coils together. Warrell suggested the puff adder (*Bitis arietans*) on the basis of true blowing and having a unique crawling motion. It is found in northern Sudan but not in Egypt today.

Para. 28: Warrell agreed with Sauneron that this is the horned viper, *Cerastes cerastes* (= *cornutus*), familiar as the phonetic hieroglyph 'f' (Gardiner sign-list I 9).

Para. 29: Sauneron proposed *Cerastes vipera*, but Warrell suggested it might also be an immature hornless *Cerastes cerastes* (para. 28).

Para. 32: Warrell questioned Sauneron's grounds for believing that this might be the Egyptian cobra (*Naja haje*) which can undoubtedly be lethal in contrast to the papyrus which says 'he who is bitten will not die'.

Para. 33: The text says 'one hears a loud noise like the blowing of a forge'. Warrell and Sauneron both raised the possibility of a species of *Echis* (see para. 27).

Para. 35: Sauneron suggested an elapid (cobra) because of the teeth, which Warrell thought could be the black desert cobra (*Walterinnesia aegyptia*) or perhaps the burrowing asp (*Atractapsis microlepidota*) as for para. 16.

Para. 36: Sauneron suggested the colubrid *Psammophis sibilans*, but Warrell did not consider the description sufficient to confirm the identification. *Echis pyramidum* is more likely to be encountered in the fields than *Echis coloratus*, which inhabits rocky and desert areas.

Para. 37: Sauneron suggested the colubrid *Psammophis sibilans*, but Warrell did not consider the description sufficient to confirm the identification.

Para. 38: Sauneron and Warrell were agreed that this must be the chameleon (*Chamaeleo africanus C. chamaeleon*) which, however, is harmless in spite of what is said in the papyrus.

The second section of the papyri, concerned with treatment, refers to many of the snakes listed in the first section (Table 8.3) and to five named snakes which are not listed (*sekhtef* (46 and 50), *garsha* (49), *heby* (54), *ka-nay* (57) and *arat* (82)), the numbers in parentheses indicating the paragraphs covering specific treatment described in the second section of the papyri. It seems likely that these snakes were described in the lost paragraphs 1–13. Identification of the species from the very limited information in the second section is not possible.

The effects of a bite

The paragraphs in the first section contain a very brief description of the effects of a bite by each particular snake and this is followed by the prognosis. Numbers below refer to paragraphs of the Brooklyn papyri and may be related to specific snakes by reference to Table 8.3 and the notes above.

The most important local symptom of snake bite is intense and spreading pain. Surprisingly, this is seldom mentioned in the papyri: perhaps it was too well known to require repeated mention. There is certainly nothing comparable to the description of the distress of the unfortunate cat who was stung by a scorpion on the lonely road, and whose cries reached those in heaven (Metternich stela; Spruch III; Sander-Hansen, 1956). Absence of pain receives comment in 36 and 37. Other local symptoms at the area of the bite include swelling (e.g. 14, 31) and hardening (19). Swelling was probably so common that its absence is specially noted in the bite of the relatively harmless snake (36): 'there is not any harm from it: the bite does not swell'. There is no mention of local bleeding, which is to be expected with certain vipers, but its absence is noted in the cases of 31 and 36. The bite of the viper *ka-en-am* is compared to a dried raisin and this may indicate local tissue necrosis (18).

General symptoms receive more attention. Fever of duration seven, nine or eleven days is specified in seven cases (18, 22, 23, 24, 25, 26, 28). Several cases refer to weakness or weariness, using the Egyptian words *bag* or *bedesh* (14, 20, 24, 25, 28). There are other cases in which there appears to be hyperactivity of the muscular system – limbs shaking (*neha*) (26), quivering (*ketket*) (29) and twitching of the eyes and eyebrows (33). In paragraph 25 the patient is said to *tehes* from head to feet. The word *tehes* is otherwise unknown and Sauneron translates it as tetanisation. Vomiting is an important prognostic sign indicating severe systemic envenoming by elapids and some vipers. It is described in paragraphs 23 and 24, in both cases an unfavourable prognostic sign. Nevertheless, vomiting was induced therapeutically in some cases (see below).

In the case of the *arar* cobra (32) there is the following remarkable passage:

If it bites a man, he suffers in that half where he was not bitten.
He will not suffer in his half bearing the bite.

Although the meaning of the text is perfectly clear, it is difficult to understand the basis for these statements other than to emphasise that the pain is not confined to the area of the bite. However, it might conceivably refer to numbness around the bite.

A generalised bleeding tendency results from the procoagulant effect of some viper venom causing defibrinogenation (Warrell, personal communication, 1994). The likelihood of bleeding seems to have been recognised in paragraph 63a, which unfortunately does not specify any particular snake – 'If the bite is high (*khy*), blood flows from all his members/limbs'. In fact, bleeding is usually from gums, nose, gastrointestinal and urinary tracts after bites by *Echis* species in Egypt. Further recognition of bleeding appears in treatment (see below).

Intense thirst is a feature of the bite of certain vipers, and this symptom may be recognised in a 'remedy for thirst (*ib*) in the victim of a bite by any snake' (77a). Sweating and hypothermia also result from the bite of certain vipers, and paragraph 20 (*Echis coloratus* – a viper) contains the phrase 'his face sweats (*fedet*)'.

Difficulty in breathing is an effect of cobra venom which, like curare, blocks transmission from nerves to muscles, including those concerned with breathing. These effects seem to be recognised in two remedies, one to 'cause the throat to breathe' (43a) and one to 'open the throat' (69). Coma and impending death are implied in the phrase 'his head is not knowing and he is blind' (92). Loss of speech is implied in the phrase 'he will speak immediately' in response to receiving a remedy (92).

Prognosis

The prognoses are described in a series of phrases such as the following:

One does not die because of it (21)
He will live (22, 25, 26, 28)
He who is bitten by it will not die (32, 33, 37)
One can save (*nehem*) him (18, 20, 24, 27, 29, 30, 31, 33, 34, 38)
Death hastens very quickly (19)
If it bites someone, he will die immediately (*her-awy*) (15, 16, 17)

Sometimes the prognosis is conditional on the number of days which have elapsed (presumably since the bite) or on treatment, either rational or magical:

One can save from it up to the seventh day (38)
One can save from it if three days have passed (18)
One can save from it by magic [and/or] remedies (27)

Survival is sometimes said to be related to vomiting:

If he vomits, he will die (23)
If he does not vomit he will live (24)

Somewhat similar is a remarkable prognostic test in the second section of the papyrus (40):

Will he die? Will he live? To know what will happen with him – *kady*-animal, *djais*-plant, water, crushed and taken by the man bitten by the snake. If it remains in his belly, he will live. If he vomits he will die.

Treatment

The essential directions of treatment are threefold – local treatment of the bite, treatment with drugs (mainly herbal) and magical incantations. It is possible to detect four separate approaches to therapy. The first is specific treatment for a total of thirteen named snakes. Nine of these are listed in surviving parts of the first section, and references to their specific therapy in the second section are shown in the last column of Table 8.3. The remaining five snakes with specific therapy were presumably listed in the missing part of the first section of the papyri (see above). The second approach comprises a large number of remedies which are intended to be used with any snake. The third approach is therapy depending on what is found when the patient is examined (51, 63, 64, 87). Finally there are a series of treatments for specific symptoms.

Local treatment of the bite was apparently directed primarily toward the relief of local symptoms rather than to prevent the generalised absorption of the venom. There is no reference to sucking the bite or using a tourniquet to prevent the spread of the venom. There are several recommendations that a bandage be applied (e.g. 44c, 62c, 63a, 63b, 64a) but this appears to be to retain specified local medication rather than that it should be tight enough to restrict the circulation.

Incision or excision of the wound might be useful to remove necrotic tissue or, if early enough, to limit absorption of the venom. The relevant phrase *ir nek nef djua*, usually translated as 'you should use the knife treatment for him', is used throughout the medical papyri when simple surgery is required, as for incision of an abscess. This phrase appears in 31 (the male viper) and 32 (the cobra *arar*). More detail is given for the bite of an unidentified male snake in 81:

What is to be done for the bite of the male snake. Incise (*teshtesh*) his wound/bite with the knife treatment (*djua*) many times. Then you should apply a bandage to it, red natron . . . salt, etc. . . .

This approach is clearly used for the relief of oedema (accumulation of tissue fluid) in 72a:

Another [remedy] to drive out the swelling. Incise (*teshtesh*) his wound/bite with the *des*-knife many times on the first day. Apply salt 1/8 or natron. Bandage the wound with it.

The osmotic effect of the salt or natron (p. 145) would reduce the swelling in the same way that Glauber's salts (magnesium sulphate) is used today. The outward flow of tissue fluid might further impede the absorption of the venom, but the treatment would have to be very early to be effective and we note the emphasis 'on the first day'. There is a common phrase literally translated as 'hasten for it the technique/skill', implying that there was an accepted procedure ready to be used at the earliest opportunity.

The papyri contain remedies with almost a hundred herbal ingredients, mixed with typical Egyptian polypharmacy. By far the most commonly recommended ingredient is the onion, often compounded with other ingredients such as salt and sweet beer in specified proportions. The onion-like bulb of the lily *Crinum yuccaeflorum* is still widely used for snake bite throughout West Africa. Far less commonly prescribed were *djaret* (probably carob), various leaves and grain, and terebinth.

Emetics are prescribed on twenty-four occasions, mostly using the unequivocal causative verb *sebesh* – to cause vomiting. The rationale is to expel the venom with the vomitus but this is a false hypothesis because the venom is not in the stomach. However, vomiting might distract the patient's attention from his bite and make him feel that something was being done.

> An emetic to be made for a man bitten by the blowing *fy*-snake (para. 27):
> onion 1, salt 1, *sam*-plant 1: grind finely with sweet beer 1 or fermented liquid.
> Swallow and reject. (73)

On several occasions the prescription ends with instructions to fumigate (*kap*) the patient, but this was always in addition to some other form of therapy and appeared to be an adjuvant.

This exceptionally pragmatic papyrus is by no means free from magic. Paragraph 27 clearly states 'If one reads [a spell] for him, he will live, for it is exorcised by magic'. The use of the onion is specifically linked to incantations invoking Ra, Horus and Serqet in paragraphs 41 and 42. There are twelve incantations, most of which are intended for use with particular remedies. A number of these follow in the tradition of the Horus legend outlined in Chapter 5.

The remarkable Brooklyn papyrus has revolutionised our knowledge of the ancient Egyptian approach to the treatment of snake bite. It has also given firm evidence that the *kherep* priests of Serqet practised what we would call conventional medicine and were not solely concerned with magic.

Scorpion stings

Scorpions are an order to the class Arachnida, which otherwise contains spiders, ticks and mites. The sting, which is in the tail of the animal, was much feared by the ancient Egyptians and features in mythology as outlined in Chapter 5. The stinging of Horus is described in detail on the Metternich stela, Spruch VII and IX (Sander-Hansen, 1956). Spruch III provides a dramatic account of the stinging of a cat. In both cases the treatment is predominantly magical and based on the mythology (pp. 108–10). It is not easy to discern any pragmatic treatment of a scorpion sting on the Metternich stela although Horus' mother Isis does 'open the wound' (191) and places her nose in Horus' mouth. However, this appears to be for the purpose of detecting the poison by its smell rather than for giving some form of artificial respiration. Paragraph 193 says that Isis clasps Horus and 'leaps with him like fishes thrown on a fire', which may indicate a form of stimulation to avert coma and respiratory depression.

The Brooklyn papyrus (see above) specifically states in paragraph 39 that it will include remedies for bites of scorpions, but sadly they are not to be found in that part of the papyrus which has survived. The main medical papyri are remarkably silent on the subject of scorpion stings although Ebers (200) compares stomach pain with what might be felt by 'one who has been bitten' (*khery demet*). The *Grundriss* suggests that this might refer to a scorpion, but the phrase *khery demet* is also used to describe snake bite and the word for scorpion does not appear in Ebers 200.

Berlin 78 gives a solitary remedy for 'driving out the sting of a scorpion' using the unusual word *djanary* for scorpion instead of the more usual *wehat*, which does not appear at all in the *Grundriss Wörterbuch*. Apart from wax, the nature of the ingredients remains unknown.

Crocodile bites (*Crocodylus niloticus*)

The crocodile attempts to drag its prey below water to drown, as described clearly in the Westcar papyrus. In ancient Egypt this would confer membership of an elite group, the *hesyu* or the blessed drowned ones. However, some victims escaped with extensive injuries and their treatment received attention in Ebers 436:

> What is to be done for the bite (*tep-r*) of a crocodile. If you examine the bite of a crocodile and you find it [with] his flesh piled up and its two sides being separated, then you should bandage it with fresh meat on the first day, likewise all wounds of a man.

A crocodile bite is also specified in Hearst 239:

> Another remedy for the bite (*peseh*) of a crocodile in all limbs of a man. You should bandage it with [fresh] meat on the first day.

Bandaging with fresh meat on the first day was a standard Egyptian remedy for any major flesh wound. Identical or very similar wording appears in at least thirteen cases in the Edwin Smith papyrus (see above).

Human bites

Human bites appear to have been a problem sufficient to merit four paragraphs of the Ebers papyrus. The section commences at paragraph 432 (parallel to Hearst 21):

> Another [remedy] for the bite of mankind. A measure of dough (*shedet*, Hearst only) which is in a jar (*andju*) and a leek. Pound and make into one mass, and bandage with it.

Two other remedies follow in the Ebers papyrus (433 and 434) and these include terebinth (*senetjer*). The final remedy for human bites (Ebers 435) reverts to bandaging with fresh meat on the first day and then following with oil/fat, honey and wax.

Mankind is written as the usual and very common word *remetj*, which usually refers to Egyptians rather than foreigners. Nevertheless it seems strange that a human bite should be the only mammalian bite to be considered in the papyri. The *Grundriss* (IV 2, 161) considers that *remetj* is a mistaken writing for *rer* meaning pig, although the writing is the same in both Ebers 432 and Hearst 21.

Conclusion

The Edwin Smith papyrus shows a logical and impressive approach to the management of trauma in ancient Egypt. However, other surviving papyri give only a very fragmentary picture of surgery outside the field of trauma, and no surgical instruments have been found. Planned surgery may well have matched their management of trauma, but this must remain conjectural until we find surgical instruments or papyri which go further than the final section of the Ebers papyrus in describing surgical practice.

CHAPTER **NINE**

Specialised branches of medicine

Herodotus (II, 83) remarked on the degree of specialisation of Egyptian doctors:

> The practice of medicine they split up into separate parts, each doctor being responsible for the treatment of only one disease. There are, in consequence, innumerable doctors, some specialising in diseases of the eyes, others of the head, others of the teeth, others of the stomach and so on.

No doubt this statement is an exaggeration, but the titles of some specialists are known to us, particularly dentists, ophthalmologists, doctors of the belly and also 'herdsmen of the anus' (Chapter 6).

Gynaecology and obstetrics

It is difficult to say who practised in the fields of gynaecology and obstetrics. There are no known words for midwife, gynaecologist or obstetrician, and no documentary evidence has survived to indicate the involvement of the *swnw* in childbirth. It might be suspected that modesty would have introduced a certain reluctance for women to subject themselves to some of the bizarre treatments recommended in the gynaecological papyri, although concepts of modesty might have been very different in ancient Egypt. The following extract from Hyginus, cited by von Staden (1989), may well relate to the Herophilus who practised in Alexandria in the Ptolemaic Period (see Chapter 10):

> The ancients had no midwives, and therefore women died [in childbirth], led on by their sense of shame. For the Athenians had taken heed that no slave or woman should learn the science of medicine. A certain girl, Hagnodice, as a young woman desired to learn the science of medicine. Because of this desire, she cut her hair, put on male clothing, and entrusted herself to a certain Herophilus for her training. After learning this science, when she heard that a woman was having labour-pains, she used to go to her. And when the woman refused to entrust herself [to Hagnodice], thinking that she was a man, Hagnodice lifted her undergarment and revéaled that she was a woman. In this way she used to cure women.

Fertility and pregnancy testing

Kahun (19–27), Berlin (193–9) and the Carlsberg papyri contain an extraordinary series of tests for fertility, pregnancy and to determine the sex of the unborn child. The usual introduction is in the sense 'to distinguish between who will bear a child and who will not bear a child', so it is not easy to distinguish between fertility and pregnancy tests. The tests cover a wide range of procedures, including the induction of vomiting and examination of the eyes. Perhaps the most famous test is in Berlin 199, with a much damaged parallel in Carlsberg III (1, 6–x+3). This is so often paraphrased that a literal translation may be helpful:

> Another [test] to see [if] a woman will bear a child or [if] she will not bear a child. Emmer (*bedet*) and barley (*it*), the lady should moisten with her urine

every day, like dates and like sand in two bags. If they all grow, she will bear a child. If the barley grows, it means a male. If the emmer grows, it means a female. If they do not grow, she will not bear a child.

This would seem to be a test for pregnancy rather than fertility, and something very similar was being practised in Germany in the eighteenth century AD (Westendorf, 1992). The technique was put to the test by Ghaliounghui, Khalil and Ammar (1963), who showed no growth of either seed when watered with male or female (non-pregnant) urine. With forty specimens from pregnant women there was growth of one or both species in twenty-eight cases. Thus growth seemed to be a good indicator of pregnancy, but no growth failed to exclude pregnancy in 30 per cent of cases. When only one species germinated, the prediction of sex was correct in seven cases and incorrect in sixteen.

At least two of the pregnancy tests have loose parallels in the Hippocratic corpus, and provide some of the very few links between Egyptian and Greek medicine. One of these appears to be based on examination of the blood vessels over the breasts, as in Berlin 193. The title is missing from Berlin 193 and is therefore taken from the parallel passage Kahun 26:

To recognise who will be pregnant and who will not be pregnant.
She lies down [while] you smear her breast and her two arms and her two
    shoulders with new oil. You rise early in the morning to examine her.
[If] you find her blood vessels (metu) fresh and good, none being collapsed
    (lit. sunken), bearing children will be happy (or satisfactory – hetep).
[If] you find them collapsed like the skin of her limbs, this means bened
    (meaning unknown).
If you find them green and dark at the time of investigating them, she will bear
    children late.

Dilated veins over the breasts are well known as an early sign of pregnancy. Hippocratic aphorisms v, 37 and 53 refer to the breasts becoming lax or regressing as a sign of impending miscarriage.

Carlsberg IV (1,x+4–x+6) and Kahun 28, in a very badly damaged state, describe a test which also appears in a modified form in the Hippocratic aphorism v, 59:

[To determine] who will [bear children] and who will not [bear children], you
    should then cause the bulb of an onion to spend the night in her flesh (iuf) until
    dawn. If the odour appears in her mouth, she will bear [children]. If [it does
    not], she will never [bear children].

The reconstructions are partly taken from Kahun 28. The word iuf (lit. flesh) is often used to mean vagina. The Hippocratic aphorism uses burning incense but the object is again to see whether the odour 'passes through the body to the nose and mouth'.

Obstetrics

The medical papyri say nothing about the normal conduct of labour, and we have only representations of magical births of pharaohs (fig. 9.1), together with an account in the Westcar papyrus. In the latter, the lady Red-djedet was pregnant with triplets, the father being the god Ra to the consternation of her husband Ra-user. The children were destined to be the first three kings of the Fifth Dynasty (Userkaf, Sahura and Neferirkara), and the purpose of the story was to establish their divine origin. The obstetric team in this case comprised the goddesses Isis, Nephthys, Meskhenet and Heqet (see Chapter 5):

9.1 (right) Mythical representation of Cleopatra giving birth (Ptolemaic Period) with goddesses in attendance, as recorded by the Napoleonic expedition (1798–1801) in the birth house at Armant which is now destroyed. (From *Description de l'Égypte*, 1809) (below) Ptolemaic birthing scene from Dendera, with Hathors in attendance. (Cairo Museum, 40627)

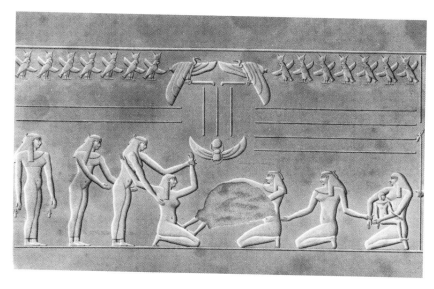

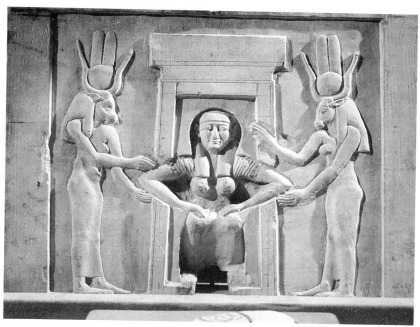

Then these deities set forth, having transformed themselves into female musicians, Khnum with them as their porter. [Ra-user said:] 'My ladies! Behold, it is the lady who is sick and her parturition is painful.' Then they said: 'Allow us to see her. Behold, we know how to bring her to birth.' Then he said to them: 'Proceed'. Then they set forth and entered into the presence of Red-djedet. Then they sealed the room with her [and them] in it. Isis placed herself in front of her, Nephthys behind her (see fig. 9.1a) and Heqet hastened the birth. Then said Isis:

'Be not strong (*user*) in her womb (lit. belly) in this your name as a powerful man (*user*) indeed' (word play on the name Userkaf). The child rushed forth into her two arms, as a child of one cubit (i.e. 52 cm), his bones strong, his limbs covered in gold, his headdress of real lapis lazuli. Then they washed him and his umbilical cord (*khepa*) was cut (*shad*). He was placed in cloth on [a couch of] brick. Then Meskhenet presented [herself] to him . . . Then Red-djedet purified [herself] with a purification of fourteen days.

The accounts of the next two births are very similar, but in each case the words addressed to the child are a word play on the name of the future king. There is a tantalising lack of obstetrical detail but the scene accords well with that shown for Cleopatra in fig. 9.1a. It would seem that the woman in labour normally squatted on a birthing stool, for which the Egyptian word *meskhenet* differs from the name of the goddess Meskhenet only in the determinative. The birth hieroglyph suggests that the vertex presentation was regarded as normal (fig. 9.2).

There is a group of remedies in the Ebers papyrus (800–7) and an incantation in Ramesseum IV (C, 28–30) to 'release a child from the belly of a woman' and a further group, Ebers 797–9, to cause a woman to 'give to the earth' (*redi r ta*) which means to give birth or, perhaps, to abort. These would appear to be intended to hasten birth but no more precise indications are given. Some remedies are to be bandaged on the abdomen, a few to be taken by mouth and others were to be placed in the vagina. Many components of these remedies (Table 9.1) remain unknown but those which can be translated are not known to contract the uterus, which would have been as well if the delivery was obstructed.

Problems after birth

Ebers 823 is a remedy to 'pull together' or contract the uterus but it is not clear whether this was intended to hasten birth, to expel the placenta or to assist the return of the uterus to normal size after delivery:

> Another [remedy] to contract (*saq*) the uterus (*hemet*): *kheper-wer*-plant, 1; honey, 1; water of carob (*djaret*), 1; milk, 1; strain and place in the vagina (*iuf*).

Unfortunately the identity of the *kheper-wer*-plant is unknown.

Kahun 4 would be compatible with a birth injury to the perineum:

> Instructions for a lady [suffering in] her pubic region, her vagina and the region (*djadjat*) of her vagina which is between her buttocks. You shall say concerning her/it: Very swollen due to giving birth. You should then prepare for her/it: new oil, 1 *henu* (450 ml), to be soaked into her vagina.

Assessment and treatment of the neonate

Ebers 838 says that if, on the day a child is born, it says '*ny*' it will live and if it says '*mebi*' it will die. An unfavourable verdict is also given if the child's voice is moaning, or if it bends its face downwards (Ebers 839).

Ramesseum IV (the Mother and Child papyrus) gives 'another thing to be done for him (i.e. the child) on the day when he is born' (C, 17–24) and 'protection to be made for the child on the day when he is born' (C, 15–16). Unfortunately, these passages are much damaged. The former provides only an incantation, and what remains of the latter contains the ominous phrase 'a lump of faeces as something which has gone down into the vagina (*kat*) of his mother'. If this is not some form of ill-advised medication, it is the first recorded account of a fistula between rectum and vagina.

phonetics

mswt: birth

9.2 The full hieroglyphic writing of the word for birth, with a determinative showing a normal vertex delivery and the mother in the squatting position.

Table 9.1 Drugs which were probably intended to contract the uterus

'It is a contraction (*saq*) of the uterus'

placed in vagina	ground seed corn of emmer (Ebers 820)
	cyperus grass ground in oil/fat (Ebers 820)
	hemp ground in honey (Ebers 821)
	senetjer-resin (Ebers 822)
	celery ground in cow's milk (Ebers 822)
	kheper-wer-plant (Ebers 823)
	honey (Ebers 823)
	water of carob (Ebers 823)
	milk (Ebers 823)
	water of *mesta* (Ebers 824)
	juice of *Potamogeton lucens* (*neshau*) (Ebers 825)
	juice of *qetqetu* (Ebers 826)
	juice of *niaia*-plant (Ebers 827)

'To cause a woman to give to earth'

to be sat upon	*niaia*-plant (Ebers 797)

'To cause all that is in a woman's belly to come down'

taken by mouth	date juice (Ebers 799)
	Lower Egyptian salt (Ebers 799)
	oil/fat (Ebers 799)
placed in vagina	sherds of new *henu*-jar ground in oil/fat (Ebers 798)

To release (*sefekh*) a child from the belly of a woman (or from his mother)

taken by mouth	fresh salt of Lower Egypt (Ebers 801)
	honey (Ebers 801)
	niaia-plant (Ebers 804)
	qesnet-mineral (Ebers 804)
	wine (Ebers 804)
placed in vagina	*besbes*-plant (Ebers 802)
	senetjer-resin (Ebers 802)
	onion (Ebers 802)
	djesret-beer (Ebers 802, 805)
	fresh salt of Lower Egypt (Ebers 802)
	fly's excrement (Ebers 802)
	ished-fruit (Ebers 805)
	juniper berries (Ebers 806)
	niaia-plant (Ebers 806)
	resin of fir tree (Ebers 806)
applied to abdomen (or bandaged therewith)	salt of Lower Egypt (Ebers 800)
	white emmer (Ebers 800)
	sut-hemet-plant (Ebers 800)
	senetjer-resin (Ebers 803)
	nis-part of tortoise (Ebers 807)
	hekun-beetle (Ebers 807)
	pine oil (Ebers 807)
	djesret beer (Ebers 807)
	oil/fat (Ebers 807)
incantations	Ramesseum IV (C, 25–30)

See Tables 7.3, 7.4, 7.5 and 7.6 for identity of drugs.

Contraception

It was recommended that various materials or extracts of materials should be placed in the vagina. Ebers 783 explains the objective in no uncertain terms:

> Beginning of the prescriptions prepared for women/wives (*hemut*) to allow a woman (*set*) to cease conceiving (*iur*) for one year, two years or three years: *qaa* part of acacia, carob (*djaret*), dates; grind with one *henu* (450 ml) of honey, lint is moistened with it and placed in her flesh (*iuf*).*
>
> **Hemet*, singular of *hemut*, is a homophone meaning both woman and uterus; however, the determinatives are different, and the meaning is seldom in doubt.

All contraceptives are for local application by the woman: Kahun 22 specifies the vagina (*kat*) and Ramesseum IV (c, 2–3) that 'the lint should be placed at the mouth of the uterus'. Honey also features in Kahun 22, which might be spermicidal by means of its osmotic effect. One has unpleasant suspicions that some ingredients might be intended to deter the man. Ramesseum IV (c, 2–3) and Kahun 21 both recommend the excrement of crocodile! Riddle (1992) has reviewed contraception and abortion in the ancient world.

Gynaecology

Surgery plays a major role in modern gynaecology but there is no recommendation for surgical intervention in any of the gynaecological papyri. Treatment is confined to oral medication and materials for local application, mainly in the vagina. The possibility of cancer of the uterus has been considered in Chapter 4 in relation to 'eating' of the uterus.

Prolapse of the uterus is known from human remains (Smith and Jones, 1910; Harer, 1993) and is suggested in remedies to 'cause the uterus to go down (*ha*) to its place' (Ebers 789–95), but there are linguistic problems. Both Ebers 789 and 795 use the word *ha* which normally implies 'descent' and seems inappropriate to describe the restoration of a prolapsed uterus. However, both passages unequivocally say 'to its place'. Ebers 795 uses the word *hemet* for uterus, which is not open to doubt. However, Ebers 789 uses the phrase *mut remetj* (lit. mother of mankind), which usually means placenta (*Grundriss*), although logically it would be difficult to deny the meaning 'uterus', which is favoured by Weeks (1970). Ebers 790–4 are simply 'other remedies' for the condition described in Ebers 789. Remedies are to be drunk, smeared on the pubic region, applied to the umbilicus, used for fumigating the vagina, rubbed on the limbs or sat upon. Their components give no clue to the meaning of the indication for their use.

There are many remedies for 'cooling the uterus' and 'driving out heat'. One assumes that this must refer to some type of inflammation but the pathology is not at all clear. Both Kahun 24 and Ebers 812 refer to *setet* of the uterus. There is the unresolved problem of whether *setet* means mucus ('Schleimstoffe' of the *Grundriss*) or shooting pains as suggested by Dawson (1934b) and supported by the determinative which depicts an arrow piercing an animal skin (see Chapter 3). Again the treatments give no clue to the condition.

Recognition of amenorrhoea is clearly defined in Ebers 833:

> If you examine a woman who has spent many years without her menstruation (*hesmen*) coming. She spits out something like *hebeb*. Her belly is like that which is on fire. It ceases when she has vomited. Then you shall say concerning it/her: It is a raising up (*akhet*) of blood in her uterus.

A complex but innocuous remedy is then prescribed to be drunk for four days.

Excessive bleeding (menorrhagia) is not clearly defined but there are remedies 'to draw out (*iteh*) the blood of a woman' (Ebers 828–30). The rationale is that drawing out the blood would stop the bleeding. Kahun 9 sounds like instructions for a victim of rape:

> Instructions for a woman suffering in her vagina, and all her limbs likewise, having been beaten. You shall say concerning it/her: 'This has loosened (? *fekh*) her uterus'. You should then prepare for her: oil to be eaten (sic) until she is well.

Discharges

The declaration in Kahun 3, 7 and 10 states: 'you shall then say concerning it/her: "it is a *khaau* of the uterus"'. The verb *khaa* has the general meaning of 'throw, cast off, eject or excrete' and the plural noun *khaau* has been translated as 'discharges' (Faulkner, 1962), 'excrementa' (Griffith, 1898) and 'defluxations' (Stevens, 1975). The *Grundriss* remained uncommitted with '*khaau*-symptom'. Innocuous drinks and smearing of feet and calves with mud are prescribed. No other parts of these passages throw light on the meaning of *khaau* in this context.

Urinary problems

Interpretation of Kahun 34 is critically dependent on translation. I favour the following, which is close to that of Stevens (1975):

> [Remedy for] a woman whose urine is in an irksome (*qesen*) place (*set*). If [her] urine comes . . . she is aware of it, will be likewise for ever.

The decisive factor is the translation of *set*, which most commonly means 'place'. However, the *Grundriss* translates the phrase as '. . . a woman, the urine is in a bad condition' which is linguistically feasible and makes sense, implying a diagnosis of cystitis. However, if *set* is assigned its usual meaning indicating location, the reading strongly suggests a fistula between bladder and vagina, which has been observed in human remains (Derry, 1935; Harer, 1993).

The breasts

There is a sequence of remedies for the breast which is embedded within the gynaecological section of the Ebers papyrus. However, the order of the sections makes little sense. Ebers 808 is 'the beginning of remedies to prevent the breasts going down (presumably sagging)'. The recommended treatment is that the breasts, the belly and the thighs should be smeared with (literally 'drink') the blood (*senef*) of one whose menstruation has just begun, clearly a sympathetic remedy. It then goes on to say that 'the *gesu* will not appear against her'. There are no further remedies for sagging breasts but 809 is 'to prevent the *gesu* against a woman'. Ebers 810 is 'another remedy for the breast if it is diseased (*mer*)' although without giving any clues as to the nature of the disease. Finally, 811 is an incantation for the breasts, including the words 'Do not make discharge (*wesesh*): do not make any eating (*weshau*): do not make blood'. If 'eating' is a euphemism for cancer (p. 81), this trio suggests carcinoma of the breast, arising from milk ducts.

Diseases of the eyes

The eye plays a major part in Egyptian mythology. The eye of Horus was torn out by Seth, but magically restored (see Chapter 5). The restored and healthy (*wedjat*) eye then became a potent symbol for protection and cure, and is the subject of innumerable amulets. Its component parts were used to define fractions between 1/2 and 1/64 (see fig. 7.3) and were used extensively in prescriptions.

The ancient Egyptian doctors were renowned for their skill in the treatment of eyes. Herodotus (III, 1) wrote that Cyrus sent to Ahmose II (Amasis, Twenty-sixth Dynasty) to ask for the services of the best ophthalmologist in Egypt, an incident which, according to Herodotus, played a part in the Persian invasion of Egypt in 525 BC. Ophthalmologists were designated *swnw irty*, the doctor of the eyes, and this was well shown in the stela of Ir-en-akhty (see fig. 6.8). There is virtually no archaeological evidence of eye disease and artificial eyes often replaced mummies' eyes. However, there are many representations of blindness, particularly of harpists (fig. 9.3). The best sources of information are the medical papyri, almost exclusively the compact section of the Ebers papyrus, 336–431. This section starts as follows, giving a selection of remedies for *wekhedu*, the unknown but all pervasive pathological factor discussed in Chapter 3:

9.3 Typical representation of blindness in a harpist. This example is from the tomb of Pa-aten-em-heb in Saqqara (Amarna Period of the 18th Dynasty). (Rijksmuseum van Oudheden, Leiden, AMT 1–35)

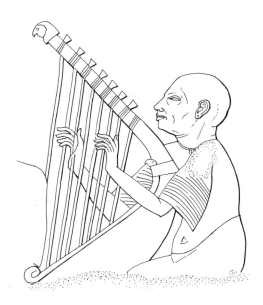

Beginning of the collection of remedies for the eyes.
a) What is to be done for a growth (*redet*) of *wekhedu*, with blood in the eyes: *sia* (? orpiment) from Upper Egypt, 1; honey, 1; *senen*, 1; *nehed*, 1.
b) Treatment of its water: incense (*senetjer*), 1; incense (*antyu*), 1; *tentem*, 1; ochre, 1.
c) Treatment of the growth: *sia* from Lower Egypt, 1; red ochre (*menshet*), 1; green eye-paint, 1; honey, 1.
d) Afterwards: you should prepare for him oil/fat, 1.
Beginning of the after [treatment]: wax, 1; *gesfen* (? decomposing chalcopyrite), 1; *khenetet* from incense (*senetjer*), 1; ochre, 1.
Completion of after [treatment]: *khet-awa*, 1; incense (*senetjer*), 1; fat of goose, 1.
End of after [treatment]: ochre, 1; black eye-paint, 1; oil/fat, 1; Bandage with it on four days. You should not disturb it at all. (Ebers 336)

Table 9.2 Terms of uncertain meaning for diseases of the eyes, with their recommended treatments

wehat-disease	black eye-paint, red ochre, ochre, red natron, applied to outside (*sa*) of both eyes (Ebers 346)
pedset in the eye	black eye-paint, green eye-paint, carob, *khet-awa*, *gesfen*, applied to outside of both eyes (Ebers 355)
	black eye-paint, *senen*-balm, *khet-awa*, both eyes painted therewith (Ebers 423 = 430)
nehat-disease	bile of tortoise, ladanum (*iber*), applied to both eyes (Ebers 350)
	leaves of acacia, flour of carob, granite, ground, bandaged on both eyes (Ebers 383)
	black eye-paint, red ochre, ochre, red natron, ground, applied to outside of both eyes (Ebers 407)*
sharu-disease	roasted ox liver, pressed, applied thereon, really effective (Ebers 351)
khesefu of the flesh	green eye-paint, *senetjer*-resin, red ochre, ground and applied to both eyes (Ebers 421)
khenet-disease	black eye-paint, *senen*-balm, *hetem*-mineral, *tjeru*-mineral, fresh *antyu*-resin, Upper Egyptian *sia*-mineral, ground and introduced into both eyes (Ebers 367)
bid-disease	black eye-paint, fat of goose, milk from one who has borne a male child, *antyu*-resin, both eyes painted with it (Ebers 368)
tekhen-injury	dried faeces from belly of infant, honey, vegetable mucilage, applied to outside of both eyes (Ebers 349)
	cooked *shasha* (? valerian), carob, honey, finely ground, bandaged on both eyes (Ebers 381)
	see text for Ebers 337
qenit-injury	green eye-paint, *tjeru*-mineral, black eye-paint, natron, ochre, ground in water and applied to outside of both eyes (Ebers 416)
	red ochre, fat of goose, anoint exterior of both eyes (Ebers 417)

* This treatment is identical to Ebers 346 (*wehat*-disease).

The Egyptian word *sa*, usually meaning 'back' is here translated as 'outside'.

Khenet-disease of the head features in Ebers 391, and of the nose in Ebers 418.

See Tables 7.3, 7.4, 7.5 and 7.6 for identity of drugs.

The word for growth (*red*) should not be interpreted as a synonym for tumour as in English. Other remedies for *wekhedu* of the eye appear in Ebers 341 and 386.

The treatments in this section of the Ebers papyrus consist entirely of medication, mostly to be applied externally to the eye. Many of the prescriptions include black and green eye-paint, probably sympathetic remedies (Table 9.2). The pigments in these are respectively galena (lead sulphide) and finely powdered malachite (copper carbonate/hydroxide). Both would be mechanical irritants, but it is conceivable that the latter would exert an anti-bacterial effect (see Chapter 7). There is no mention of any type of surgical intervention.

General treatments for blindness and poor eyesight

The Egyptian word for blindness – *shepet* – is well attested, and there are a group of non-specific remedies (Ebers 356–8 and 420) which are simply designated 'another [remedy] for blindness' or '. . . for driving out blindness' without any indication of the cause of the blindness. Ebers 356 includes the water of a pig's eyes, but the remedy is to be poured into the ear, which is linked to the eye in the vessel book. Ebers 359 is for treating, and 393 for strengthening, the sight in the two eyes. Several sections are to 'open (*weba*) the eyesight (*maa*)', which may be a quite literal reference to an eye closed by swelling and dried pus, although many idioms refer to 'opening the face'. Ebers 392 is for 'an eye in which any evil (*dju*) thing has appeared' and includes pig bile. This may relate to the entry of a disease-demon into the eye. Many of the remedies seem highly unlikely to be beneficial in any way. They include black and green eye-paint, honey and fragments of an earthenware jar.

Chapter 7 cited the use of liver in the treatment of blindness: this raises the question of whether it was an attempt to treat night blindness with vitamin A, for which liver is a rich source. Kahun 1 is a difficult text, which opens the 'gynaecological treatise'. The involvement of the uterus here seems to be entirely spurious and irrelevant, perhaps because of the unfortunate lacunae in the text:

> Instructions for a woman -LACUNA- [with] sickness [so that] she cannot see and with (OR on account of) pain in her neck. You shall say concerning her: It is -LACUNA- of her uterus with/in her two eyes. You shall then do for her/it: Fumigate her with incense and fresh oil. Fumigate her vagina with it. Fumigate her eyes with the shanks of the *genyu*-bird. Then you shall cause her to eat fresh liver of an ass.

Discounting the fumigations, we may concentrate on the last instruction. There is no doubt of the reading 'Then you shall cause her to eat'. The following phrase is *miset net aa wadjet*, literally 'liver of ass (*aa*) raw (*wadjet*). The adjective *wadjet* (fresh, raw, green) has the feminine termination which agrees with the feminine noun for 'liver', and therefore applies to the 'liver' rather than the masculine noun for 'ass', although separated from *miset* by the indirect genitive. Thus we have a recommendation for raw liver for an unspecified condition of the eyes, but with no mention of impaired night vision.

The second reference to the use of liver for a disorder of the eyes is Ebers 351:

> Another for *sharu*-disease in both eyes: liver of ox, roasted and pressed. Apply to it. Really effective.

The word *sharu* (written *shau* in Ebers 351) also appears in London 34 and 36. Ebbell (1937) translated it as 'night blindness', perhaps because of the use of liver in treatment. However, there is no collateral evidence to support the interpretation as night blindness, and the ideogram for 'night' does not appear in the word. It should be noted that local application of liver to the eye could not cure night blindness, and roasting would have reduced the vitamin A content. The *Grundriss* and Ghaliounghui (1987) do not commit themselves beyond 'eye disease', but in 1992 Westendorf gave 'night blindness'.

Cloudiness and watering of the eye

Ebers 339–40 are remedies to 'drive out cloudiness (*hati*) in the eye', while Ebers 415 extends the indication to include darkness (*keku*). These are well attested words and are fully supported by the determinatives employed. Cloudiness and darkness could well be used to describe opacities in the cornea or the lens (cataract). The remedies to be used are not remarkable, but in Ebers 339 there is 'another statement' that 'you should pour it [into the eye] with a feather of a vulture'. Ghaliounghui (1987) posed the question whether the quill could be modified to function as an eye dropper. Nowhere is there any reference to surgical treatment of cataract.

The word *djefdjefet*, related to *defdef* (to drip) would appear to mean excessive lachrymation (Ebers 376), which can arise from many causes, including blocked tear ducts. Ebers 378 is a remedy to 'drive out the raising up of the water in the eyes', which may well mean the same thing. The remedy included real lapis lazuli (presumably powdered) and 'earth of crocodile' (? dung), neither of which would seem likely to have improved watering eyes! Ebers 385 is an incantation to be used in combination with a local application for the same condition. Westendorf (1992), however, raises the question whether *djefdjefet* is yet another reference to Nile shipping with a flooding of the river presenting problems to shipping. He points out that the modern word cataract means both a torrent of water and an opacity of the lens.

Trachoma

This is a chronic granulomatous conjunctivitis, due to infection with *Chlamydia trachomatis*, giving a characteristic roughened appearance, and constituting a grave hazard to eyesight. The condition was probably endemic in ancient Egypt, although no archaeological evidence can be expected. Ebers 350, 383 and 407 all refer to the *nehat*-disease. The adjective *neha*, used in other contexts, has various meanings such as uneven, restless, troubled, shaking or terrible. The Greek word *trachoma* has similar meaning, and Ebbell (1937) suggested that *nehat*, with pustule determinative, meant trachoma, an interpretation which was accepted by Ghaliounghui (1987) and Westendorf (1992). Remedies include bile of tortoise, ladanum, acacia leaves, carob, ground up granite, black eye-paint, ochre, red ochre and red natron.

Foreign bodies and eye injuries

Something looking very like removal of a foreign body from the eye is shown in Ipwy's tomb (see fig. 3.6). Westendorf (1992) interprets Ebers 337 as directions for treatment of a foreign body, and *tekhen* here has a striking arm determinative, which is commonly associated with some act of violence. The instructions are in four stages.

> Another made for the *tekhen*-injury of the eye.
> Day one: marsh water.
> Day two: honey, 1; black eye-paint, 1; on one day.
> If it bleeds: honey, 1; black eye-paint, 1; bandaged with it for two days.
> If, however, much liquid flows down from it, you should prepare for it a remedy
> *aafs* (? wrung out): *iau*, 1; green eye-paint, 1; incense (*senetjer*), 1; top of
> *heden*-plant; cooked.

The *tekhen*-injury appears also in Ebers 349 where it has 'attached (*tjes*) itself in the eye'. Ebers 381 says that what is *tekhen*-injured is outside (*her-sa*) the eye. Ebers 416–17 concern the *qenit*-injury, a word which is used in relation to the eye injury of Horus.

Troublesome eyelashes

The Ebers papyrus is quite specific on troublesome eyelashes which grow inwards to irritate the cornea (Ebers 424):

> Another [remedy] to drive out curling up of the hair in the eye: incense (*antyu*),
> 1; blood of lizard, 1; blood of bat, 1. Pull out the hair. Apply to it so that it gets
> well.

Also Ebers 425:

> Another [remedy] for not allowing hair to grow in the eye after it has been pulled out. ... To be applied to the place of this hair after it has been pulled out. It will not grow [again].

The second remedy is similar to the first but includes blood of ox, ass, pig, hound and goat.

Spots on the eyes

A number of remedies are to drive out *sehedju* which appear in the eyes. The *Grundriss* translates *sehedju* as white spots but it is not clear whether these are corneal opacities or pterygia (small nodules of yellowish tissue on the conjunctiva which may invade the edge of the cornea) or pingueculae (yellowish spots on either side of the cornea which look fatty and appear in the aged). The last is quite likely for Ebers 354 and 431, which contain remedies to drive out fat from the eyes. Remedies for *sehedju* occur in Ebers 347, 382 and 402–6. Ebers 360 is an incantation to be recited over bile of tortoise, beaten with honey and applied to the upper eyelid. Perhaps more specific is a *pedset* of the eye (Ebers 355). The usual meaning is a pellet and there is wide agreement that it means 'sty' in this context. However, a Meibomian cyst would also fit the description.

Blood in the eye

It is unambiguously stated in Ebers 348, 352 and 384 that each is 'another [remedy] to drive out blood from the eyes'. Ebers 387 is 'another [remedy] to drive out vessels (*metu*) of blood from the eyes'. Ebbell (1937) translated this as 'blood extravasation', and subconjunctival haemorrhage would seem to be the most likely meaning.

Inflammation

Heat (*tjau*) in the eye may mean inflammation, although alternatively it may mean irritation. Remedies include black eye-paint and ground-up tooth of an ass, neither of which would be soothing.

Unidentified eye diseases

There remain many Egyptian words apparently denoting eye diseases which cannot be translated (Table 9.2). Conversely there are many diseases of the eye which must have existed in pharaonic times for which we do not know the Egyptian words.

The teeth

A wealth of skulls has survived to give a clear picture of dental health in ancient Egypt, from the Predynastic to the Roman Period. Teeth and jaws are highly resistant to decay, especially in the dry conditions of Egypt and, unlike soft tissues, were generally undamaged by the processes of mummification. Radiographs show detail which is hardly inferior to that obtained with living patients today (Leek, 1979; Baldock *et al.*, 1994).

Care of the teeth was clearly a major problem and the dentist was designated *ibhy*, some of whom were also *swnw*. Hieroglyphs for this word could be abbreviated simply to the tusk-sign, the determinative of *ibhy*, as seen for Hesy-ra (see fig. 6.4), who was the first recorded doctor and dentist. It is unfortunate that human remains have revealed almost no evidence of the practical work of the *ibhy*, which might have been expected from the excellent preservation of teeth.

Attrition

Most mature adult teeth from the earliest times show attrition due to hard particulate matter in food, partly as a result of grinding corn with stone and partly from contamination of grain with wind-blown sand. Leek (1979) proposed four classes to describe the progression of the condition (fig. 9.4). Class I is flattening of the enamel cusps which would have been asymptomatic. Dentine is exposed in Class II and this would have been associated with some discomfort. The rate of abrasion of primary dentine often exceeded the rate of deposition of secondary dentine and this resulted

9.4 Internal structure of a tooth, showing the classes of attrition described by Leek (1979). Classes III and IV would have resulted in considerable pain.

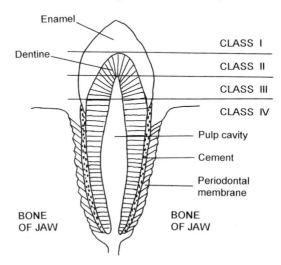

Enamel

Dentine

CLASS I

CLASS II

CLASS III

CLASS IV

Pulp cavity

Cement

Periodontal membrane

BONE OF JAW

BONE OF JAW

in exposure of the pulp cavity (Class III). Nerves would then be exposed to mechanical, thermal and osmotic stimuli, and there would have been considerable discomfort. Class IV denotes advanced wear of the body of the tooth.

Leek reported Class II–III attrition in all mummies and heads examined from the Twelfth to the Twenty-fifth Dynasties. Attrition was a very prominent feature found in nearly every one of forty skulls from the period approximately 1069–715 BC (Smith, 1986). A modest decrease in incidence between 4000 BC and AD 1000, first reported by Ruffer (1921) and confirmed by Thornton (1990), was probably due to improved techniques of grinding corn.

Caries

All investigators have reported a remarkably low incidence of caries extending from the earliest times until the first millennium BC (Smith and Jones, 1910; Leek, 1972; Grilletto, 1973). This is almost certainly attributable to the absence of sugars in the diet. Honey was available but was too scarce and expensive to be a major factor. Tetracycline in food or beer (see Chapter 7) may have been a factor in the prevention of caries (Rose, Armelagos and Perry, 1993). Thornton showed an increase in the incidence of caries from about 3 per cent in the Predynastic Period to 20 per cent in the early Christian Period. Leek (1979) found only one small cavity in material prior to 1000 BC, and Smith found an incidence of only 6.9 per cent of 691 teeth. There is general agreement that caries increased during the Ptolemaic Period and reached high levels in the Christian era. It seems likely that increasing foreign influence led to dietary changes which encouraged caries formation.

ANCIENT EGYPTIAN MEDICINE

Dental abscesses

Leek found twenty-five abscesses in six mummies out of a total of eighteen adult mummies and heads examined. The infection arose from caries (Leek, 1979) or through the pulp exposed by attrition (Smith, 1986). A root abscess would have been difficult to treat, and it is questionable whether the hole shown in fig. 9.5 is a natural sinus or whether it was drilled. This could have been accomplished with available techniques, but would have been extremely painful and therefore very difficult to accomplish. Furthermore, in view of the prevalence of dental abscesses, had the operation been current practice, one might have expected to see more examples of drilling in the large number of well preserved jaw bones.

9.5 Two sinuses, close to the roots of the molar tooth (on either side of the fracture line), may be natural or could have been drilled for the relief of a root abscess. In front of them is seen the normal mental foramen, through which the mental nerve emerges to provide the sensory innervation of the chin and lower lip. (Old Kingdom, case presented by Breasted, 1930)

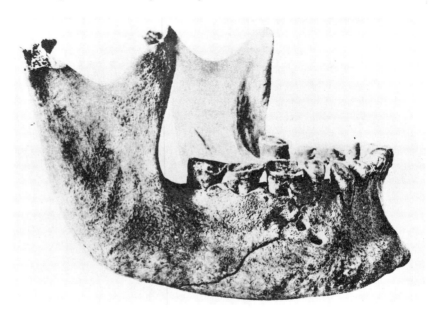

Periodontal disease

Both Leek and Smith reported widespread periodontal disease, leading to loss of alveolar supporting bone. This often progressed to the point at which teeth became loose and either fell out or could be removed with minimal effort. The abrasive material which caused attrition (see above) should have stimulated the gums and removed hard tartar, both factors militating against periodontal disease.

The removal of teeth

With advanced periodontal disease, teeth can be removed with the fingers alone. Otherwise it is necessary to use either forceps or levers. No such instruments have been identified from the pharaonic period, and the medical papyri are silent on the extraction of teeth. Nevertheless, Leek (1979) reached the conclusion, from the skulls which he examined, that some teeth must have been removed from strong and well developed arches. He believed that some method of removal of teeth was known and practised, although we do not know how this was accomplished.

Dislocated jaw

Chapter 8 cites Edwin Smith 25, which gives a superb description of a dislocated jaw, followed by an account of its reduction which differs little from modern practice.

Dental care in the medical papyri

The papyri are silent on all operative aspects of dental care, and Smith and Jones (1910) found no evidence of 'the dentist's handiwork' in some 6000 bodies and skeletons at any of the periods covered by the Nubian cemeteries. However, some dental remedies are found, mainly in Ebers 553–5 and 739–49. As usual, the translation of the pathological entities presents difficulties.

There are five remedies to make firm or strengthen the teeth. Ebers 739 and 743 use the causative verb *smen* with the very well attested meaning of make firm, make fast, make to endure and so on. Ebers 748 uses the equally well attested causative verb *serudj* with the meaning of strengthen or make secure. What is unclear is whether these remedies were directed towards a tooth which was loose due to periodontal disease or a tooth which was crumbling from caries. However, caries only became a major problem long after the papyrus was written, and the former, therefore, seems the more likely interpretation. The remedies include scrapings of a millstone (a sympathetic remedy), and malachite which might have a favourable effect on sepsis (see Chapter 7). Two remedies include honey which would hardly have helped with caries.

The remedy in Ebers 553 is for driving out 'crushing' of ulcers in the teeth, and in Ebers 554 for driving out ulcers in the teeth and to strengthen the flesh. It is unclear whether 'teeth' are here taken to include the periodontal tissue or if the 'ulcers of the teeth' might perhaps mean 'caries'. The treatment includes unknown plants, carob and honey to be applied locally.

Ebers 741 is to drive out growth of *wekhedu*, the untranslatable disease principle discussed in Chapter 3, and 745 is to treat a tooth with 'chewing' (*khepau*). It is unclear whether this might refer to attrition (see above). Ebers 742 is 'another to treat a tooth which is eating at the mouth (or opening) of the flesh'. This suggests a sharp projection on a damaged tooth which is causing ulceration of tongue or cheek. The remedy comprised cumin, incense (*senetjer*) and carob (*djaret*) applied as a powder.

CHAPTER **TEN**

Epilogue

There is no evidence of major changes in the format or content of classical Egyptian medicine between the Old Kingdom and the end of the Twenty-sixth Dynasty, covering the years 2600 to 525 BC. This may be ascribed to the innate conservatism of the Egyptians, their geographical isolation and their relative freedom from foreign domination. Irreversible changes commenced with the Persian invasion of 525 BC, when the Egyptians found themselves governed by people with a level of sophistication comparable to their own. Simultaneously, Greek medicine was acquiring an international reputation and challenging the supremacy of Egyptian medicine to which Homer had referred in the Odyssey (pp. 131–2).

During the Twenty-seventh Dynasty, Egypt was under the domination of the Persian kings whose names were represented in cartouches after the manner of the pharaohs. Wedja-hor-resnet (p. 129) is the only Egyptian doctor whose name has survived from this period. He held powerful administrative posts under Cambyses, but still made repeated reference to the fact that he was a *wer swnw*. Darius I, the second king of the Persian Dynasty, commanded Wedja-hor-resnet to restore the house of life (*per ankh*) with particular reference to the 'art to revive all that are sick'. This is also the period of the visit of Herodotus to Egypt, and his description of the practice of Egyptian medicine (II, 76–83), stressing their great reluctance to adopt foreign practices. However, they were not universally successful in treating their Persian conquerors. According to Herodotus (III, 129), Darius I dislocated his ankle and his Egyptian physicians failed to relieve his pain. Eventually he coerced a captive Greek doctor, Democedes, into treating him. He was so successful that not only was he richly rewarded but he was also able to dissuade Darius from impaling his Egyptian physicians.

Greek mercenaries and traders were permitted to establish the city of Naucratis in the Delta during the Twenty-sixth Dynasty (664–525 BC), a time which coincided with the birth of Greek medical science and natural philosophy. There was considerable interchange of information and technology at that time. However, Greek medicine came to Egypt in strength during the Ptolemaic Period, following Alexander's conquest of the country in 332 BC. The Ptolemies (305–30 BC) may have been depicted in the classical guise of pharaohs in the temples they built in Egypt, but otherwise they maintained their Hellenistic culture, language and outlook. Only gradually did the native Egyptian influence penetrate the court, and Cleopatra VII, the last of the Ptolemies, was the first to speak Egyptian.

The Greek settlers in Alexandria included physicians, particularly from the Hippocratic school at Cos. It seems likely that Greek and Egyptian medicine initially followed separate lines, Greek physicians probably concentrating their attention on the Greek ruling classes, while Egyptian physicians continued to treat the indigenous population. Nevertheless the Greek rulers patronised the Egyptian gods of healing. Ptolemy VIII Euergetes II built a shrine to Imhotep in Deir el-Bahri, and the Greeks identified him with Asklepios (Chapter 6).

Alexander himself established the new town of Alexandria in 331 BC and it rapidly became the major cultural and scientific centre of the Hellenistic world. Ptolemy I Soter I (305–282 BC) and Ptolemy II Philadelphus (284–246 BC) established the museion ('house of muses') and the immense library, providing powerful patronage for science and letters. They developed an exceptionally fertile field and climate for scientific innovation, which attracted Greeks from a wide area. Egyptian input to the Alexandrian scientific and cultural centres seems to have been minimal in the third century BC, the most important exception being Manetho of Sebennytos, a native Egyptian and the first known to have written in Greek. He was commissioned by Ptolemy II to write an account of Egyptian history about 280 BC, and has been quoted as a source for information on legendary doctors in Chapter 6.

It is not clear whether medicine was an integral part of the museion, although there is no doubt that Alexandria developed an outstanding medical school, where Galen studied in the second century AD (Nutton, 1993). Royal patronage and support made possible the work of Herophilus who, early in the third century BC, moved to Egypt to practise medicine in Alexandria. He was born about 325 BC in Calcedon, on the Asiatic side of the Bosporus, and had been a pupil of Praxagoras of Cos (von Staden, 1989), and so a follower of the Hippocratic school.

The most dramatic aspect of Herophilus' research was in human anatomy, for which he broke both Greek and Egyptian taboos on defilement of the dead. In his pioneer studies of human dissection, and probably also vivisection, he used bodies and, it seems, living criminals supplied by the kings (probably Ptolemy I and II). Celsus wrote as follows (Loeb edition, I Prooemium 23):

> Moreover, as pains, and also various kinds of diseases, arise in the more internal parts, they [the Rationalists] hold that no one can apply remedies for these who is ignorant about the parts themselves; hence it becomes necessary to scrutinize their viscera and intestines. They hold that Herophilus and Erasistratus did this in the best way by far, when they laid open men whilst alive – criminals received out of prison from the kings – and whilst they were still breathing.

Although these methods were subsequently deemed improper, if not barbarous, Herophilus made major contributions on anatomy, particularly of the brain. He discovered at least seven of the cranial nerves and paid particular attention to the fourth ventricle, lying between the cerebellum and the brain stem, which he correctly identified as the main controlling centre of the brain.

He distinguished motor and sensory functions of the nerves, although occasionally confusing nerves with ligaments and tendons, as did the ancient Egyptians in their description of the *metu* (see Chapter 3). His name is still perpetuated in the torcula Herophili, the posterior confluence of the venous sinuses draining the brain. The first section of the small bowel is named the duodenum because Herophilus observed that its length was equal to the width of twelve fingers. He also made major advances in identifying the structure of the eye and the reproductive organs of both sexes.

In the field of physiology, Herophilus correctly supported Aristotle's earlier view that the pulse reflected activity of the heart, and was not due to intrinsic rhythmic contraction of the arteries. In this he rejected the prevailing view of his teacher Praxagoras. Herophilus was the first to time the pulse using a portable klepsydra (water clock), calibrated for different ages of his patients. He was perhaps the first to bring measurement into clinical investigation.

Although far from recognising the circulation of the blood, he noted that arteries had walls six times thicker than veins and he may have hinted that arteries contained blood as well as air (*pneuma*). At the time it was widely believed, among both Greeks and Egyptians, that arteries contained only air, a view which prevailed until the work of Galen in the second half of the second century AD. Erasistratus, a contemporary of Herophilus, who may also have worked in Alexandria, described the tricuspid and mitral valves of the human heart, and came closer than anyone before Harvey to discovering the circulation of the blood. Furthermore, he recognised the threefold distribution of arteries, veins and nerves to various organs and tissues.

Herophilus was a staunch rationalist and so attracted the criticisms of the empiricists, who were more concerned with observational experience than the causal explanation of disease. His books have survived only in fragments quoted by other authors, but he was cited extensively by many later physicians, particularly Galen. These sources together with those of early Christian writers and others have been comprehensively reviewed by von Staden (1989).

On his death (*c.* 255 BC), Herophilus was followed by a group of Greek Alexandrian physicians termed the Herophileans. They abandoned human dissection but pursued the other interests of Herophilus in study of the pulse, gynaecology and therapeutics. They made major contributions and were frequently cited, although all their own writings are lost, no doubt in part as a result of the great fire of the library of Alexandria in 47 BC and its final loss in AD 389. The Herophileans also devoted major attention to the philology of the Hippocratic corpus. They survived the expulsion of the intelligentsia in 145–144 BC under Ptolemy VIII Euergetes II and, a century later, set up a daughter school in Laodicea in Asia Minor, which lasted until about AD 50 (von Staden, 1989).

In general, Herophilus and his followers remained aloof from the Ptolemaic court, with its dangerous intrigues. There were, however, two exceptions. Andreas became personal physician to Ptolemy IV Philopator (*c.* 244–205) and was killed in the fourth Syrian war against Antiochus III (Polybius Hist. 5.58.87). Dioscurides Phacas was closely associated with the court of Ptolemy XII Auletes (80–51 BC) and Ptolemy XIII. An ambiguous passage by Julius Caesar (*de bello civili* 3. 109, 3–6) suggests he may have survived a murderous attack in 48 BC to become influential in the court of Antony and Cleopatra (41–30 BC). In spite of these involvements, both Andreas and Dioscurides undertook valuable research, which was extensively cited by later authors.

Greek and Egyptian medical practice followed relatively separate courses in the early Ptolemaic Period but, in due course, the two systems of medicine learned from one another. The extant copy of the P. Vindob, D 6257, from Crocodilopolis (see Chapter 2) is second century AD, but the original is thought to be early Ptolemaic. It is written in demotic and much is in the traditional format of the Egyptian medical papyri of the New Kingdom. However, 59 of the 201 named drugs are not attested in pharaonic times and must be presumed to have come to Egypt during the Late and Ptolemaic Periods. All have Egyptian names. Perhaps most remarkable of all is the total absence of any magical spells in the Crocodilopolis papyrus. This is contrary to the general trend for the relative role of magic in medicine to increase with time, which is also discernible in Mesopotamian medicine.

The Romans exerted direct rule of Egypt after Octavian's defeat of Mark Antony in the battle of Actium in 31 BC, although Greek remained the language of government. Roman medicine was dominated by Greeks or Romans who practised in the Greek manner (Jackson, 1988). Therefore, Roman rule would have had little influence on medical practice in a country where Greek influence was already very strong. From the third century AD, we have the medical and magical papyrus of London and Leiden (see Chapter 2), one of the last known papyri written in demotic. The text is freely embellished with Greek inserts and glosses which were very helpful in identifying obscure demotic words in the medical section. Parts are in the general format of the earlier medical papyri although entirely new drugs are introduced, in particular the mandrake for inducing sleep. However, this papyrus is predominantly magical and shows no advance in medical science which might have been expected from its late date.

Christianity was established very early in Egypt, and Coptic became the main language of the country until the Arab conquest of AD 640, and still remains the liturgical language of the Coptic church. Coptic evolved from ancient Egyptian, enriched with Greek words, and was written from the third century AD in a script which was basically Greek with the addition of seven demotic characters. A major consequence of Christianity was the closing of the Egyptian temples, which led directly to loss of understanding of the ancient Egyptian language during the fifth century AD. Egyptian then remained a dead language until the work of Åkerblad and Thomas Young, but particularly Champollion in 1822.

Coptic medicine was predominantly Greek, though containing many Egyptian remedies (see Till, 1951). It was, furthermore, partly written in a format reminiscent of classical Egyptian medicine. With time it became increasingly influenced by Arabic medicine, which grew in strength to reach its climax at the end of the first millennium AD. With the loss of understanding of the Egyptian language, and the second great fire of the Alexandrian library in AD 389, Egyptian medicine became difficult to study. Coptic medicine was a dead end, and pharaonic Egyptian medicine remained sequestered in buried and unintelligible papyri until their discovery and interpretation commenced in the last century.

The mainstream of transmission of medical knowledge was from Greece to Rome and thence into the mainstream of European medicine. However, an important route was the exodus of the Nestorians from Christendom, following the condemnation of their leader at the Council of Ephesus in AD 431. The Nestorians carried their learning and their manuscripts with them on their journeys to the east, becoming a major factor in the development of Arabic medicine, particularly in Baghdad. This knowledge returned to Europe in the Renaissance.

Chronological table

PREDYNASTIC PERIOD		
Badarian	c. 5000–4000 BC	
Naqada I	c. 4000–3600	
Naqada II	c. 3600–3100	
EARLY DYNASTIC PERIOD		
1st Dynasty	c. 3100–2890	Djer supposedly a physician
2nd Dynasty	c. 2890–2686	(according to Manetho)
OLD KINGDOM		Breasted's date for original of Edwin Smith papyrus
3rd Dynasty	c. 2686–2613	Imhotep, Hesy-ra (first known *swnw*)
4th Dynasty	c. 2613–2494	
5th Dynasty	c. 2494–2345	Peseshet (*swnwt*)
6th Dynasty	c. 2345–2181	Mereruka, Ankh (*swnw*); Ankh-ma-hor
FIRST INTERMEDIATE PERIOD		
7th/8th Dynasties	c. 2181–2125	
9th/10th Dynasties	c. 2160–2025	Ir-en-akhty (*swnw*)
11th Dynasty (early)	c. 2125–2040	
MIDDLE KINGDOM		
11th Dynasty (late)	c. 2040–1985	Gua, Seni (*swnw*)
12th Dynasty	c. 1985–1795	Ref-seneb (*swnw*), Hery-shef-nakht (*swnw*); Kahun papyrus
SECOND INTERMEDIATE PERIOD		
13th–17th Dynasties	c. 1795–1550	Ramesseum papyri
NEW KINGDOM		
18th Dynasty	c. 1550–1295	Ebers and Edwin Smith papyri
19th Dynasty	c. 1295–1186	Hearst, London and Carlsberg papyri
20th Dynasty	c. 1186–1069	Chester Beatty and Berlin papyri
THIRD INTERMEDIATE PERIOD		
21st–25th Dynasties	c. 1069–656	
LATE PERIOD		
26th Dynasty (Saite)	664–525	
27th Dynasty (Persian)	525–404	Wedja-hor-resnet (*swnw*) Herodotus in Egypt
28th Dynasty	404–399	Hippocrates in Cos
29th Dynasty	399–380	
30th Dynasty	380–343	
Persian reconquest	343–332	
GRAECO-ROMAN PERIOD		
Macedonian	332–305	
Ptolemaic	305–30	Alexandrian museion; Herophilus; Erasistratus; Brooklyn papyrus on snake bite (may be 30th Dynasty); Diodorus Siculus in Egypt
Roman	30 BC–AD 323	Galen in Alexandria Crocodilopolis papyrus
BYZANTINE PERIOD	AD 323–642	
ARAB CONQUEST	AD 642	

The Third Dynasty is sometimes assigned to the Early Dynastic Period.
There is no agreement on the limits of the First Intermediate Period. It is often limited to the Ninth and Tenth Dynasties.

Concordance of tabulations of known doctors (*swnw*)

NO.	NAME OF *SWNW*	DYNASTY, RULER	J 1958	W M 1973	G 1983	M 1986 AND P	PRIMARY REFERENCES IN PRESENT BOOK
Old Kingdom and First Intermediate Periods							
1	Akh-hotep	5	–	E1	1	–	–
2	Akhi	–	–	E2	2	–	–
3	Iy-nefer	–	–	–	3	–	–
4	Ipi(1)	4	2	–	4	–	p. 99
5	Ipi(2)	6	3	–	5	–	–
6	Ir-en-akhty(1)	5 Isesi ?	7	–	6	–	–
7	Ir-en-akhty(2)	10 ?	8	–	7	–	pp. 126–7: fig. 6.8
8	Ir-en-akhty(3)	–	9	–	8	–	–
9	Isi-ankh	5	–	D7	9	–	–
10	Idu	–	–	–	10	–	–
11	Aperef	5 Isesi	–	–	add 1	–	–
12	Ankh(1)	6 Teti	10	–	11	–	p. 126: fig. 6.7
13	Ankh(2)	–	11	–	12	–	–
14	Ankh(3)	–	12	–	13	–	–
15	Wash-duaw	5	15	–	14	–	p. 134
16	Wa	4/5	16	–	15	–	–
17	Wenen-nefer(1)	5	18	–	16	–	p. 120
18	Wenen-nefer(2)	5	19	–	17	–	–
19	Bebi	–	21	–	18	–	–
20	Peseshet	5/6	30	–	19	–	pp. 124–5: fig. 6.5
21	Ptah-hotep	5	31	–	20	–	–
22	Men-kaw-ra-ankh	5 Sahura	33	–	21	–	–
23	Memi	6	–	–	22	–	–
24	Mer-pepi	6	34	–	23	–	–
25	Mereruka	6 Teti	35	–	(133)	–	p. 125: fig. 6.6
26	Mehu	6	–	–	–	A1	–
27	Metjen	4 Sneferu	37	–	–	–	–
28	Medu-nefer	–	38	–	24	–	p. 116
29	Ny...ra	4/5	Ba	–	25	–	–
30	Ny-ankh-ra	5	39	–	26	–	pp. 99, 100
31	Ny-ankh-khnum	6 Pepi 2	40	–	27	–	–
32	Ny-ankh-sekhmet	5 Sahura	41	–	28	–	–
33	Ny-ankh-duaw	5 ?	42	–	29	–	–
34	Ny-shepsesu-nesu	5	–	D9	30	–	–
35	Ny-ka-teti	–	–	–	–	P2	–
36	Nefer-irtes	–	45	–	31	–	–
37	Nefer-her-en-ptah	–	47	–	32	–	–
38	Nefer-tjes	–	48	–	33	–	–
39	Nakht-hedjes	–	50	–	34	–	–
40	Nes-em-naw	4/5	52	–	35	–	–
41	Ra-aperef	–	–	–	36	–	–
42	Ra-khuf(1)[1]	5 Isi	–	D6	37	–	–
43	Ra-khuf(2)[1]	–	–	–	38	–	–

Concordance of tabulations of known doctors (*swnw*) continued

NO.	NAME OF *SWNW*	DYNASTY, RULER	J 1958	W M 1973	G 1983	M 1986 AND P	PRIMARY REFERENCES IN PRESENT BOOK
Old Kingdom and First Intermediate Periods continued							
44	Ra-khuf-kakai	5 Neferirkara	–	–	add 2	–	–
45	Redi-en-ptah	5	57	–	39	–	–
46	Hesy-ra	3 Netjerkhet	63	–	40	–	p. 124: fig. 6.4
47	Heka	5	–	D8	41	–	–
48	Hetep-akhty	–	65	–	42	–	–
49	Khuy	–	69	–	43	–	pp. 100, 120
50	Khnum-ankh	6	70	–	44	–	–
51	Sankhu-ptah	6	–	–	–	–	p. 134
52	Seshem-nefer	–	73	–	45	–	–
53	Ka-wedja(1)	5	75	–	46	–	–
54	Ka-wedja(2)	5	76	–	47	–	–
55	Tjau	6	–	–	–	–	p. 134
56	Tjenty	–	–	–	–	P1	–
57	Djaw(1)	–	79	–	48	–	–
58	Djaw(2)	–	80	–	49	–	–
59	Djuaw-khuf	5	–	–	–	–	p. 134
60	...m...	6	Bb	–	50	–	–
61	Anon, ? Iry[2]	5/6 Unas/Teti	NN1	–	51	–	–
62	Anon	6	–	–	52	–	–
Middle Kingdom							
63	Impy	–	4	–	53	–	–
64	Imny	–	5	–	54	–	–
65	Iw	–	–	–	–	A2	–
66	Nemty-em-hat	–	13	–	55	–	pp. 100, 120
67	Akmu	12 Amenemhat III	14	–	56	–	pp. 99, 120, 128
68	Wah-ka	–	–	D2	57	–	–
69	Wepay	–	–	D1	58	–	–
70	Min-em-sehnet	–	–	D10	59	–	p. 44
71	Nefery	12	44	–	60	–	–
72	Nakht	–	49	–	61	–	–
73	Nedjemu	12	53	–	62	–	p. 120
74	Renef-seneb	12 Amenemhat III	56	–	63	–	p. 128
75	Hery-shef-nakht	12	62	–	64	–	pp. 128–9: fig. 6.10
76	Hetep	12 Senusret I	64	–	65	–	–
77	Sankh-khnum	12	71	–	66	–	–
78	Seni	11/12	72	–	67	–	pp. 127–8
79	Senebef	–	–	–	68	–	–
80	Gua	11/12	77	–	69	–	pp. 127–8: fig. 6.9
81	Anon	12 Senusret I	NN2	–	70	–	–
82	Anon	12 Amenemhat III	NN3	–	71	–	pp. 99, 120, 128
83	Anon	–	NN4	–	72	–	pp. 100, 120

Concordance of tabulations of known doctors (*swnw*) continued

NO.	NAME OF *SWNW*	DYNASTY, RULER	J 1958	W M 1973	G 1983	M 1986 AND P	PRIMARY REFERENCES IN PRESENT BOOK
Second Intermediate Period and New Kingdom							
84	Iuti	18/19	1	–	73	–	–
85	Amen-hotep (1)	18/19	6	–	74	–	p. 120
86	Amen-hotep (2)	–	–	–	75	–	p. 120
87	Innay	20	–	D13	76	–	p. 120
88	Ibi-meh	–	–	–	–	A3	–
89	Wia-em-shutef?	–	–	–	–	P4	–
90	Ben-antjit	20	–	–	–	A4	–
91	Pa(?neh)si	–	–	–	77	–	–
92	Pa-ra-em-hat[3]	19 Ramses II	24	–	78	–	p. 131
93	Pahatyu	20 Ramses IX	25	–	79	–	p. 120
94	Pentju	18 Akhenaten	26	–	80	–	–
95	Pu-ra	19/20	27	–	81	–	pp. 117, 120
96	Men/Menna	18 Amenhotep III	32	–	82	–	–
97	Men-...	–	–	–	–	A5	–
98	Mahu	18 Amenhotep III	36	–	83	–	–
99	Nay	14	–	–	84	–	–
100	Neb-amen	18 Amenhotep III	43	–	85	–	p. 131
101	Nefer	18	–	D11	86	–	–
102	Nefer-en-maat	–	–	–	–	A6	–
103	Nefer-hebef (1)	18	–	E3	87	–	–
104	Nefer-hebef (2)	–	–	–	–	A7	–
105	Nefer-hor	19	46	–	88	–	–
106	Nefer-sekheru	–	–	–	–	A8	–
107	Ra	–	54	–	89	–	–
108	Ra-em-wia	–	–	–	90	–	–
109	Ra-mes	–	55	–	91	–	–
110	Huy(1)	–	58	–	92	–	p. 130: figs 6.12–13
111	Huy(2)	–	–	–	–	A9	–
112	Hor-mes	20 Ramses V	61	–	93	–	–
113	Khay	–	66	–	94	–	p. 130: fig. 6.12
114	Khay-min (1)	20 Ramses IX	67	–	95	–	–
115	Khay-min (2)	20 Ramses IX	68	–	96	–	–
116	Kha-em-waset	19	–	–	–	A10	pp. 130–31: fig. 6.13
117	Sa-wadjet?	–	–	D4	97	–	–
118	Ta	–	–	–	–	P3	–
119	Tjener	20	–	D12	98	–	–
120	Tjutju	–	78	–	99	–	–
121	Djehuty-mes	19	–	D3	100	–	–
122	Djehuty-hotep	–	–	–	101	–	–
123	Anon	18 Hatshepsut	NN5	–	102	–	–
124	Anon	18 Hatshepsut	NN6	–	103	–	–
125	Anon	18 Hatshepsut	NN7	–	104	–	–

Concordance of tabulations of known doctors (*swnw*) continued

NO.	NAME OF *SWNW*	DYNASTY, RULER	J 1958	W M 1973	G 1983	M 1986 AND P	PRIMARY REFERENCES IN PRESENT BOOK
Second Intermediate Period and New Kingdom continued							
126	Anon (Babylonian)	18 Amenhotep III	NN8	–	105	–	p. 132
127	Anon (Babylonian)	19 Ramses II	NN9	–	106	–	p. 132
128	Anon (Babylonian)	19 Ramses II ?	NN10	–	107	–	p. 132
129	Anon (Babylonian)	19 Ramses II ?	NN11	–	108	–	p. 132
130	Anon	19	NN12	–	109	–	–
131	Anon	20 Ramses IX	NN14	–	110	–	–
132	Anon	20	NN15	–	111	–	p. 135
133	Anon	20 Ramses III	NN13	–	112	–	–
134	Anon	–	–	–	–	–	p. 134
Third Intermediate and Late Periods							
135	Ir-hor-sekheru	–	–	D5	113	–	–
136	Wa (or Ipi)	–	17	–	114	–	–
137	Wedja-hor-mehnet	26	–	E4	115	–	–
138	Wedja-hor-resnet	27 Cambyses	20	–	116	–	p. 129: fig. 6.11
139	Bak-en-khonsu	22/24	suppl 2	–	117	–	–
140	Pef-tjaw-a-neith	26 Apries	22	C1	118	–	–
141	Pa-an-meniu	22/25	23	C2	119	–	–
142	Pa-di	26	suppl 3	–	120	–	–
143	Pa-di-amen	–	–	–	–	A11	–
144	Psamtek	26 Amasis	28	–	121	–	–
145	Psamtek-soneb	26	29	C3	122	–	pp. 100, 120
146	Nes-pa-medu	26	51	–	123	–	–
147	Huy(3)	22	59	–	124	–	pp. 99, 120
148	Hor-akhbit	26	60	C4	125	–	–
149	Shed-su-hor	22	74	–	126	–	–
150	Anon	26 Amasis	NN16	–	127	–	–

The listing is in the conventional order of the Egyptian phonetic alphabet as followed by Jonckheere and Ghaliounghui.

There are no inflexible rules for anglicisation of proper names and, in many cases, alternative forms are in common use. Hyphenation has been used to simplify pronunciation, but also indicates the division between Egyptian words in the names.

J   Jonckheere (1958)
W M   van der Walle and de Meulenaere (1973)
G   Ghaliounghui (1983)
M (A)   de Meulenaere (1986)
   (P)   de Meulenaere: personal communication to the author (1994)

1 van der Walle and de Meulenaere believe these may be the same individual.

2 Ghaliounghui also lists this *swnw* as 5b.

3 Known from Akkadian texts as Pariamakhu, which may represent the Egyptian name Pa-ra-em-hat or Pa-ra-em-heb.

Addenda at reprinting (1997), all four reported by Miss Carol Andrews:

Old Kingdom
Iry (*swnw per aa*): On stela of unknown origin

Middle Kingdom
Ii-seneb (*swnw*), Renef-seneb (*swnw*), Sen-wosret (*wr swnw*): All on stela in Cairo Museum (JdE 91253) (Simpson, W K. 1995. *The Inscribed Material from the Pennsylvania-Yale Excavations at Abydos.* Yale University Press/University of Pennsylvania Press, New Haven/Philadelphia.)

Pharmacological properties which are currently attributed to extracts from some of the more clearly identifiable botanical species used in pharaonic medicine (see Tables 7.4 and 7.5)

Abies cilicica	other *Abies* species are antiseptic, diuretic and carminative[1]
Acacia nilotica	other African species of *Acacia* are bulk laxatives[8] and demulcents[1,6,7]
*Allium cepa**	antibiotic, expectorant, diuretic[1]; reduces platelet aggregation, reduces plasma cholesterol[7]
Allium kurrat / porum	–
Ambrosia maritima	–
Anacyclus pyrethrum	–
*Anethum graveolens**	carminative[1,3,7,8]
Apium graveolens	diuretic[1,4,5]; antirheumatic[2,5]; carminative[1,5]; spasmolytic[5]
*Artemisia absinthum**	antihelminthic (especially nematodes)[1,3]; antiseptic, antipyretic[1]
Balanites aegyptica	–
*Bryonia dioica**	powerful purgative[1,3]; irritant[1]; emetic, antihelminthic[3]
*Cannabis sativa**	complex psychotropic effects[6,7]
*Ceratonia siliqua**	antidiarrhoeal, anti-emetic[7]
*Cinnamonium zeylanicum** (=*Laurus cinnamonium*)	carminative[1-3,7,8]; astringent[1,2,7]; stimulant[1]; spasmolytic, antihelminthic, antimicrobial, antidiarrhoeal[3]
Cistus creticus	–
Citrullus lanatus	–
*Coriandrum sativum**	stimulant[1]; carminative[1,7]
Cucumis melo	–
Cuminum cyminum	carminative, stimulant, antidiarrhoeal[1]
Cyperus esculentus	–
Cyperus papyrus	–
Erigeron aegypticus	–
*Ferula foetida**	expectorant[1,3,5,7]; carminative[3,5,7]; spasmolytic[3,4]; used for hysteria and neuroses[1,5]
*Ficus carica**	purgative[1,2,7]; demulcent[8]
Ficus sycomorus	–
*Hedera helix**	antispasmodic[1]
*Hordeum vulgare**	demulcent[1]; nutritive and vehicle[7]
*Juniperus phoenicea**	antiseptic, diuretic[1-3,7]; carminative[1,3,7]; stimulant, styptic[1]; anodyne[3]
*Lactuca virosa**	sedative[1,3-5]; hypnotic[1]; antitussive[5]
*Linum usitatissimum**	purgative, anti-inflammatory[1]; antibacterial[2]; laxative, antitussive, anodyne[3]; demulcent[7,8]
Mimusops laurifolis	–
Moringa ptergosperma	–
Myrtus communis	astringent, antiseptic (external use, especially for haemorrhoids)[1]
Nymphaea lotus	anti-aphrodisiac, antiseptic, astringent[1] (see also Harer, 1985)
*Papaver somniferum**	powerful narcotic and analgesic (morphine)[1,6-8]
Phoenix dactilifera	–
*Pimpinella anisum**	carminative[1-3,7,8]; expectorant[1,3,7]; diuretic, purgative[1]; spasmolytic[3]

Pharmacological properties continued

Pinus pinea	–
Pisum sativum	–
*Punica granatum**	antihelminthic[1,7]; antibacterial (in root bark), antidiarrhoeal[1]; astringent (in rind of fruit)[1,2]
*Ricinus communis**	powerful purgative, also external application as demulcent[1,2,6-8]
Salix safsaf	analgesic, antipyretic, anti-inflammatory (in powdered bark, due to salicin)[2-6]
Tamarix nilotica	–
*Trigonella foenum-graecum**	carminative, tonic[1]; laxative, expectorant[3]; appetite stimulant[7]
Triticum dicoccum	–
Vigna sinensis	–
*Vitis agnus-castus**	anti-aphrodisiac[1]
*Vitis vinifera**	–
Zizyphus spina-Christi	–

Species likely to have been used medicinally but which does not appear in the medical papyri under its usual Egyptian name (*khetem*)

*Allium sativum**	antibacterial, expectorant[1]; hypotensive[1,5]; reduces blood lipids, antimicrobial[4,5,7]; anti-inflammatory, antihelminthic[5]

Species possibly used medicinally but without a known Egyptian name

*Citrellus colocynthus**	powerful cathartic[2,7]
*Melilotus officinalis**	carminative, expectorant, antibiotic[1]
*Valeriana officinalis**	sedative[1,4,5,7,8]; antispasmodic[1,2,5]; carminative[1,7]; relaxant, hypotensive[5]

None of these botanical species is now indexed in the *British Pharmacopoeia*, but pharmacological properties of extracts are listed as under note 8 (see below).

From the above list, only drugs extracted from *Papaver somniferum* appear in the British National Formulary (number 28, September 1994).

* The species is mentioned in *The Extra Pharmacopoeia* of 1993, but pharmacological properties are only listed as under note 7 (see below).

1 *The Encyclopaedia of Herbs and Herbalism* (Stuart, 1979).
2 *Trease and Evans' Pharmacognosy* (Evans, 1989).
3 *British Herbal Pharmacopoeia* (1983).
4 *British Herbal Pharmacopoeia* (1990).
5 *British Herbal Compendium* (Bradley, 1992).
6 *The Pharmacological Basis of Medical Therapeutics* (Gilman et al., 1985).
7 *Martindale: The Extra Pharmacopoeia*, 30th edition (Reynolds, 1993).
8 *British Pharmacopoeia* (1993).

– Indicates there was no mention of pharmacological properties in any of the listed references.

Glossary

analgesic	relieving pain
anodyne	relieving pain (but less potent than an analgesic)
antibacterial	killing or preventing growth of bacteria
antihelminthic	killing and expelling intestinal worms
antimicrobial	killing bacteria
antipyretic	reducing fever
antitussive	relieving cough
astringent	causing contraction of tissues and prevention of bleeding and secretion
carminative	facilitating eructation of gas from the stomach
cathartic	an especially powerful purgative
cholesterol	a high molecular weight alcohol which may be deposited in the lining of blood vessels, causing obstruction
demulcent	soothing and relieving irritation
diuretic	increasing the amount of urine
expectorant	increasing fluidity of bronchial secretions and thereby facilitating their expulsion
hypotensive	reducing blood pressure
lipids	a term including fats, fatty acids and their salts
styptic	astringent (see above)

Reduction of platelet aggregation interferes with blood clotting.

Transliteration, hieroglyphs and probable meaning (if known) for some of the more important words which appear in the text in an anglicised version of the supposed vocalisation of the Egyptian word. See also figs 3.3, 3.4, 4.3, 6.1 and 9.2.

aaa	ꜥ3ꜥ		unidentified toxic substance, disease or manifestation of disease (see Chap. 3)
aat	ꜥ3t		swelling or tumour
adj	ꜥd̲		fat
ais	3is		viscera (especially brain)
akut	3kwt		unidentified disease or manifestation of disease
amem	ꜥmm		brain (this word only appears as a remedy in the medical texts)
anaret	ꜥnꜥrt		unidentified worm
andju	ꜥnd̲w		a jar or pot
antyu	ꜥntyw		resin, formerly thought to be myrrh but now probably resins in general
anut	ꜥnwt		swelling or tumour
arar	ꜥrꜥr		unidentified snake (see Chap. 8)
arat	ꜥrꜥt		unidentified snake (see Chap. 8)
ashaut	ꜥš3wt		crying (excessively)
ashyt	3šyt		unidentified disease (especially appearing in wounds)
at	ꜥt		limb or other part of the body

Transliteration, hieroglyphs and probable meaning continued

atekh	ꜥtẖ		to strain or filter
awy	ꜣwy		bandages (a pair)
bag	bꜣg		weary or exhausted
baq	bꜣḳ		moringa (oil)
bedesh	bdš		weary or weak
bened	bnd		meaning unknown
benef	bnf		bile (this word only appears as a remedy in the medical texts)
benut	bnwt		ulcer
besen	bsn		gypsum
besh	bš		to vomit
besy	bsy	(?)	swelling
betju	bṯw		real or metaphorical intestinal worm
bid	bid		unidentified eye disease
bit	bit		honey
da	dꜣ		to copulate
debdeb	dbdb		abnormal action of the heart

Transliteration, hieroglyphs and probable meaning continued

degem	dgm		castor-oil plant
des	ds		unidentified type of knife
dewen	dwn		to stretch out or apart
djanary	ḏnȝry		scorpion (an unusual word for scorpion, appears in Berlin 78)
djaret	ḏȝrt		plant, probably carob, previously thought to be colocynth
djedfet	ḏdft		generic term for snakes and intestinal worms
djefdjefet	ḏfḏft		tears or drop (related to *defdef*, meaning to drip)
djennet	ḏnnt		skull
djeret	ḏrt		hand
djua	ḏwˤ		knife-treatment or knife
fedet	fdt		sweat
fenet	fnt		real or metaphorical intestinal worm
fy	fy		viper
gab	gȝb		upper arm or humerus bone
gany	gȝny		snake, perhaps black desert cobra or burrowing asp (see Chap. 8)
garsha	gȝršȝ		unidentified snake (see Chap. 8)

Transliteration, hieroglyphs and probable meaning continued

ges	gs		smear, anoint
ges-tep	gs-tp		'half a head' (as in migraine)
gesu	gsw		ointment
ha	ḥꜥ		flesh (usually as plural in the medical texts)
hayt	ḥꜣyt		bandage
heby	ḥby		unidentified snake (See Chap. 8)
hefaw	ḥfꜣw		snakes in general
hekay	ḥkꜣy		magician
hemat	ḥmꜣt		common salt
hemem	ḥmm		unidentified type of knife or other surgical instrument
henepu	ḥnpw		unidentified snake (see Chap. 8)
henqet	ḥnḳt		beer (many varieties existed)
henu	hnw		unidentified surgical instrument
heqat	ḥḳꜣt		volume measure (single *heqat* was approx. 4.5 litres)
hes	ḥs		faeces or excrement
hesbet	ḥsbt		real or metaphorical intestinal worm

Transliteration, hieroglyphs and probable meaning continued

heseq	ḥsḳ		disease-demon, especially 'cutting'
hesmen	ḥsmn		menstruation
hewau	ḥw3w		unidentified disease or manifestation of disease, probably skin
inem	inm		skin
irep	irp		wine
irtet	irtt		milk
itjetjet	iṯṯt		unidentified disease or manifestation of disease, probably of the skin
iuf	iwf		flesh, but may be used to mean vagina
iweh	iwḥ		pour
ka-en-am	k3-n-ᶜm		snake, probably *Pseudocerastes persicus* (see Chap. 8)
ka-nay	k3-nᶜy		unidentified snake (see Chap. 8)
kakaut	k3k3wt		probably blister or pustule, as suggested by similar Coptic word
kap	k3p		fumigate
kefet	kft		gash or gaping wound
khaau	ḫ3ᶜw		uterine manifestation of disease, probably discharge

Transliteration, hieroglyphs and probable meaning continued

khenet	ḫnt		probably catarrh
khenmet	ḫnmt		dry nurse
khery demet	ḫry-dmt		to be bitten or stung
khery-hebet	ḫry-ḥbt		lector priest
khet	ḫt		belly, body or abdomen (also uterus)
m khet wat	m ḫt wˁt		as one thing
maa	mȝȝ		to see
maa	mȝˁ		true, real
mer	mr		ill, sick or in pain
merhet	mrḥt		oil or fat
met	mt		vessels, ducts, tendons, etc. (see Chap. 3)
mu	mw		water
nebed	nbd		snake, possibly *Psammophis* or *Philothamnyus* (see Chap. 3)
nedj	nḏ		to grind or crush
neg	ng		to break
neha	nhȝ		uneven, restless, troubled or terrible

Transliteration, hieroglyphs and probable meaning continued

nehat	nḫ3t		unidentified disease (may involve eyes)
nehep	nhp		to copulate
nek	nk		to copulate
nekhebkheb	nḫbḫb		possibly an onomatopoeic word for crepitus (see Chap. 8)
neki	nki		snake, possibly *Naja pallida* (see Chap. 8)
nerut	nrwt		sprain or joint injury
neser	nsr		inflammation or to be inflamed
nesiet	nsyt		unknown disease caused by disease-demon
netnet	ntnt		membrane over the brain
pedset	pdst		eye disease, probably a stye
pehedj	pḥd		to sever, split or crack
pekha	pḫ3		to purge or open
pekhret	pḫrt		remedy or prescription
pes	ps		to cook
peseg	psg		to spit out
peseh	psḥ		to bite or sting

Transliteration, hieroglyphs and probable meaning continued

pesesh-kef	psš-kf		instrument for 'opening the mouth'
peshen	pšn		to split or crack
qa, qas	ḳ˓, ḳ3s		to vomit
qenit	ḳnit		type of eye injury
qesen	ḳsn		irksome, difficult or bad (of illness)
redet	rdt		growth (not synonymous with tumour)
redi	rdi		to place or give
rekh kaw	rḫ k3w		veterinary surgeon (or one who 'knows the bulls')
resh	rš		unidentified disease of nose
ryt	ryt		pus
sa	s3		unidentified worm
sau	s3w		magician
sed	sd		to break or smash
sedbu	sdbw		snake of uncertain identity (see Chap. 8)
sedjer	sḏr		to spend the night, lie or sleep
sehem	sḥm		to crush, bruise or pinch

Transliteration, hieroglyphs and probable meaning continued

seher	sḥr		swelling, tumour or abscess
sekhtef	sḫtf		unidentified snake (see Chap. 8)
senef	snf		blood
senetjer	snṯr		incense, probably terebinth
sereq	srḳ		to cause to breathe
seryt	sryt		cough
seshed	sšd		type of bandage
setet	stt		unidentified pathological condition, perhaps mucus or shooting pains
sharu	šꜣrw		unidentified eye disease
shefut	šfwt		swelling
shena	šnꜥ		obstruction
shesau	šsꜣw		collection of medical knowledge
tau	ꜣw		heat, hence inflammation
tehem	thm		perforation or puncture
tekhen	tḫn		type of eye injury
tepau	tpꜣw		part of skull, also a disease of the head

Transliteration, hieroglyphs and probable meaning continued

teshtesh	tštš		to incise
tjau	ṯȝw		breath, air, wind or blowing
tjes	ṯs		vertebra
wab	wˁb		pure
wadju	wȝḏw		green eye-paint
webdet	wbdt		a burn
webnu	wbnw		a wound
wedeh	wdḥ		to pour
wedja	wḏȝ		healthy, whole or unhurt
wehat	wḥˁt		scorpion
wehau	wḥȝw		unidentified skin disease or rash
wekhedu	wḫdw		unidentified disease state or factor (see Chap. 3)
wenekh	wnḫ		dislocation or abnormal movement
wesesh	wsš		discharge, elimination or excretion (non-specific)
wet	wt		bandage

Words are alphabetised according to the anglicised spelling. Note that there are two different hieroglyphs that are anglicised as 'a', 'h' and 'kh'.

Transliteration follows the style of Gardiner (1957) and Faulkner (1972).

The hieroglyphs are according to the sign-list of Gardiner (1957) and prepared with Inscribe software.

The Egyptian writing for the words is seldom unique and the fuller version has generally been selected.

For more detail, reference should be made to the *Grundriss* (see Table 2.2). Not all of the words listed here appear in the medical papyri.

BIBLIOGRAPHY AND RECOMMENDED READING

NOTE: Bardinet's new (1995) French translation of the medical papyri (see below) was received too late for inclusion in the present work. This is a publication of his doctoral thesis at the Ecole Pratique des Hautes Etude and includes the Papyrus Rubensohn and Papyrus Zagreb 881, which are neither in the *Grundriss* nor the work of Sauneron (1989).

ÅKERBLAD, J D. 1802. *Lettre à M. de Sacy*. L'Imprimerie de la République, Paris.

ALDRED, C. 1988. *Akhenaten: King of Egypt*. Thames and Hudson, London.

ALLEN, J P. 1994. 'Nefertiti and Smenkh-ka-ra', *Göttinger Miszellen*. 141: 7–17.

ANDREWS, C A R. 1984. *Egyptian Mummies*. British Museum Publications, London.

ANDREWS, C A R. 1994. *Amulets of Ancient Egypt*. British Museum Press, London.

ANTHES, R. 1928. *Die Felseninschriften von Hatnub*. Hinrichs, Leipzig.

ARMELAGOS, G J and MILLS, J O. 1993. 'Palaeopathology as science: the contribution of Egyptology', in: *Biological Anthropology and the Study of Ancient Egypt*. Ed: Davies, W V and Walker, R. British Museum Press, London.

AUFRÈRE, S. 1984. 'Études de lexicologie et d'histoire naturelle IV–VI', *Bulletin de l'Institut Français d'Archéologie Orientale*. 84: 1–21.

AUFRÈRE, S. 1986. 'Études de lexicologie et d'histoire naturelle VIII–XVII', *Bulletin de l'Institut Français d'Archéologie Orientale*. 86: 1–32.

AUFRÈRE, S. 1987. 'Études de lexicologie et d'histoire naturelle XVIII–XXVI', *Bulletin de l'Institut Français d'Archéologie Orientale*. 87: 21–44.

BADAWY, A. 1978. *The Tomb of Nyhetep-Ptah at Giza and the Tomb of Ankhmahor at Saqqara*. University of California Press, Berkeley.

BAER, K. 1960. *Rank and Title in the Old Kingdom*. University of Chicago Press, Chicago.

BALANDRIN, F M, KLOCKE, J A, WURTELE, E S and BOLLINGER, W H. 1985. 'Natural plant chemicals: sources of industrial and medicinal materials', *Science*. 228: 1154–60.

BALDOCK, C, HUGHES, S W, WHITTAKER, D K, TAYLOR, J, DAVIS, R, SPENCER, A J, TONGE, K and SOFAT, A. 1994. 'Reconstruction of an ancient Egyptian mummy using X-ray computer tomography', *Journal of the Royal Society of Medicine*. 87: 806–8.

BARDINET, T. 1995. *Les Papyrus Médicaux de l'Égypte Pharaonique*. Fayard, Paris.

BARNS, J W B. 1956. *Five Ramesseum Papyri*. Oxford University Press, Oxford.

BEECHER, H K, KEATS, A S, MOSTELLER, F and LASAGNA, L. 1953. 'The effectiveness of oral analgesics (morphine, codeine, acetylsalicylic acid) and the problem of placebo "reactors" and "non-reactors"', *Journal of Pharmacology and Experimental Therapeutics*. 109: 393–400.

BENITEZ, J T. 1988. 'Otopathology of Egyptian mummy Pum II: final report', *Journal of Laryngology and Otology*. 102: 485–90.

BERGER, E. 1970. *Das Basler Arztrelief*. Archäologischer Verlag, Basel.

BERGMAN, A, YANAI, J, WEISS, J, BELL, D and DAVID, M P. 1983. 'Acceleration of wound healing by topical application of honey', *American Journal of Surgery*. 145: 374–6.

BIERBRIER, M. 1982. *The Tomb-builders of the Pharaohs*. British Museum Publications, London.

BILHARZ, T M. 1852. 'Ein Beitrag zur Helminthographia humana aus breiflichen Mittheilungen des Dr. Bilharz in Cairo, nebst Bermerkungen von C. T. v. Siebold', *Zeitschrift für wissenschaftliche Zoologie*. 4: 53–76.

BISSET, N G, BRUHN, J G, CURTO, S, HOLMSTEDT, B, NYMAN, U and ZENK, M H. 1994. 'Was opium known in 18th dynasty ancient Egypt? An examination of materials from the tomb of the chief royal architect Kha', *Journal of Ethnopharmacology*. 41: 99–114.

BRADLEY, P R. 1992. *British Herbal Compendium*. vol 1. British Herbal Medicine Association, Bournemouth.

BREASTED, J H. 1906. *Ancient Records of Egypt*. University of Chicago Press, Chicago.

BREASTED, J H. 1930. *The Edwin Smith Surgical Papyrus*. (two volumes) University of Chicago Press, Chicago.

BREWER, D J and FRIEDMAN, R F. 1989. *Fish and Fishing in Ancient Egypt*. Aris and Philips, Warminster.

British Herbal Pharmacopoeia. 1983. British Herbal Medicine Association, Bournemouth.

British Herbal Pharmacopoeia. vol 1. 1990. British Herbal Medicine Association, Bournemouth.

British Pharmacopoeia. 1993. (two volumes) Her Majesty's Stationery Office, London.

BROTHWELL, D R and CHIARELLI, B A. 1973. *Population Biology of the Ancient Egyptians*. Academic Press, London.

BROTHWELL, D and SANDISON, A T. 1967. (editors) *Diseases in Antiquity*. Charles C Thomas, Springfield.

BRUGSCH, H F K. 1853. 'Mémoire sur la médicine de l'Ancienne Égypte', *Allgemeine Monatschrift für Wissenschaft und Lit'*, pp. 44–56.

BRYAN, C P. 1930. *The Papyrus Ebers*. Geoffrey Bles, London.

BUIKSTRA, J E, BAKER, B J and COOK, D C. 1993. 'What diseases plagued the ancient Egyptians? A century of controversy considered', in: *Biological Anthropology and the Study of Ancient Egypt*. Ed: Davies, W V and Walker, R. British Museum Press, London.

BUTZER, K W. 1976. *Early Hydraulic Civilization in Egypt: a study of cultural ecology*. University of Chicago Press, Chicago.

CASSAR, P. 1974 'Surgical instruments on a tomb slab in Roman Malta', *Medical History*. 18: 89–92.

CERNY, M J. 1927. 'Quelques ostraca hiératiques inédits de Thèbes au Musée du Caire', *Annales du Service des*

Antiquités de l'Égypte. 27: 183–210.

CERNY, J and GARDINER, A H. 1957. *Hieratic Ostraca*. Griffith Institute, Oxford.

CHAMPOLLION, J F. 1822. *Lettre à M. Dacier*. Firmin Didot Père et Fils, Paris.

CHAPMAN, P H. 1992. 'Case seven of the Smith surgical papyrus: the meaning of *tp3w*', *Journal of the American Research Centre in Egypt*. 29: 35–42.

CHARPENTIER, G. 1981. *Recueil de Matériaux Épigraphiques Relatifs à la Botanique de l'Égypte Antique*. Trismégiste, Paris.

COCKBURN, A and COCKBURN, E. (editors) 1980. *Mummies, Disease and Ancient Cultures*. Cambridge University Press, Cambridge.

COCKBURN, A, BARRACO, R A, REYMAN, T A and PECK, W H. 1975. 'Autopsy of an Egyptian Mummy', *Science*. 187: 1155–60.

DARBY, W J, GHALIOUNGHUI, P and GRIVETTI, L. 1977. *Food: the Gift of Osiris*. (two volumes) Academic Press, London.

DASEN, V. 1993. *Dwarfs in Ancient Egypt and Greece*. Clarendon Press, Oxford.

DAVID, A R. 1979. (editor) *The Manchester Museum Mummy Project*. Manchester University Press, Manchester.

DAVID, A R and TAPP, E. 1992. *The Mummy's Tale*. Michael O'Mara Books, London.

DAVIES, N de G. 1927. *Two Ramesside Tombs at Thebes*. Metropolitan Museum of Art, New York.

DAVIES, W V and WALKER, R. 1993. (editors) *Biological Anthropology and the Study of Ancient Egypt*. British Museum Press, London.

DAWSON, W R. 1924. 'The mouse in Egyptian and later medicine', *Proceedings of the Royal Society of Medicine*. 10: 83–6.

DAWSON, W R. 1929. *Magician and Leech*. Methuen, London.

DAWSON, W R. 1933. 'Studies in the Egyptian medical texts – II', *Journal of Egyptian Archaeology*. 19: 133–7.

DAWSON, W R. 1934a. 'Studies in the Egyptian medical texts – III', *Journal of Egyptian Archaeology*. 20: 41–6.

DAWSON, W R. 1934b. 'Studies in the Egyptian medical texts – IV', *Journal of Egyptian Archaeology*. 20: 185–8.

DAWSON, W R. 1938. 'Pygmies and dwarfs in ancient Egypt', *Journal of Egyptian Archaeology*. 24: 185–9.

DAWSON, W R and GRAY, P H K. 1968. *Catalogue of Egyptian Antiquities in the British Museum. I. Mummies and Human Remains*. Trustees of the British Museum, London.

DAWSON, W R and UPHILL, E P. 1972. *Who Was Who in Egyptology*. Egypt Exploration Society, London.

DEELDER, A M, MILLER, R L, DE JONGE, N and KRIJGER, F W. 1990. 'Detection of schistosome antigen in mummies', *Lancet*. 335: 724–5.

DERRY, D E. 1912–13. 'A case of hydrocephalus in an Egyptian of the Roman Period', *Journal of Anatomy and Physiology*, London. 47: 436–58.

DERRY, D E. 1935. 'Notes on five pelves of women of the Eleventh Dynasty in Egypt', *Journal of Obstetrics and Gynaecology of the British Empire*. 43: 490–8.

DERRY, D E. 1938. 'Pott's disease in ancient Egypt', *Medical Press and Circular*. 197: 196–9.

Description de l'Égypte. 1809. Publié par les ordres de sa Majesté l'Empereur Napoléon le Grand, Imprimerie Impériale, Paris.

DOLLERY, C. 1994. 'Medicine and the pharmacological revolution', *Journal of the Royal College of Physicians*. 28: 59–69.

DOLS, M W. 1974 'Plague in early Islamic history', *Journal of the Oriental Society*. 3: 371–84.

EBBELL, B. 1937. *The Papyrus Ebers*. Oxford University Press, London.

EBERS, G M. 1875. *Papyros Ebers*. (two volumes) Englemann, Leipzig.

EDELSTEIN, E J and EDELSTEIN, L. 1945. *Asclepius: a Collection and Interpretation of the Testimonies*. (two volumes) Williams and Wilkins, Baltimore.

EDITORIAL. 1994. 'Pharmaceuticals from plants: great potential, few finds', *Lancet*. 343: 1513–15.

EDWARDS, I E S. 1938. *Handbook to the Egyptian Mummies and Coffins Exhibited in the British Museum*. British Museum, London.

EGGEBRECHT, A. 1984. *Das Alte Ägypten*. C Bertelsmann, Munich.

ELLIOT SMITH: see SMITH, G E.

ERMAN, A and GRAPOW, H. 1926–31. *Wörterbuch der ägyptischen Sprache*. (five volumes) Hinrichs, Leipzig.

ESTES, J W. 1989. *The Medical Skills of Ancient Egypt*. Science History Publications, Canton.

EVANS, W C. 1989. *Trease and Evans' Pharmacognosy*. 13th ed. Baillière Tindall, London.

FAULKNER, R O. 1962. *A Concise Dictionary of Middle Egyptian*. University Press, Oxford.

FAULKNER, R O. 1972. *The Ancient Egyptian Book of the Dead*. British Museum Publications, London.

FIRTH, C M. 1915. *The Archaeological Survey of Nubia, Report for 1909–1910*. Government Press, Cairo.

FIRTH, C M and GUNN, B. 1926. *Excavations at Saqqara: Teti Pyramid Cemeteries*. Imprimerie de l'Institut Français d'Archéologie Orientale, Cairo.

FLEMING, S and FISHMAN, B. 1980. *The Egyptian Mummy: secrets and science, 21. University Museum Handbook 1*. University Museum, Philadelphia.

FORBES, D C. 1993. 'The Rameses II legacy', *KMT*. 4: 52–9.

GARDINER, A H. 1935. *Hieratic Papyri in the British Museum*. British Museum, London.

GARDINER, A H. 1938. 'The house of life', *Journal of Egyptian Archaeology*. 24: 157–79.

GARDINER, A H. 1955. *The Ramesseum Papyri*. University Press, Oxford.

GARDINER, A H. 1957. *Egyptian Grammar*. 3rd ed. Oxford

University Press, London.

GARDINER, A H, PEET, T E and CERNY, J. 1952. *The Inscriptions of Sinai*. Oxford University Press, London.

GARNER, R. 1979. 'Experimental mummification', in: *The Manchester Museum Mummy Project*. Ed: David, A R. Manchester University Press, Manchester.

GERMER, R. 1979. *Untersuchung über Arzneimittelpflanzen in Altern Ägypten*. PhD thesis. University of Hamburg.

GERMER, R. 1991. *Mumien: Zeugen des Pharaonenreiches*, Artemis and Winkler, Zurich and Munich.

GERMER, R. 1993. 'Ancient Egyptian pharmaceutical plants and the eastern Mediterranean', in: *The Healing Past*. Ed: Jacob, I and Jacob, W. E J Brill, Leiden.

GHALIOUNGHUI, P. 1949. 'Sur deux formes d'obésité représentées dans l'Égypte ancienne', *Annales du Service des Antiquitiès de l'Égypte*, 49: 303–16.

GHALIOUNGHUI, P. 1973. *Magic and Medical Science in Ancient Egypt*. 2nd ed. B.M. Israël, Amsterdam.

GHALIOUNGHUI, P. 1983. *The Physicians of Pharaonic Egypt*. Al-Ahram Center for Scientific Translations, Cairo.

GHALIOUNGHUI, P. 1987. *The Ebers Papyrus*. Academy of Scientific Research and Technology. Cairo.

GHALIOUNGHUI, P, KHALIL, S and AMMAR, A R. 1963. 'On an ancient Egyptian method of diagnosing pregnancy and determining foetal sex', *Medical Historian*. 7: 241–6.

GILMAN, A G, GOODMAN, L S, RALL, T W and MURAD, F. 1985. *Goodman and Gilman's The Pharmacological Basis of Therapeutics*. 7th ed. Macmillan, New York.

GRANVILLE, A B. 1825. An essay on Egyptian mummies with observations on the art of embalming among the ancient Egyptians', *Philosophical Transactions of the Royal Society*, 115: 269–319.

GRIFFITH, F Ll. 1898. *Hieratic Papyri from Kahun and Garob*. Bernard Quaritch, London.

GRIFFITH, F Ll and THOMPSON, H. 1904. *The Demotic Magical Papyrus of London and Leiden*. H. Grevel & Co., London.

GRIFFITHS, J G. 1970. *Plutarch's de Iside et Osiride*. University of Wales Press, Cardiff.

GRILLETTO, R. 1973. 'Caries and dental attrition in the early Egyptians as seen in the Turin collections', in: *Population Biology of the Ancient Egyptians*. Ed: Brothwell, D R and Chiarelli, B A. Academic Press, London.

Grundriss: see Table 2.2.

HABRICH, C, KÜNZL, E and ZIMMERMAN, S. 1991. *Theodor Meyer-Steineg (1873–1936) – Artz Historiker, Sammler*. Deutsches Medizinhistorisches Museum, Ingolstadt.

HAFFEJEE, I E and MOOSA, A. 1985. 'Honey in the treatment of infantile gastroenteritis', *British Medical Journal*. 290: 1866–7.

HALL, R. 1986. *Egyptian Textiles*. Shire Publications, Princes Risborough.

HARE, R. 1967. 'The antiquity of disease caused by bacteria and viruses', in: *Diseases in Antiquity*. Ed: Brothwell, D and Sandison, A T. Charles C Thomas, Springfield.

HARER, W B. 1985. 'Pharmacological and biological properties of the Egyptian lotus', *Journal of the American Research Center in Egypt*. 22: 49–54.

HARER, W B. 1993. 'Health in pharaonic Egypt', in: *Biological Anthropology and the Study of Ancient Egypt*. Ed: Davies, W V and Walker, R. British Museum Press, London.

HARER, W B. 1994. 'Peseshkef: the first special-purpose surgical instrument', *Obstetrics and Gynecology*. 83: 1053–5.

HARER, W B and TAYLOR, J H. (in preparation) *Irty Senu: Granville's Egyptian Female Mummy: The Autopsies of 1824 and 1994*. British Museum Press, London.

HARRIS, J E and WENTE, E S. 1980. (editors) *An Atlas of the Royal Mummies*. University of Chicago, Chicago and London.

HARRISON, R G. 1966. 'An anatomical examination of the pharaonic remains purported to be Akhenaten', *Journal of Egyptian Archaeology*. 52: 95–119.

HART, G. 1986. *A Dictionary of Egyptian Gods and Goddesses*. Routledge & Kegan Paul, London.

HART, G D, MILLET, N B, RIDEOUT, D F, SCOTT, J W, LYNN, G E, REYMAN, T A, DE BONI, U, HORNE, P D, BARRACO, R A and others. 1977. 'Autopsy of an Egyptian Mummy (Nakht – ROM I)', *Canadian Medical Association Journal*. 117: 461–76.

HASSAN, S. 1932. *The Egyptian University Excavations at Giza (1929–1930)*. Oxford University Press, Oxford.

HASSAN, S. 1960. *Excavations at Giza, Season 1936–37–38*. VOI IX. *The Mastabas of the Eighth Season and their Description*. General Organisation for Government Printing Offices, Cairo.

HAYES, C. 1962. 'The world's oldest surgery', *Africana*. 1: 14–15.

HEDGES, R E M and Sykes, B A. 1993. 'The extraction and isolation of DNA from archaeological bone', in: *Biological Anthropology and the Study of Ancient Egypt*. Ed: Davies, W V and Walker, R. British Museum Press, London.

HEPPER, F N. 1990. *Pharaoh's Flowers*. Her Majesty's Stationery Office, London.

HICKS, R M. 1983. 'The canopic worm: role of bilharziasis in the aetiology of human bladder cancer', *Journal of the Royal Society of Medicine*. 76: 16–22.

HUSSEIN, M K. 1949–50. 'Quelques spécimens de pathologie osseuse chez les anciens Égyptiens', *Bulletin de l'Institut d'Égypte*. 32: 11–17.

ISHERWOOD, I and HART, C W. 1992. 'The radiological examination', in: *The Mummy's Tale*. Ed: David, A R and Tapp, E. Michael O'Mara Books, London.

ISHERWOOD, I, JARVIS, H and FAWCITT, R A. 1979. 'Radiology of the Manchester mummies', in: *The*

Manchester Museum Mummy Project. Ed: David, A R. Manchester University Press, Manchester.

IVERSEN, E. 1939. *Papyrus Carlsberg, no VIII*. Munksgaard, Copenhagen.

IVERSEN, E. 1947. 'Some remarks on the terms *ʾmm* and *ais*', *Journal of Egyptian Archaeology*. 33: 47–51.

JACKSON, R. 1986. 'A set of Roman instruments from Italy', *Britannia*. 17: 119–67.

JACKSON, R. 1988. *Doctors and Diseases in the Roman Empire*. British Museum Press, London.

JACKSON, R. 1990. 'Roman doctors and their instruments: recent research into ancient practice', *Journal of Roman Archaeology*. 3: 5–27.

JANSSEN, J J. 1975. *Commodity Prices from the Ramessid Period*. E J Brill, Leiden.

JOACHIM, H. 1890. *Papyros Ebers*. G Reimer, Berlin.

JONCKHEERE, F. 1944. *Une Maladie Égyptienne, l'Hématurie Parasitaire*. Fondation Égyptologique Reine Élizabeth, Brussels.

JONCKHEERE, F. 1947. *Le Papyrus Médical Chester Beatty*. Fondation Égyptologique Reine Élizabeth, Brussels.

JONCKHEERE, F. 1954. *Prescriptions Médicales sur Ostraca Hiératiques*. Fondation Égyptologique Reine Élizabeth, Brussels.

JONCKHEERE, F. 1958. *Les Médecins de l'Égypte Pharaonique*. Fondation Égyptologique Reine Élizabeth, Brussels.

JONES, F W. 1908. 'Some lessons from ancient fractures', *British Medical Journal*. 455–8.

JUNKER, H. 1928. 'Die Stele des Hofarztes *ʾIry*', *Zeitschrift für ägyptische Sprache*. 63: 53–70.

KANAWATI, N. 1985. *The Rock Tombs of El-Hawawish: the cemetery of Akhmin*. Macquarie Ancient History Foundation. Canberra.

VON KÄNEL, F. 1984. *Les Prêtes-ouâb de Sekhmet et les Conjurateurs de Serket*. Presses Universitaires de France, Paris.

KATZ, S H and VOIGT, M M. 1986. 'Bread and beer: the earliest use of cereals in the human diet', *Expedition (University of Pennsylvania)*. 28: 23–34.

KITCHEN, K A. 1975. *Ramesside Inscriptions, Historical and Biographical*, I. Blackwell, Oxford.

KITCHEN, K A. 1982. *Pharaoh Triumphant: the Life and Times of Ramesses II*. Aris and Philips, Warminster.

KITCHEN, K A. 1986. *Ramesside Inscriptions, Historical and Biographical*, VII:2. Blackwell, Oxford.

KITCHEN, K A. 1987. *Ramesside Inscriptions, Historical and Biographical*, VII:7. Blackwell, Oxford.

KROGMAN, W M and BAER, M J. 1980. 'Age at death of pharaohs of the New Kingdom, determined from X-ray film', in: *An X-ray Atlas of the Royal Mummies*. Ed: Harris, J E and Wente, E F. University of Chicago Press, Chicago.

KÜNZL, E. 1983. *Medizinische Instrumente aus Sepulkralfunden der Römischen Kaiserzeit*. Reinland Verlag, Köln.

LECA, A-P. 1988. *La Médecine Égyptienne au temps des pharaons*. Roger Dacosta, Paris.

LEEK, F F. 1972. 'Bite, attrition and associated oral conditions as seen in ancient Egyptian skulls', *Journal of Human Evolution*. 1: 289–95.

LEEK, F F. 1979. 'The dental history of the Manchester mummies', in: *The Manchester Museum Mummy Project*. Ed: David, A R. Manchester University Press, Manchester.

LEFEBVRE, M G. 1924. *Le Tombeau de Petosiris*. Imprimerie de l'Institut Français d'Archéologie Orientale, Cairo.

LEFEBVRE, G. 1956. *Essai sur la Médecine Égyptienne de l'Époque Pharaonique*. Presses Universitaires de France, Paris.

LESKO, L H. 1982–90. *A Dictionary of Late Egyptian*. (five volumes) B C Scribe Publications, Providence.

LICHTHEIM, M. 1980. *Ancient Egyptian Literature*, vol 3: *The Late Period*. University of California Press, Berkeley.

LONGRIGG, J. 1992. *Greek Rational Medicine: Philosophy and Medicine from Alcmaeon to the Alexandrians*. Routledge, London.

LORET, V. 1892. *La Flore pharaonique*. 2nd ed. Ernest Leroux, Paris.

LUCAS, A and HARRIS, J R. 1989. *Ancient Egyptian Materials and Industries*. Histories and Mysteries of Man, London.

MAJNO, G. 1975. *The Healing Hand*. Harvard University Press, Cambridge, Mass.

MALEK, J. 1993. *The Cat in Ancient Egypt*. British Museum Press, London.

MANNICHE, L. 1989. *An Ancient Egyptian Herbal*. British Museum Publications, London.

MARGANNE-MÉLARD, M-H. 1987. *Les Instruments Chirurgicaux de l'Égypte Gréco-Romaine*. Editions APDCA, Juan-les-Pins.

MARIETTE, A. 1889. *Les Mastabas de l'Ancien Empire, Mastaba D 62, Le Tombeau de Ptah-Hotep*. Vieweg, Paris.

MASALI, M and CHIARELLI, B. 1972. 'Demographic data on the remains of ancient Egyptians', *Journal of Human Evolution*. 1: 161–9.

MATHIEU, B. 1993. 'Sur quelques ostraca hiératiques littéraire, récemment publiés', *Bulletin de l'Institut Français d'Archéologie Orientale*. 93: 335–47.

MAYS, B, PARFITT, A and HERSHMAN, M J. 1994. 'Treatment of arrow wounds by nineteenth century USA army surgeons', *Journal of the Royal Society of Medicine*. 87: 102–3.

MERRILLEES, R S. 1962. Opium trade in the Bronze Age Levant. *Antiquity*. 36: 287–92.

DE MEULENAERE, H. 1986. 'Review of *The Physicians of Pharaonic Egypt*', by Ghaliounghui, P. (1983), *Chronique d'Égypte*. 61: 239–42.

MILLER, R L. 1989. '*Dqr*, spinning and treatment of

guinea worm in P. Ebers 875', *Journal of Egyptian Archaeology*. 75: 249–54.

MILLER, R L. 1991a. 'Counting calories in Egyptian ration texts', *Journal of the Economic and Social History of the Orient*. 34: 257–69.

MILLER, R L. 1991b. 'Palaeoepidemiology, literacy and medical tradition among necropolis workmen in New Kingdom Egypt', *Medical History*. 35: 1–24.

MILLER, R L, ARMELAGOS, G J, IKRAM, S, DE JONGE, N, KRIJGER, F W and DEELDER, A M. 1992. 'Palaeoepidemiology of schistosoma infection in mummies', *British Medical Journal*. 304: 555–6.

MILLER, R L, DE JONGE, N, KRIJGER, F W and DEELDER, A M. 1993. 'Predynastic schistosomiasis', in: *Biological Anthropology and the Study of Ancient Egypt*. Ed: Davies, W V and Walker, R. British Museum Press, London.

MILLER, R L, IKRAM, S, ARMELAGOS, G J, WALKER, R, HARER, W B, SHIFF, C J, BAGGETT, D, CARRIGAN, M and MARET, S M. 1994. 'Diagnosis of *Plasmodium falciparum* infections in mummies using the rapid manual *Para*Sight™-F test', *Transactions of the Royal Society of Tropical Medicine and Hygiene*. 88: 31–2.

MILLET, N B, HART, D G, REYMAN, T A, ZIMMERMAN, M R and LEWIN, P K. 1980. 'ROM I: mummification for the common people', in: *Mummies, Disease and Ancient Cultures*. Ed: Cockburn, A and Cockburn, E. Cambridge University Press, Cambridge.

MØLLER-CHRISTENSEN, V. 1967. 'Evidence of leprosy in earlier people', in: *Diseases in Antiquity*. Ed: Brothwell, D and Sandison, A T. Charles C Thomas, Springfield.

MOLLESON, T I. 1993. 'The Nubian pathological collection in the Natural History Museum', in: *Biological Anthropology and the Study of Ancient Egypt*. Ed: Davies, W V and Walker, R. British Museum Press, London.

MORSE, D, BROTHWELL, D R and UCKO, P J. 1964. 'Tuberculosis in ancient Egypt', *American Review of Respiratory Diseases*. 90: 524–41.

MUZIO, I. 1925. 'Su di un olio medicato della tomba di Cha', *Atti della Società Liguistica di Scienze e Lettere*. 4: 249–53.

NUTTON, V. 1993. 'Galen and Egypt', in: *Galen und das Ellenistische Erbe*. Franz Steiner, Stuttgart.

OMLIN, J A. 1968. *Der Papyrus 55001*. Edizioni d'Arte Fratelli Pozzo, Turin.

PÄÄBO, S. 1985. 'Molecular cloning of Ancient Egyptian mummy DNA', *Nature*. 314: 644–5.

PARANT, R. 1982. *L'Affaire Sinouhé*. Aurillac, Paris.

PARKINSON, R and QUIRKE, S. 1995. *Papyrus*. British Museum Press, London.

PESTMAN, P W. 1982. 'Who were the owners, in the 'community of workmen', of the Chester Beatty papyri', in: *Gleanings from Deir el-Medina*. Ed: Demareé, R J and Janssen, J J. Nederlands Instituut voor het Nabije Oosten, Leiden.

PETRIE, W M F. 1907. *Gizeh and Rifeh*. Bernard Quaritch, London.

PETRIE, W M F. 1914. *Amulets*. Constable, London.

PETRIE, W M F. 1917. *Tools and Weapons*. Constable, London.

PETRIE, W M F and MACKAY, E. 1915. *Heliopolis, Kfar Ammar and Shurafa*. Bernard Quaritch, London.

PETTIGREW, T J. 1834. *A History of Egyptian Mummies*. Longmans, London.

PORTER, B and MOSS, R. 1981. *Memphis, Saqqara to Dashur*. III². Griffith Institute, Ashmolean Museum, Oxford.

QUIBELL, J E. 1913. *Excavations at Saqqara (1911–12): the Tomb of Hesy*. Imprimerie de l'Institut Français d'Archéologie Orientale, Cairo.

QUIRKE, S G J. 1992. *Ancient Egyptian Religion*. British Museum Press, London.

REEVES, C. 1992. *Egyptian Medicine*. Shire Publications, Princes Risborough.

REEVES, C N. 1990. *The Valley of the Kings*. Kegan Paul International, London.

REISNER, G A. 1905. *The Hearst Medical Papyrus*. Hinrichs, Leipzig.

RETSAS, S. 1986. *Palaeo-oncology: the Antiquity of Cancer*. Farrand Press, London.

REYMOND, E A E. 1976. *A Medical Book from Crocodilopolis*. Verlag Brüder Hollinek, Vienna.

REYNOLDS, J E F. 1993. *Martindale: The Extra Pharmacopoeia*. 30th ed. Pharmaceutical Press. London.

RIDDLE, J M. 1992. *Contraception and Abortion from the Ancient World to the Renaissance*. Harvard University Press. Cambridge, Mass.

ROSE, J C, ARMELAGOS, G J and PERRY, L S. 1993. 'Dental anthropology of the Nile Valley', in: *Biological Anthropology and the Study of Ancient Egypt*. Ed: Davies, W V and Walker, R. British Museum Press, London.

ROTH, A M. 1991. *Egyptian Phyles in the Old Kingdom*. Oriental Institute of the University of Chicago, Chicago.

ROTH, A M. 1992. 'The *pss-kf* and the "opening of the mouth" ceremony: a ritual of birth and rebirth', *Journal of Egyptian Archaeology*. 78: 113–47.

ROWLING, J T. 1961a. *Some Observations on the Pathological Changes Found in Mummies*. MD thesis. University of Cambridge.

ROWLING, J T. 1961b. 'Pathological changes in mummies', *Proceedings of the Royal Society of Medicine*. 54: 409–15.

ROWLING, J T. 1967. 'Hernia in Egypt', in: *Diseases in Antiquity*. Ed: Brothwell, D and Sandison, A T. Charles C Thomas, Springfield.

ROWLING, J T. 1989. 'The rise and decline of surgery in dynastic Egypt', *Antiquity*. 63: 312–19.

RUFFER, M A. 1910a. 'Note on the presence of 'Bilharzia

haematobia' in Egyptian mummies of the xxth Dynasty', *British Medical Journal*. 1: 16.

RUFFER, M A. 1910b. *Potts'che Krankheit an einer ägyptischer Mumie aus der Zeit der 21 Dynastie. Zur historischen Biologie der Krankheitserreger*. 3 Heft Giessen.

RUFFER, M A. 1921. *Studies in Palaeopathology of Egypt*. Ed: Moodie, R L. University of Chicago Press, Chicago.

RUFFER, M A and FERGUSON, A R. 1911. 'Note on an eruption resembling that of variola in the skin of a mummy of the XXth Dynasty', *Journal of Pathology and Bacteriology*. 15: 1–3.

SAFFIRIO, L. 1972. 'Food and dietary habits in ancient Egypt', *Journal of Human Evolution*. 1: 297–305.

SAMUEL, D. 1993. 'Ancient Egyptian bread and beer: an interdisciplinary approach', in: *Biological Anthropology and the Study of Ancient Egypt*. Ed: Davies, W V and Walker, R. British Museum Press, London.

SANDER-HANSEN, C E. 1956. *Analecta Aegyptiaca*: vol VIII: *die Texte der Metternichstele*. Munksgaard, Copenhagen.

SANDISON, A T. 1967a. 'Diseases of the skin', in: *Diseases in Antiquity*. Ed: Brothwell, D and Sandison, A T. Charles C Thomas, Springfield.

SANDISON, A T. 1967b. 'Diseases of the eyes', in: *Diseases in Antiquity*. Ed: Brothwell, D and Sandison, A T. Charles C Thomas, Springfield.

SANDISON, A T. 1972. 'Evidence of infective diseases', *Journal of Human Evolution*. 1: 213–24.

SANDISON, A T. 1980. 'Diseases in ancient Egypt', in: *Mummies, Disease, and Ancient Cultures*. Ed: Cockburn, A and Cockburn, E. Cambridge University Press, Cambridge.

SATINOFF, M I. 1972. 'Study of the squatting facets of the talus and tibia in ancient Egyptians', *Journal of Human Evolution*. 1: 209–12.

SAUNDERS, J B DE C M. 1963. *The Transitions from Ancient Egyptian to Greek Medicine*. University of Kansas Press, Lawrence.

SAUNERON, S. 1989. *Un Traité Égyptien d'Ophiologie*. L'Institut Français d'Archéologie Orientale, Cairo.

SCHIAPARELLI, E. 1927. *Relazione sui Lavori della Missione Archeologica Italiana in Egitto (anni 1903–1920)*. vol 2: *La Tomba Intatta dell'Architetto Cha*. R. Museo di Antichita, Turin.

SCOTT, N E. 1951. 'The Metternich stela', *Bulletin of the Metropolitan Museum of Art*. 9: 201–17.

SMITH, G E. 1908. 'The most ancient splints', *British Medical Journal*. 732–4.

SMITH, G E. 1912. *The Royal Mummies*. Imprimerie de l'Institut Français d'Archéologie Orientale, Cairo.

SMITH, G E and DAWSON, W R. 1924. *Egyptian Mummies*. George Allen and Unwin, London.

SMITH, G E and DERRY, D E. 1910. Anatomical report. *Archaeological Survey of Nubia. Bulletin 6*. National Printing Department, Cairo.

SMITH, G E and JONES, F W. 1910. *The Archaeological Survey of Nubia: Report for 1907–1908*. vol II: *Report on the human remains*. National Printing Department, Cairo.

SMITH, N J D. 1986. 'Dental pathology in an ancient Egyptian population', in: *Science in Egyptology*. Ed: David A R. Manchester University Press, Manchester.

SPENCER, A J. 1993. *Early Egypt*. British Museum Publications, London.

VON STADEN, H. 1989. *Herophilus: the Art of Medicine in Early Alexandria*. Cambridge University Press, Cambridge.

STEAD, M. 1986. *Egyptian Life*. British Museum Press, London.

STEUER, R O. 1948. '*Wḥdw*: aetiological principle of pyaemia in ancient Egyptian medicine', *Bulletin of History of Medicine*. Supplement 10.

STEUER, R O and SAUNDERS, J B DE C M. 1959. *Ancient Egyptian and Cnidian Medicine*. University of California Press, Berkeley.

STEVENS, J M. 1975. 'Gynaecology from ancient Egypt: the Papyrus Kahun', *Medical Journal of Australia*. 2: 949–52.

STROUHAL, E. 1992. *Life in Ancient Egypt*. University of Oklahoma Press, Norman.

STUART, M. 1979. *The Encyclopaedia of Herbs and Herbalism*. Guild, London.

SYKES, R. 1994. 'Innovation in the pharmaceutical industry', *British Medical Journal*. 309: 422–3.

TABANELLI, M. 1958. *Lo Strumento Chirurgico e la sua Storia*. Milan.

TAPP, E. 1979. 'Disease in the Manchester mummies', in: *Science in Egyptology*. Ed: David, A R. Manchester University Press, Manchester.

TAPP, E and WILDSMITH, K. 1992. 'The autopsy and endoscopy of the Leeds mummy'. in: *The Mummy's Tale*. Ed: David, A R and Tapp, E. Michael O'Mara Books, London.

THORNTON, F. 1990. *Oral Pathological Comparison of Discrete Ancient Nile Valley and Concurrent Populations*. MPhil dissertation, University of Bradford.

TILL, W C. 1951. *Die Arzneikunde der Kopten*. Akademie-Verlag, Berlin.

TRIGGER, B G, KEMP, B J, O'CONNOR, D and LLOYD, A B. 1983. *Ancient Egypt: a Social History*. Cambridge University Press, Cambridge.

VIGNARD, M E. 1923. 'Une nouvelle industrie lithique. Le Sebilien', *Bulletin de l'Institut Français d'Archéologie Orientale*. 22: 1–76.

VIKENTIEFF, W. 1949–50. 'Deux rites du jubilé royal à l'époque protodynastique', *Bulletin de l'Institut d'Égypte*. 32: 171–228.

VAN DE WALLE, B and DE MEULENAERE, H. 1973. 'Compléments à la prosopographie médicale', *Revue d'Égyptologie*. 25: 58–83.

WARD, W A. 1982. *Index of Egyptian Administrative and Religious Titles of the Middle Kingdom*. American University of Beirut, Beirut.

WEEKS, K R. 1970. *The Anatomical Knowledge of the Ancient Egyptians and the Representation of the Human Figure in Egyptian Art*. PhD thesis. Yale University.

WELLS, C. 1963. 'Ancient Egyptian pathology', *Journal of Laryngology and Otology*. 77: 261–5.

WESLEY, J. 1747. *Primitive Physic*. John Smith, London.

WESTENDORF, W. 1966. *Papyrus Edwin Smith*. Verlag Hans Huber, Berne and Stuttgart.

WESTENDORF, W. 1992. *Erwachen der Heilkunst: die Medizin im Alten Ägypten*. Artemis und Winkler, Zürich.

WHITE, C. 1991. *Isotopic Analysis of Multiple Human Tissues from Three Ancient Nubian Populations*. PhD thesis, University of Toronto.

WILDUNG, D. 1977a. *Egyptian Saints: Deification in Pharaonic Egypt*. New York University Press, New York.

WILDUNG, D. 1977b. *Imhotep und Amenhotep*. Deutscher Kunstverlag, Munich.

WILDUNG, D. 1984. *L'Age d'Or de l'Égypte: le Moyen Empire*. Office du livre, S.A., Fribourg.

WILSON, H. 1988. *Egyptian Food and Drink*. Shire Publications, Princes Risborough.

WINLOCK, H E. 1945. *The Slain Soldiers of Neb-hetep-re Mentu-hotpe*. Metropolitan Museum of Art, New York.

WOOD JONES: see JONES, F W.

WRESZINSKI, W. 1909. *Der Grosse Medizinische Papyrus des Berliner Museums*. Hinrichs, Leipzig.

WRESZINSKI, W. 1912. *Der Londoner Medizinische Papyrus (British Museum No. 1005) und der Papyrus Hearst in Transkription, Übersetzung, und Kommentar*. Hinrichs, Leipzig.

WRESZINSKI, W. 1913. *Der Papyrus Ebers*. I Teil: *Umschrift*. Hinrichs, Leipzig.

YOUNG, T. 1816. *Letter to the Archduke John of Austria*.

YOUNG, T. 1819. 'Egypt', in: *Supplement* to Encyclopedia *Britannica*.

ŽÁBA, Z. 1956. *Les Maximes de Ptahhotep*. Éditions de l'académie Tchécoslovaque des Sciences, Prague.

ZORAB, P A. 1961. The historical and prehistorical background of ankylosing spondylitis', *Proceedings of the Royal Society of Medicine*. 54: 415–20.

ZUMLA, A and LULAT, A. 1989. 'Honey – a remedy rediscovered', *Journal of the Royal Society of Medicine*. 82: 384–5.

GENERAL INDEX